The medical renaissance of
the sixteenth century

The medical renaissance of the sixteenth century

EDITED BY

A. WEAR, R. K. FRENCH AND I. M. LONIE

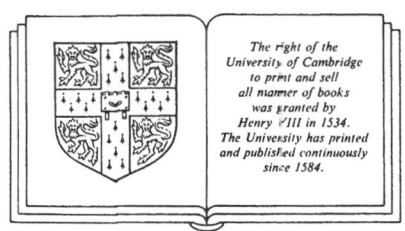

The right of the
University of Cambridge
to print and sell
all manner of books
was granted by
Henry VIII in 1534.
The University has printed
and published continuously
since 1584.

CAMBRIDGE UNIVERSITY PRESS
CAMBRIDGE
LONDON   NEW YORK   NEW ROCHELLE
MELBOURNE   SYDNEY

CAMBRIDGE UNIVERSITY PRESS
Cambridge, New York, Melbourne, Madrid, Cape Town, Singapore, São Paulo, Delhi

Cambridge University Press
The Edinburgh Building, Cambridge CB2 8RU, UK

Published in the United States of America by Cambridge University Press, New York

www.cambridge.org
Information on this title: www.cambridge.org/9780521104562

First published 1985
This digitally printed version 2009

A catalogue record for this publication is available from the British Library

Library of Congress Catalogue Card Number: 84-14973

ISBN 978-0-521-30112-1 hardback
ISBN 978-0-521-10456-2 paperback

Contents

Contributors

G. Baader, *Institut für Geschichte der Medizin, Augustastrasse 37, 1000 Berlin 45. W. Germany*

J. J. Bylebyl, *Institute for the History of Medicine, 1900 East Monument Street, Johns Hopkins University, Baltimore, Maryland 21205, USA*

A. Cunningham, *Wellcome Unit for the History of Medicine, Department of History and Philosophy of Science, Cambridge University, Free School Lane, Cambridge CB2 3EL, UK*

R. K. French, *Wellcome Unit for the History of Medicine, Department of History and Philosophy of Science, Cambridge University, Free School Lane, Cambridge CB2 3EL, UK*

L. García-Ballester, *Departamento de Historia de la Medicina, Santander, Spain*

I. M. Lonie, *48 Duncan Street, Dunedin, New Zealand*

V. Nutton, *Wellcome Institute for the History of Medicine, 183 Euston Road, London NW1 2BP, UK*

R. Palmer, *Wellcome Institute for the History of Medicine, 183 Euston Road, London NW1 2BP, UK*

L. Deer Richardson, *33 High Street, Roydon, Harlow, Essex, UK*

C. B. Schmitt, *Warburg Institute, Woburn Square, London WC1 UK*

N. Siraisi, *Hunter College, City University of New York, Department of History, 695 Park Avenue, New York 10021, USA*

A. Wear, *Department of History and Philosophy of Science, King's College, University of Aberdeen AB9 2UB, Scotland, UK*

Acknowledgements

We would like to thank the Wellcome Trust for generously funding the conference which gave rise to this book. Indeed, without Wellcome support and encouragement the history of medicine would be in a poor state in this country. The financial help of the British Academy is also gratefully acknowledged. Our thanks also go to Dr Vivian Nutton who gave valuable advice at various stages of planning; to the Wellcome Unit for the History of Medicine at Cambridge which provided invaluable administrative support and helped to entertain the members of the conference; to Dr J. A. Bennett, Curator of the Whipple Science Museum for extending his Museum's hospitality to conference members; and to Corpus Christi College for providing ideal surroundings, hospitality and sustenance.

Introduction

When planning the conference on sixteenth century medicine that took place at Corpus Christi College, Cambridge in September 1983, the organisers did not intend to present a refined version of the usual picture of medicine steered by a number of heroes through a time of change that saw the origins of modern medicine. Rather, the intention was to develop an alternative picture of a less heroic but perhaps more real medicine as it was taught and practised within the context of other features of sixteenth century life. Such medicine is largely a *terra incognita* for the historian-at-large, and the historian of medicine who is familiar with one or two of its aspects – anatomy has received some attention – has made little attempt to compare medicine with other sources of renaissance knowledge, shared by medical men, men of letters, philosophers and often priests.

Nor was the sixteenth century an arbitrary choice. Few would deny that it was a period of radical and rapid change – broadly, the renaissance – and it was hoped that by bringing together a number of historians working in related but distinct fields this change could be related to changes with the theory and practice of medicine and to those within the society in which it was taught.

The links between medicine and the rest of renaissance intellectual life were intimate. Together with theology and law, medicine stood at the top of the university curriculum in the northern universities, requiring as a precondition a full arts education, which included the scientific elements of natural philosophy on which medicine was based. The medical degree was necessary for recognition as a 'proper' physician, and nothing served more readily than a lack of it to mark out the uneducated empiric. In the universities of the south – particularly Italy – arts and medicine were read together and were as closely related as in the north.

Medicine was, then, a subject of high academic status. Its teachers often possessed formidable linguistic skills in Greek and Latin together with detailed knowledge of the works of Hippocrates, Galen and the lesser classical (and often medieval and Arabic) authors. There is no reason to suppose that the teachers of medicine were inferior to their colleagues in other disciplines in point of scholarship; and in addition they were professional men teaching a vocational subject and combining their learning with actual practice of medicine. It is one of the aims of this book to see how this was done.

Although we can speak of 'renaissance medicine' because it continued to be taught and practised during the period we may wish (for other reasons) to call the renaissance, it is not so easy to describe the essential nature of renaissance medicine. Certainly in the eyes of many people at the time, medicine in the sixteenth century was undergoing changes more rapid than those of earlier centuries, and by and large as historians we can agree with this impression. But these changes occurred late in the period we commonly call the renaissance. Was medicine in some way resistant to changes occurring in other areas? What features did renaissance medicine share with other renaissance activities? How can the renaissance love of all things Greek, visible in sixteenth century medicine, be reconciled with the vigour of the form and content of surviving Arabic and medieval medicine?

These and many related questions are tackled by the contributors to this volume. Nancy Siraisi shows how Avicenna's *Canon* remained a popular text throughout the century and beyond, Gerhard Baader describes how the arch-humanist Jacques Dubois (Sylvius) incorporated Arabic elements into his practical works and Andrew Wear brings forward evidence to show that Arabic and medieval textbooks on practical medicine were by no means redundant in the renaissance. What seem to have been especially valued were the practical instructions and the prescriptions of the Arabs and medieval writers, no doubt because they were of use in the actual practice of medicine, distant from but not necessarily incompatible with the carefully restored Greek texts. Sometimes, as in the case of the *Canon* and the *practica* (textbooks on practical medicine) attempts were made to reconcile the usefulness of such texts with the aims of humanist scholarship by 'humanizing' them, either by correcting the translation or by purging the language of barbarisms.

As suggested above, the historians' notions of 'renaissance' and 'humanism' have been generated without particular, or any, reference to medicine; and we should, then, be careful about applying these terms too easily to the medicine of the time and its practitioners. Roger French shows that in the late fifteenth and early sixteenth century much of what we call 'humanism' was seen by medical contemporaries as 'Hellenism'. The Hellenists viewed Latin merely as the language in which Greek ideas were transmitted and were very different from the humanists of the previous century, who praised and emulated the classical Roman authors. It is further argued in his chapter that while the earlier humanists had been concerned to put their texts into an historical setting, Hellenists like Leoniceno went straight to the Greek and received Greek medical knowl-

edge not only uncritically but unhistorically. In contrast an academic like
Berengario da Carpi, opposing these features of Hellenism, displayed a
textual sensitivity (even to Arabic sources) and an historical awareness
which we would associate with humanism but which he made characteristic of the work of the *scholastici*. Clearly the 'scholasticism' and 'humanism'
of renaissance studies do not translate easily into medical terms.

The meaning of these terms in a medical context is rounded out by the
different emphases put on them by Iain Lonie in his chapter on the Paris
Hippocratics, and by Vivian Nutton's discussion of how so practical an
arm of medicine as surgery could be 'humanised'. A rather different aspect
of practical medicine, that of the writers of the *practica*, discussed by
Andrew Wear, again shows us a combination of textual and historical
sensitivities with practical application.

Despite the obvious usefulness of old techniques and *materia medica*, and
despite the attempts to retain this usefulness by modernizing them it is
clear that the sixteenth century medical writers felt that they were making
a break with their Arabic and medieval past. They believed that they were
creating a Reformation for medicine of which the central feature was the
purification and assimilation of Greek knowledge. But the spirit of a
Reformation is a more radical thing than its practice, and in looking at the
topics of the conference – the teaching and practice of medicine – the
participants agreed that the most obvious signs of change lay in the
rhetoric and the ideological positions adopted by the medical men of the
sixteenth century.

Associated with the issue of continuity and change is the question of
progress. The whig historian looking for the origins of modern medicine
in a progress of human knowledge 'ever upward and onward' would find
little to enthuse over in the sixteenth century as a whole. Only in anatomy
was there progress in this sense, and it is no accident that this is the area into
which historians have delved the most. Indeed, in looking for progress
historians have been inclined to jump from Vesalius, as a kind of progressive signpost to Harvey, to Harvey himself, without examining closely the
ground they have passed over. It is no accident that this book does not
include an account of Vesalius' work and does not extend its time scale to
cover Harvey's. Instead it shows that 'progress' meant different things to
different medical men in the sixteenth century, and that their notions of
progress were different from our own. We, like them, believe that
progress is *making medicine better*; but our view is predominantly that this
will continue to happen only from the acquisition of new knowledge –
research and discovery. But in the sixteenth century making medicine
better might be seen in addition, as a question of making it more rational,
or more observational, or closer to its pure and original sources, or freer
from the dependence on authority. The contemporaries of Houllier and
the other Paris Hippocratics did not praise them for their discoveries but

for their wide knowledge of classical sources, for integrating it with their wide experience and bringing this unity of scholarship and experience to bear upon contemporary medical problems: 'erudition in the service of practice' in Iain Lonie's phrase. The Paris Hippocratics and the physicians and surgeons described by Wear and Nutton did not merely 'go back to the Greeks' but sought to manipulate Greek knowledge into the circumstances of sixteenth century practice: their scholarship, although important to them in its own right, was primarily important in making available a better standard of medicine.

What unites the medical men described in these chapters is their common attempt to improve medicine. The differences between them relate to the faults they found in contemporary medicine and in the ways they chose to remedy them; and for this book it is important that these differences become clear at the level of teaching and practice. Thus behind the Venetian apothecaries' practical, step-by-step attempts (described by Richard Palmer) to reconstitute the ancient theriac is the notion of the superiority of classical remedies. Others, like the Parisians and Sylvius, found it necessary not only to restore Greek medicine but to make it apply to the new circumstances of sixteenth century Europe. Where this involved modification to the medicine of the ancients the means of doing so was often found within ancient medicine itself. For example, well-read anatomists knew that Galen had laid down rules for procedure that provided for anatomy to be extended beyond Galen himself. And as Andrew Cunningham shows, in engaging in an Aristotelian enterprise to find Aristotelean answers, Fabricius of Aquapendente expected nevertheless to go further than Aristotle had done. In fact, the chapter of Jerome Bylebyl on the pulse controversy and that of Andrew Cunningham analyse the fine structure of anatomical and physiological thought. They illustrate the wide range of factors: methodological, observational, textual and authoritarian that, in Bylebyl's phrase, helped to make up the fabric of renaissance physiology. The two chapters show that progress, even in anatomy, was very different from the modern concept.

Naturally, sixteenth century physicians were sometimes faced with problems that appeared difficult to solve on a basis of humanised Arabic or reconstituted Greek medicine. For example, medicine seemed largely inefficient against plague and certain skin conditions, and on the other hand, *new* diseases like syphilis had no classical precedent or authority and so they did not always seem to fit into the dominant theory of disease which was based on the theory of temperaments. Linda Deer Richardson discusses how Jean Fernel became dissatisfied with the theory of temperaments as an explanation of certain diseases and developed the idea that there were hidden or occult causes of disease together with diseases of the 'total substance'. Fernel's theory was not so radical as it might seem, for it had been suggested by Galen and was known to Fernel's contemporaries.

This can be seen as another and extreme example of the refining of Greek medicine with Greek materials. The process allowed for flexibility of approach to traditional medicine, and the extent to which Fernel uses that flexibility reflects the urgency of the problems posed by syphilis. That few followed Fernel was not merely because most of his contemporaries were orthodox Galenists but because they felt, after due consideration, that Fernel's solution was inappropriate and unintelligible. Of course (to put it another way), the training of physicians was based upon Hippocrates and Galen and these authors defined in one sense what was rational and intelligible for university-trained physicians. However, there still remained in the orthodox mind a space for critical awareness: the variability of patients and of conditions which physicians and surgeons came across every day meant that there was a constant need to keep a place for learning by observation and experience. As Vivian Nutton writes, the success or failure of a surgical technique was more obvious than the effects of a drug in internal medicine.

The academic training of physicians did not only consist in reading medical writers like Hippocrates and Galen. It was Galen who had written that the 'best doctor is also a philosopher', and many sixteenth century university teachers of medicine had a sophisticated grasp both of the techniques and content of philosophy. The traditional method of dialectical argument for and against an opinion was frequently used by medical writers (though, as Bylebyl shows, in the seventeenth century dialectical argument was falling into dispute even in the eyes of a traditionalist like Jean Riolan, the Younger). Also a high level of philosophical awareness in the minds of medical writers was ensured by the continuing debates between the followers of Aristotle and Galen.

Charles Schmitt has looked at the relationship between medicine and philosophy, not from the point of view of how physicians used philosophy but rather from that of how philosophers thought their subject could be of use in the education of physicians. It seems that philosophers often saw their subject as an end itself rather than as a stage in the education of physicians. However, there was an awareness on the part of some philosophers and physicians (and this was enshrined in university statutes) that certain branches of philosophy should be taught as necessary preliminaries to the study of medicine. Schmitt's chapter also throws light on the relative status of teachers of philosophy and medicine and reminds us that in the sixteenth century medicine was held in greater esteem than philosophy when measured by the internal university ranking and by the salaries of the teachers of the two subjects.

One practical aspect of medicine, that relates closely to other aspects of sixteenth century society, and was taught to all physicians was pharmacology. It was also the business of the botanist and the pharmacist. Richard Palmer's chapter opens up for us a vivid vista of the activities of Venetian doctors, botanists and pharmacists as they relate to pharmacy. Drawing upon contemporary archival sources, Palmer describes the development of botanical research in the light of the renewed interest in Greek botany, the growing influence of Paracelsian chemical remedies in the second half of the sixteenth century and the relationship, both intellectual and commercial, between doctors and pharmacists. The closeness of this relationship should counter the idea put forward by older histories of medicine that there was a rigid separation between doctors and pharmacists.

Although this book has a necessarily limited focus and is mainly concerned with intellectual aspects of sixteenth century medicine there are some other glimpses of the way in which academic medicine was located in society. Vivian Nutton, while describing how surgery was 'humanized' and given a Greek basis, depicts the flourishing, if frantic, world of renaissance academic publishing. Gerhard Baader's chapter on Jacques Dubois illustrates how the desperate social condition of contemporary France and the reaction of the State to starvation and poverty stimulated men like Dubois to write books on diet for the poor.

At this point it may be useful to turn to aspects of sixteenth century medicine not touched upon in this book except in one important chapter. This will help to put the book into a larger perspective.

Medicine for the sixteenth century, as for most periods, was concerned with preserving health and with curing illness. Such is the hunger for these two commodities that there has nearly always been a buyers' market for them. However, suppliers, buyers and, indeed, markets have varied enormously not only over time but also within a country in any one period; with different groups and classes of patients patronizing different types of medical practitioners. In the sixteenth century there was a wide variety of medical expertise available ranging from wise-women, charmers, wizards or magicians, astrologers, priests and ministers and their wives, herbalists, empirics and barbers to pharmacists, surgeons and physicians. In terms of articulateness and literary remains the latter group appear to predominate. However, only a small minority of people used the services of the trained and educated pharmacists, surgeons and physicians. In sixteenth century Europe most people would have had recourse to practitioners who had not been formally trained and whose knowledge was part of the oral culture of the period. The village wise-woman or the clergyman's wife was unlikely to publish anything about her skills, while the possibility that anything written could be used as evidence in a prosecution by Church or State discouraged publication by anyone practising magical healing. As is usual, the written word – in this case that of the educated physician – attempted to suppress the oral culture and to assert its own values instead. Unlike the late nineteenth and twentieth centuries the attacks of the trained practitioners against the empirics were not necessarily made from a position of strength; for the protection given to them by licensing was still very weak in the sixteenth century and they were, in numerical terms, in a minority. The chapters by French, Nutton, Deer Richardson and Wear allude to the way in which orthodox university-trained medical men condemned and derided their uneducated rivals. How far they did this because of a genuine concern to keep up standards or because of self-interest is a matter for debate. In contrast, Richard Palmer illustrates the pragmatism of the Venetian authorities in accepting and licensing empirics.

Luis Garcia Ballester, however, makes a significant contribution to our knowledge of the other side of medicine. He puts empirical practice into its cultural setting and, by describing how morisco healers survived in Spain allows us to go behind the rhetoric of orthodox physicians and to share the viewpoint of the empiric. Ballester describes the conditions that produced the morisco healers and he also shows how the Church and the academic physicians put severe pressure on them. The history of popular medicine in pre-industrial Europe has yet to be written, but contributions such as Ballester's will prepare the ground.

Finally, the radical alternative to orthodox university-based medicine must be mentioned. Paracelsus wanted to replace the books of Aristotle and Galen with a new philosophy and a new medicine. In some senses it was an attempt to place oral knowledge (craft wisdom) and secret and half-forbidden practices (alchemy and magic) into the world of literary culture. University physicians reacted to the ideas of Paracelsus in various ways. Paracelsus had put forward new theories in different areas and at different levels. Physicians could embrace all of his cosmology, natural philosophy, physiology, pathology and therapeutics, they might accept one or two bits – especially therapeutics where some were tempted to use chemical remedies in addition to, or instead of traditional herbal ones – or they could reject Paracelsus altogether. Although Paracelsus died in 1541, his followers did not exert any influence until the second half of the century and it was not until the beginning of the seventeenth century that they made a major impact on the bastions of Galenic orthodoxy in countries such as England and France.

The cosmology and medical theories of Paracelsus and his followers have been explored by historians but the practical aspects of Paracelsian medicine have received little attention. Walter Pagel had begun such a study for this book, but sadly he died before he could finish it. His preliminary finding indicated that, when stripped of its theory, Paracelsian medicine in practice – that is in diagnosis and treatment – was very similar to Galenic medicine, with the important difference that chemical drugs would have been used.

For this book, the existence of Paracelsian medicine is significant because it shows that there was a radical alternative to Galenic medicine; it provided a place for those who were so dissatisfied with Galenic medicine that they could not be content merely to modify it. On the other hand, the vast majority of medical men were happy to work in the broad framework given to them by their predecessors. They used their scholarship within that framework and their practical experience to refine and extend medicine in answer to the practical problems that they faced.

1

Aristotle among the physicians

CHARLES B. SCHMITT

It is a commonplace that medicine and philosophy were closely linked in the medical curriculum of late medieval and renaissance Italian universities.[1] Nonetheless, when one reads modern scholarly works on university philosophy in renaissance Italy – those on Pomponazzi and the immortality controversy, for example – one has the impression that the philosophers were treating their subject as an end in its own right rather than as a subaltern to medical studies, as the curricular structure would have it. Medical historians, on the other hand, with relatively few exceptions, tend to push into the background the philosophical components of medical education of the period, often treating the history of medicine as though it was entirely devoid of a philosophical element.

In order to shed more light on this question, which is more a problem for contemporary historiography than it was for philosophers and physicians of the sixteenth century themselves, I should like to consider it from a somewhat different perspective. The prevailing view is so deeply ingrained in the historical interpretations that it may seem rather pointless to discuss this relationship further. Still, it is not without interest to consider the question as it related to the medical faculties of sixteenth-century Italian universities from a slightly different angle. I should like to pose the question of how the philosophers and physicians of sixteenth-century Italy saw the relation between philosophy and medicine as it related to their teaching activities. Without doubt the statutes established a curriculum in which logic and philosophy were considered as propaedeutic to medical studies proper. This is evident in many statutory formulations such as that promulgated at Bologna in 1405. Here specific books of Aristotle are designated to be read in a particular order, after which specific medical works are required to be read, also in a particular order.[2] Was such an institutional structure consciously accepted by its practitioners or had the historical circumstances which led to the intimate relationship between medicine and philosophy of earlier times been lost sight of by the sixteenth century, and had medicine and philosophy begun to go their separate ways? Did, for example, the philosophers who were teaching the first part

1

of the arts–medicine curriculum at Padua or Bologna see themselves as providing pre-medical training to students who were doing philosophy primarily to fulfil the statutory requirements?

In this paper I should like to face the question of how the sixteenth-century philosophers and physicians saw themselves and how they viewed the individual contributions of philosophy and medicine to the education of the mature, trained physician. It is unlikely that I shall be able to deal with this question in any comprehensive way, but I hope at least to bring the issue to more general attention, and to formulate several hypotheses which may lead to its solution. The question I am raising should be distinguished from at least two other relevant and related questions which have been discussed in the literature. The first is the methodological discussions in philosophy, science and medicine which were an important feature of renaissance intellectual history.[3] The second is the problem of the superiority of Galen or Aristotle which attracted much attention at least down to Harvey.[4] These are both worth studying in their own right, but my focus will be on a different point. I want to consider simply the question of the relation of the medical and philosophical components in the education of the physician and how this relationship was viewed by those involved in the education.

Before considering the sixteenth century, we must look at the historical roots of the philosophy–medicine connection, for it is clear that whatever one finds in the sixteenth century had undergone a long historical conditioning. Though the relation between philosophy and medicine varied in different schools of medical thought among the Greeks, it is clear that for both Hippocrates and Galen, philosophy played a very important role in medical education and practice. In Hippocrates we find the ideal of the 'philosophical physician',[5] and Galen in many respects can be considered a philosopher as well as a physician. Though most of the philosophical works have been lost, enough survives to give us an insight into that part of his thought.[6] Moreover, the brief treatise *Quod optimus Medicus sit quoque Philosophus* cannot be passed over, and it had a broad renaissance distribution especially in the translation made by no less a humanist than Erasmus.[7] This point, the emphasis on philosophy as a component of the best medical training, was repeatedly made and eventually became embedded in such a fundamental reference work of early modern medicine as Bartolomeo Castelli's *Lexicon Medicum*.[8]

Aristotle was also a medical writer as well as a philosopher and scientist, even if his medical works survive only in a very fragmentary form. Yet, there is both textual and iconographical evidence that he worked extensively on anatomy and other medical subjects.[9] Though only a few lines of his *De Sanitate et Morbo* survive, embedded in the *Parva Naturalia*,[10] this work was avidly discussed in the sixteenth century when the question of Aristotle's attitude towards medicine arose, as it frequently did. I shall have more to discuss about this later, but for the moment, suffice it to say that both the ancient philosophical tradition represented by Aristotle and the ancient medical tradition represented by the *corpus Hippocraticum* and Galen saw a close and beneficial relationship between philosophy and medicine. While this tradition did not pave the way for all later develop-ments, it certainly provided a foundation for some of the dominant ones of the next centuries. Though there are disagreements over details, there seems to be no doubt about the general pattern of integration of philosophical and medical learning in the education of the Alexandrian physician.[11] The same pattern followed when Greek learning passed to the Arabic world.[12] The importance of the philosophical component is evident in both Avicenna and Averroës.[13]

Western medicine after antiquity flourished in the so-called School of Salerno. Its origins are obscure, but it seems as though the general approach of Salernitan physicians during the first century or so of the 'school' was practical in orientation with little room for the refinements of philosophy.[14] Kristeller has argued – and, I think, convincingly – that there was a gradual move towards a more theoretical approach to medicine accompanied by an increasingly philosophical component as time passed.[15] These observations are corroborated by Birkenmajer's demonstration that it was primarily the physicians who championed assimilation of Aristotle into the learned culture of the medieval West of the twelfth and early thirteenth centuries.[16] There is no reason to believe that the physicians wanted Aristotle for any reason other than to derive whatever utility they could from his works as an adjunct to medical studies.

Such is also the case in the Italian universities from the earliest days when medicine was cultivated, as we see from both Bologna and Padua, which began as and remained the most distinguished medical universities from the thirteenth to the seventeenth centuries. Both in the works of Taddeo Alderotti (*c.* 1215–95) and his school at Bologna and in those of Pietro d'Abano (1257–*c.*1315) at Padua, we find the firm conviction that philosophical studies had something very valuable to contribute to the education of the physician. As Nancy Siraisi has recently shown, Alderotti and his followers were interested in a wide range of philosophical issues, including moral philosophy, as evidenced, for example, by Taddeo's work on the *Nicomachean Ethics* and Bartolomeo da Varignana (*c.* 1260–after 1321) on the *Oeconomics*.[17]

At least as clear in its insistence of the joining of philosophy to medicine, and certainly more influential, was Pietro d'Abano's *Conciliator*, a work widely read and frequently reprinted down to the end of the sixteenth century and beyond.[18] This work sets up an intellectual structure in which philosophy and medicine are conjoined as closely as they have been anywhere. In the very first *differentia* it is clearly stated that the three most important things for efficacious medical study are logic, natural philosophy, and astrology.[19] This linking of disciplines became the general pattern for Italian medical education in succeeding centuries.

Whether the *Conciliator* is a reflection of statute and practice or the inspiration of them is difficult to determine, though one suspects that it may have been a mixture of both. Certainly, the influences impinging from all sides – Hippocrates, Galen, Aristotle, Avicenna, and Averroës – provide reason enough for medical education taking the form it did. This broad approach to medicine which characterized the Italian situation and which promoted such a wide range of learning and the development of so many ancillary disciplines was all but unique to the Italian peninsula. A very different and more restrictive pattern of education was followed in France, especially at Montpellier, but also elsewhere.[20] The early six-teenth-century programme put forward at Vienna by Martin Stainpeis certainly gives little place to philosophy in the education of the physician.[21]

This then sets the stage for a consideration of the sixteenth century. Clearly the statutes from all over Italy give the impression that the education in the arts faculties consisted in a two-tiered structure of logic and philosophy followed by medical studies. This is not to say that other subjects such as mathematical arts, Greek and Latin literature, and moral philosophy and metaphysics were absent, but the central core was logic–natural philosophy–medicine. This is evident in the Florentine statutes of 1387[22] but even more clearly set forth in those of Bologna of 1405.[23] The structure became institutionalized for Padua in the late fifteenth-century statutes, which were *in vigore* for the whole of the sixteenth century,[24] and in the Pisa statutes of 1543[25] among others. This is not to say that there was a strict uniformity in Italy, for there was not. There was a considerable variation in the precise books to be read from university to university. Sometimes all of the *Organon* was prescribed, at other times only the *Posterior Analytics*; in some cases all of the *Physics* was required, at others, only books one, two and eight. Nonetheless, statutory evidence from sixteenth-century Italy reveals a pattern in medical education in which philosophy provided a preliminary and important basis for advanced medical studies at university.

It is clear, that regardless of theoretical formulations and the actual practice of writing and teaching philosophy, socially and economically the position of the philosopher in sixteenth-century Italian universities was beneath that of the physician. There is abundant evidence for this. Professors of medicine were systematically paid more handsomely than their philosophical colleagues.[26] The normal career structure was to progress from logic, through natural philosophy, to medicine.[27] In the course of such a progression the individual moved up both in social prestige and in financial rewards. In other words, there was a pecking order: the logician at the bottom of the ladder, the natural philosopher above him, but physicians at the top, with *theoretici* being superior to *practici*. There are exceptions, of course, but such was the general pattern.

Nor have I come across any evidence of a concerted effort on the part of the physicians to denigrate the philosophical component of the curriculum and thus erode the position of philosophical studies in medical education. It remained for later centuries to produce the 'empirical, scientific' and strongly anti-philosophical medical man who is suspicious of anything smacking of theory or philosophy as necessarily deleterious to medical training. Criticisms of philosophy and its value came from other quarters, but even these were of limited consequence. For example, Gianfrancesco Pico della Mirandola (1469–1533), one of the most dedicated critics of Aristotle, found little of value in philosophy in general, and in Aristotelian philosophy in particular. Yet, even he felt that philosophical studies were of some value for the practical art of medicine. He could not give whole-hearted support to philosophical studies, but he seemed to acknowledge that they could not be completely abandoned if there were to be well-trained physicians.[28] Towards the end of the century, Francesco Patrizi (1529–97) wanted to get rid of the philosophical basis of medicine altogether. This, however, was because the institutional foundation of philosophical instruction was Aristotelian, not because it was philosophical.[29] He would have warmly approved a philosophical curriculum based on Plato for medical students, in the same way that he approved of a Platonic poetics to replace the dominant Aristotelian one of his time. Thus, even convinced anti-Aristotelians such as Pico and Patrizi were not totally opposed to a philosophical foundation for medical studies, but for differing reasons had something to criticize in the curriculum they knew. A similar position was taken by the Spaniard Juan Luis Vives (1492–1540), who had a good deal to criticize about medicine in his *De Causis Corruptarum Artium*, but was not in principle against the discipline's being rooted in philosophy.[30]

Therefore, it appears, at least from the evidence that I have discovered, that there was nearly a universal agreement that philosophy was not only *not* harmful to successful medical studies, but was indeed beneficial. This still, however, leaves us with the fundamental question with which we started: how did the academic or university philosophers themselves see their activity? Did they consider it subsidiary and, in some way, propaedeutic to medicine, or did they see philosophy as an independent discipline in its own right? Based on my reading of sixteenth-century Italian Aristotelian authors, as well as their modern commentators, I would argue that university philosophy of sixteenth-century Italy was considered a subject in its own right and not as something in the curriculum meant to give a preliminary training for some more important activity. Already in the fourteenth century Petrarch had taken the logicians to task for treating their subject as important in itself rather than merely a boyhood preparation for higher things as he thought it should be.[31] As

Siraisi notes, the distinction between those primarily involved in the teaching of medicine and those primarily involved with philosophy grew during the fourteenth century.[32] Already at that date we may see the roots of the even greater distinction which was to rise in the sixteenth century. The fourteenth century was, of course, the time when Italian scholastic culture, that is, the medical faculties of the universities, underwent a strong influence from the assimilation of the highly developed tradition of logic and natural philosophy which had flourished at Oxford.[33] This influx was notable in Italian medical faculties through the fifteenth and into the early sixteenth century. Such an orientation is already evident in the *Summa Medicinalis* of Tommaso del Garbo (fl. 1370) composed in the third quarter of the fourteenth century;[34] it became a prominent and characteristic feature of Italian theoretical medicine for a century and a half. However, in addition to the tendency to assimilate logic and natural philosophy to medicine, which had already been there from twelfth-century Salerno, but was reinforced by the new English material, there developed at the same time a strong tradition of independent philosophical thought. This can be seen in figures such as Peter of Mantua (fl. 1384–99), Paul of Venice (*c.* 1370–1429), and Blasius of Parma (*c.* 1345–1416) among others.[35] These interests were sometimes allied to a theological bent (as with Paul of Venice) and sometimes to a more scientific cluster of problems (as with Blasius).

It is therefore my suspicion that by the sixteenth century there was already a well-established tradition in the Italian medical faculties for philosophers taking their subject as a serious end in its own right in a way which the statutory evidence will not bear. Certainly in later centuries philosophy gradually became an independent discipline in its own right, reaching an apogee as the highest science in German Idealism and other nineteenth-century developments.

But what can we learn from the writings of the philosophers themselves? While there is undoubtedly much yet to be dug out of the vast number of sixteenth-century philosophical writings, my own attempts to formulate a clear and generalized picture have not been entirely successful. On the whole I think we can say that Italian philosophers were much less concerned with how their teaching and writing related to medical studies than might be expected.

Agostino Nifo (1469/70–1538), for example, whose long university career took him from Padua and Pisa in the north to Rome, Naples, and Salerno in the south, was intimately familiar with both medical and philosophical traditions of all shades. He was one of the most prolific and wide-ranging writers on philosophical topics, but at the same time a physician of eminence and author of several medical works. Yet even his voluminous commentaries on the central Aristotelian works, which were mainstays of Italian medical education, frequently reprinted and constantly

cited until the end of the century, had little to say on the philosophy–
medicine relationship.[36] His writings seem to take for granted the importance of philosophical studies for medical education, and he feels no need to
justify it in the same way which Pietro d'Abano had done two centuries
earlier.

Even in those passages where Aristotelians discussed the parts of
philosophy and of learning in general – frequently as an introduction to
commentaries on the *Physics* – we find little interest in this question. Since
one of the premises of the statutes in including natural philosophy as a part
of the curriculum must certainly have been a conviction of its relevance for
medical studies, one might justifiably expect to find the topic discussed.
The place of natural philosophy and medicine in the overall schema of arts
and the relation between the two had already been given serious attention
in many discussions from the early middle ages onward. By the time we
get to the philosophers of the sixteenth century it was a commonplace
known to all. Yet, in the *Physics* commentaries of Nifo, Ludovico Boccadiferro (1482–1545), or Giampaolo Pernumia (d. before 1564) who were
active at Padua, Bologna and elsewhere, we find essentially nothing on the
topic.[37]

The same also holds true for the popular *Solutiones* of Marcantonio
Zimara (*c.* 1475–1532), a word index based on Aristotle which was used to
organize peripatetic thought on many diverse topics.[38] Other writers such
as Girolamo Balduino (fl. mid-16th century), active in both Padua and
Salerno, and Cesare Cremonini (1552–1631), possibly the last significant
Aristotelian at Padua, take note of the question, but evidently their interest
was little more than a passing one. At the beginning of his commentary on
the *Physics* Balduino considers how that work relates to medical studies,
but fails to expand on how such an approach might produce practical
results at a medical level.[39] Cremonini's explanation of the preface to the
Physics deals with the conventional topic of the division of the various parts
of philosophy so characteristic of renaissance treatments of that text, but
gives us only a few vague generalizations on how medicine relates to
physics without ever essaying a coherent analysis of this key problem.[40]

The one sixteenth-century Aristotelian philosopher who has somewhat
more to say on the medicine–philosophy relationship is Jacopo Zabarella
(1533–89). A native of Padua, who unusually spent his whole career there,
Zabarella must stand out as one of the most acute and influential peripatetic
thinkers of his age. Throughout his works we find an abiding concern with
medical problems and the methodology surrounding them. Though so far
as I know Zabarella did not write on medicine *per se*, in his writings on
logic and natural philosophy he quite obviously kept in mind the needs of
physicians and the way in which his subjects related to medicine. For
example, in his commentary on the *De Anima* he argues that one of the
reasons to study the work is that the medical art is able to draw a good deal

from discussions of life, growth and the soul.[41] In his general compendium on the structure of knowledge, *De Naturalis Scientiae Constitutione*, he stated clearly the assumptions behind the curricular structure, which, as we have noted, were not very frequently alluded to in the sixteenth century. He argued that one cannot be a good *medicus* without being a natural philosopher, and, indeed, natural philosophy provides the theoretical structure of science (that is, knowledge, not practical efficacy) which medicine can then take over and apply to some practical end.[42] This, of course, harks back to ancient and medieval formulations and had been a commonplace in his own university (Padua) since at least the days of Pietro d'Abano. In Zabarella it is insisted upon with some emphasis

Therefore, there cannot be a good physician who is not also a natural philosopher; likewise there can be no good legislator who is not highly skilled in moral philosophy. But there is a difference between them: medicine is concerned only with accomplishing its purpose, while natural philosophy has no purpose to accomplish, but is only (theoretical) knowledge.[43]

He goes on to give further precision to this viewpoint, but from what has been quoted his position is clear enough. As Zabarella sees it, natural philosophy provides the scientific knowledge from which medicine – in this scheme, it must be remembered, a practical art – takes its starting point to bring about the desired results. In the same work he argued that medicine takes a knowledge of *physiologia* (by which I think he means something relatively close to the modern use of the term) from that part of the natural philosophy which deals with the human body and its parts.[44] This is a clear statement of the position that medical studies are founded upon a preliminary and basic knowledge of the kind of information contained in the Aristotelian zoological works. He goes on to say that physicians who wish to understand the structure of the human body should follow Aristotle's approach as found in the *De Partibus Animalium* rather than in the *De Historia Animalium*.[45] By this I think he means that the approach should be through an understanding of function and purpose, rather than through a mere knowledge of the external structure of the parts.

In his writings on logic, too, which form the basis of both his renaissance and modern reputation, Zabarella emphasized more than most other logicians of his time the application of his subject to other disciplines. This is particularly true of that part of the logic discipline deriving from the *Posterior Analytics*, which he sought to relate to a spectrum of arts and sciences ranging from literature to medicine.[46] In the schematic *De Natura Logicae*, for example, he says forthrightly 'The natural philosopher takes nothing from the physician, but the physician much from the natural philosopher.'[47] This again reinforces the position already cited that natural philosophy provides the scientific basis (that is, the theoretical knowledge) which enables the physician to produce the desired results in medical treatment. In developing the theme, he provides a cogent justification for the pre-eminent place which logic held in the medical curriculum.[48] The more interesting and innovatory *De Methodis* includes an extended discussion of the logical structure of medical thinking. He argues forcefully that the fundamental logical method employed in medical reasoning is the *methodus resolutiva*. In his lengthy discussion he is at pains to show that such a position was also held by earlier authorities of note, including Galen, Avicenna, and Averroës.[49] While this theme was an old one by Zabarella's time, his forceful reiteration of it gave theoretical substance to the 'Italian' position on the medicine–philosophy relationship which was to have an important *Nachleben*, especially in seventeenth-century Germany and Britain where his works were still widely read when medicine was entering a new age.[50]

All of this indicates, I think, that unlike most of his Aristotelian associates of renaissance Italy Zabarella held in mind both the provision of the statutes under which he was teaching and the needs of his students, who were, after all, for the most part neophyte physicians. Possibly a coherent attitude towards medicine and its relation to philosophy could be extracted from Zabarella's work. It is certainly true that he was much more conscious of his position as a teacher in the medical faculty than were most of his philosophical contemporaries, including Nifo and others. Precisely how unusual he was in this respect requires further research.

Medical authors, on the other hand, were considerably more concerned with the question than most of the philosophers, as we can see, for example, in the works of Giambattista Da Monte (or Montanus) (1489–1551) and Girolamo Capodivacca (or Capivaccio) (d. 1589), both of whom were major medical figures at Padua during the middle years of the century. In his *De Differentiis Doctrinarum sive de Methodis*, which could profitably be compared with Zabarella's *De Methodis* as a contemporary treatment of the same problem by a physician, Capodivacca faces some of the same key issues.[51] He is every bit as concerned as Zabarella to determine whether the study of method is the problem of the logician alone or whether it also comes within the province of the philosopher and physician. Possibly this work, as well as any of the century, illustrates the amalgamation of medical and philosophical themes. It, along with several of Da Monte's works touching on methodological questions,[52] requires further study before its general place in sixteenth-century medical and philosophical thought can properly be evaluated.

One of the key texts, if not *the* fundamental text, which lay at the base of the whole tradition making medical training follow on from philosophical training is to be found in Aristotle's *De Sensu et Sensato*. It was frequently referred to in many different contexts in the sixteenth century, and was in many ways a rallying cry which gave full justification for the study of philosophy in Italian universities. It was cited and discussed almost everywhere in the medico-philosophical literature of the renaissance, but to the best of my knowledge has not received the modern scholarly attention it deserves. Let us first quote it in full

It is further the duty of the natural philosopher to study the first principles of disease and health; for neither health nor disease can be properties of things deprived of life. Hence one may say that most natural philosophers, and those physicians who take a scientific interest in their art, have this in common: the former end by studying medicine, and the latter base their medical theories on the principles of natural science.[53]

The passage just cited, though brief, furnished a rationale, based upon a genuine Aristotelian text, for the whole programme of medical education which still dominated the Italian universities of the sixteenth century.

There were relatively few commentaries on the *De Sensu* from the sixteenth century, but this key text was obviously in the consciousness of nearly everyone concerned with the interaction of philosophy and medicine. It is a text – along with other parts of the *Parva Naturalia* – whose importance and influence during the middle ages and renaissance have seldom been recognized, but the evidence of its broad distribution both in manuscript and in early printed editions is unequivocal.[54] Along with the more substantial and better known works of the *libri naturales* it held a central place in Italian university education.

There are two substantial and careful commentaries on the work by sixteenth-century Italians which are worthy of attention from a number of points of view and not only for the particular issue I am considering here. In both cases the brief work was translated anew from Greek into Latin and given a minute analysis based upon a thorough knowledge of the Greek text and earlier relevant commentaries and expositions. The commentators are Mainetto Mainetti (*c.* 1515–72) of Pisa, who taught philosophy and later medicine at Pisa and Bologna, and Simone Simoni (1532–1602), who became a protestant and spent most of his mature life in Northern Europe, though his Italian education shines through in his Aristotelian works. Both recognized the importance of the passage quoted above and devoted energy to explaining it. Mainetti's main strategy is the traditional one of arguing that medicine is subaltern to natural philosophy, a method common in the middle ages and renaissance when the individual sciences were generally viewed as part of an interlocking and interrelated hierarchical scheme, which had already been put forward by Aristotle in several separate works. This conception is based upon a view of the world in which particular sciences are considered superior to others by virtue of such qualities as being capable of producing greater accuracy and having a more noble subject matter, a theme treated, for example, in the *Posterior Analytics*.[55] This theme of subalternation became standard afterwards finding its way into the well known schemes of the 'division of the sciences' in medieval writers such as Al-Farabi, Gundissalinus, and Hugh of St Victor.[56]

Mainetti and Simoni both argue that sickness and health are not alien to the concerns of the *physicus* or *physiologus* (both terms are used for the natural philosopher), since they are found in the living body which is the proper subject matter of physics, that is, the changeable physical body.[57] Simoni argues, for example: 'Let us conclude that the living body is considered by the natural philosopher in so far as it is healthy.'[58] He qualifies this, however, by saying that the *physicus* treats the subject of sickness and health only under a particular aspect. Somewhat differently from the other commentators (including Mainetti), he contends that *medicina* is not subaltern to *physiologia*, since the former is a *res artis* and cannot strictly speaking be subjected to a *res naturae*.[59] Though deviating somewhat from the usual position, he nonetheless takes a standard Aristotelian position in not mixing different categories. He emphasizes that art and science (or nature) are different categories and must not be confused.[60] In spite of making this point, however, he concludes that the subject of medicine coalesces from a number of different sciences and accepts its general principles relating to sickness and health from the *physicus*.[61] The view that medicine represents a coalescence of various disciplines and fields of knowledge is itself, of course, an old one having roots in most of the ancient writings on medicine. In the Latin tradition of the West it goes back at least to the time of Cassiodorus and Isidore of Seville.[62]

This is really the premise of the medieval and renaissance medical curriculum of Italy and, indeed, with slight variations allowing for certain alterations in the nature of the sciences involved, is the basis for more modern medical education. Mainetti puts the point clearly

Medicine then coalesces from many sciences, since from the natural philosopher (*physiologo*) indeed it has drawn anatomy itself, the elements and humours, as well as the knowledge and virtues of plants.[63]

He then goes on to illustrate how medicine also draws useful material from astronomy and mathematics.[64] This, of course, is nothing but a reiteration of a tradition laid down by Hippocrates, Galen, Avicenna, Averroës, and Pietro d'Abano, among others.

What these two commentaries illustrate above all is that the authors, when faced with the question of the relationship of philosophy to medicine came down firmly for the traditional position. This is expressed in a dictum which became a cliché in the renaissance, and may have roots much earlier. I have found it stated frequently in those contexts where the medicine–philosophy relationship is discussed, and both Simoni and Mainetti use it in support of their main point. Though one encounters minor verbal variations, it perhaps most frequently takes the crisp and clear form which Simoni gives it: 'Ubi desinit physicus, ibi medicus incipit' (Where the natural philosopher finishes, there begins the physician).[65] This becomes almost as common a programmatic statement in the medical literature as the principle of Ockham's razor became in the logical literature of the fourteenth century or the principle 'Nihil est in intellectu, quod prius non fuerit in sensu' became from Thomas Aquinas to Locke. Behind this simple statement lies the assumption that natural philosophy prepares one for medical studies and that a good foundation in those traditional areas of Aristotelian learning is essential before medical practice can even begin. Moreover, it became a sort of shorthand statement for the *De Sensu* passage I have already noted, which itself becomes much quoted and discussed, as for example in Zimara's *Quaestio* on the nobility and distinction of medicine as compared to law.[66] My research on this has not been exhaustive and I have been unable to determine the origin of this principle.

It might be well to mention some of the writers who use the dictum. Zabarella[67] and Cremonini[68] both adopt it as a well-worn principle, as do several medical writers. For example, Giambattista da Monte, whose importance as a central figure of the sixteenth-century methodological discussions involving medicine has long been recognized, follows the formula of medicine being subaltern to natural philosophy.[69] He expands the saying somewhat, clearly taking it for granted as a central directive for analysing the philosophy–medicine interface.[70] The more usual version is given by Oddo degli Oddi (1478–1558) in his commentary on the first fen of Avicenna's *Canon*.[71] In the next century Caspar Bartholin (1585–1629), a Dane who studied in Italy with Fabricio, Casserio and Iasolino, wrote a *De Studio Medico* in which he outlined a programme of medical studies where he claims 'Natural philosophy and mathematics are as much relevant to the physician as ethics is for the lawyer. *Ubi enim desinit physicus, ibi incipit medicus.*'[72]

With Da Monte and degli Oddi, as well as with a number of other writers I have mentioned this principle is tied in with another brief and relevant text from the *Parva Naturalia*. These few lines are usually placed at the end of the *De Respiratione*, but there has been a good deal of discussion of how and where this short passage fits into the *corpus Aristotelicum*. Again, it is well to quote these sentiments in their entirety

As for health and disease it is the business not only of the physician but also of the natural philosopher to discuss their causes up to a point. But the way in which these two classes of inquirers differ and consider different problems must not escape us, since the facts prove that up to a point their activities have the same scope; for those physicians who have subtle and inquiring minds have something to say about natural science, and claim to derive their principles therefrom, and the most accomplished of those who deal with natural science tend to conclude with medical principles.[73]

Several points should be made about this crucial passage at the outset. First, it has been argued that it is the beginning of a separate work of Aristotle, Περὶ νόσου καὶ ὑγίειας (*De Morbo et Sanitate*), of which the remainder is lost. Internal and external evidence provide a basis for believing that Aristotle did in fact write a work on the subject and that these may be the opening sentences.[74] Secondly, a consideration of the content tells us why the passage was thought to be so crucial by Italian philosophers and physicians. Not only does it, along with the *De Sensu* passage, face the central problem of the medicine–natural philosophy issue, but it gives much more away to the physician vis-à-vis the philosopher than any other text we can find in Aristotle. In it he goes so far as to say that 'for those physicians who have subtle and inquiring minds have something to say about natural science', which is quite a concession and must have given some comfort to the physicians who felt themselves subaltern to the *physici*. Indeed, one might say that it goes so far as to question the whole subalternation viewpoint which, as I have argued, provides the basis for the Italian medical curriculum. It goes somewhat beyond saying that the physician takes the (theoretical) results of the natural philosopher and builds upon them in his own practically oriented endeavour. Yet, in the final analysis two further things can be said. First, this is a somewhat enthusiastic statement on Aristotle's part, slightly at odds with the considered opinion expressed elsewhere. Secondly, and probably more importantly, the concessive nature of the statement 'those physicians who have subtle and enquiring minds' limits those having 'something to say about natural science' somewhat severely.

This precise passage was taken up by Simoni and by a number of others who used it to cement the relationship between physician and philosopher.[75] One can read some Italian philosophers of the sixteenth century – Pomponazzi, for example – and get little impression that they saw themselves as contributing to the education of physicians or to the advance of medical studies. The same is possibly also true of one such as Nifo, who was himself not only a practising physician, but also wrote commentaries on nearly the whole gamut of Aristotle's natural philosophy. On the other hand, in those contexts in which the question of the medicine–natural philosophy relationship specifically arose, and in many other relevant passages as well, there was a general commitment by physicians to an acceptance of natural philosophy as a basis of medicine. Usually it was rigidly in the subaltern mode, but even when liberalized, it was nearly always recognized that logic and natural philosophy were necessary preparations for medical study. This become concretized in the early seventeenth century, not only in Bartholin's work previously referred to, but also in Pietro Castelli's (*c.* 1575–1661) *De Optimo Medico*, which gives a kind of utopian programme of medical education very much in line with the encyclopedic tradition of learning characterized above all by contemporary figures such as J. H. Alsted (1588–1638) and J. A. Comenius (1592–1670).[76] Castelli's work gives us an exhaustive and detailed outline of what a good medical education should have been at the turn of the seventeenth century. Empirical knowledge – including chemistry, botany and various medical subjects such as surgery and anatomy – is much emphasized, but there is still the old stress on philosophy.[77] Castelli opens his section on the role of philosophy in medical education with a reference to Aristotle's subjection of medicine to philosophy in the *De Sanitate et Morbo* fragment and thereupon quotes the dictum 'ubi desinit physicus, incipere medicum'.[78] He then goes on to square that with Galen's position stated as 'optimum medicum esse optimum philosophum'.[79] These early seventeenth-century formulations reflect the sixteenth-century view, which had developed in Italy and then spread beyond the borders through the influence of many foreign students who had studied medicine there and taken what they had learned back home.

While it was all but universally acknowledged that logic and natural philosophy were valuable – even indispensable and essential – subjects to be studied for all physicians this acceptance did not necessarily apply to the other parts of philosophy. Both Bartholin and Castelli found other branches of philosophy to be of more limited value. Bartholin said straight out that 'Metaphysics is of no direct use to the physician',[80] though his own *Enchiridion Metaphysicum* was a great popular success as a textbook in the protestant countries.[81] Both agreed, however, on rhetoric. Though Castelli in particular emphasized the necessity of clarity and precision in medical style, he had little use for rhetoric *per se*. According to him 'non eloquentia, sed medicamentis curantur aegri'.[82] Bartholin expressed it only slightly differently in saying 'non enim verbis sed herbis aeger curatur'.[83] In both men we have a clear understanding that science is to be strictly separated from the rhetorical arts as surely as modern medical research is to be separated from the twentieth-century successor of renaissance rhetoric, commercial advertizing. Whatever use, or pretended use, rhetoric may have had in renaissance history writing, politics, or royal ceremonial, it could claim little direct relevance for medicine or the sciences other than in the purely propagandistic role to which figures such as Bacon or Galilei turned it.

The conclusion must be that it was generally assumed in sixteenth century Italy that philosophy was a valuable propaedeutic to medical studies.[84] There were few dissenting voices, though there were a number of philosophers who did not concern themselves particularly with the issue, in spite of the fact they were themselves providing this preliminary education for the student physicians. Moreover, both from the formulations of the statutes and from the theory insofar as we can know it, it seems evident that only certain branches of philosophical studies – above all logic and natural philosophy – were seen as directly relevant to medical studies.

For the most part philosophers tended to treat their own subject as an independent discipline, a development which is wholly understandable given the emphasis placed upon philosophy both in statutory and in theoretical formulations. In doing so they set the stage for the progressive emergence of philosophy as a subject in its own right in later times. Thenceforward the philosophical component of Italian universities has tended to be viewed as an independent discipline instead of one closely allied to medical studies. In similar fashion renaissance medicine has been generally seen as a scientific discipline independent of philosophical presuppositions. What is clear at this point is that historians must make a greater effort to study the philosophy (especially logic and natural philosophy) and medicine of the Italian renaissance in unison and to consider the interface of the two disciplines more carefully. The traditional approach which treats history of philosophy and history of medicine separately can give only limited results.

Since this chapter went to press I have discovered further uses of the phrase 'ubi desinit physicus, ibi medicus incipit'. It occurs, for example, in the prologue to the 1604 recension of Christopher Marlowe's *Doctor Faustus*, but is not included in the 1616 revision of the play. See W. W. Greg, *Marlowe's Doctor Faustus, 1604–1616* (Oxford, 1950; repr. 1968), 165, a reference to which I am indebted to Richard Gaskin. It is also included, with a discussion of its meaning, in Gratianus Montfortius, *Axiomata philosophica, quae passim ex Aristotele circumferri et in disputionem circulis ventilari solent . . .* (Antwerp, 1926), 409. The scholarly discussion of the meaning of this axiom is concluded as follows: 'Vera manet igitur haec sententia: *Ibi medicus incipit, ubi physicus desinit*. Sed verior est haec altera: *Ibi incipit Parochus (seu sacerdos funereus), ubi desinit medicus.*'

Also relevant to the point of this chapter is the discussion entitled 'De differentia inter medicum et physicum, et an medicina subalternetur physicae, et cuius sit ponere discrimen inter scientias, which appears in lib. II, cap. 4 (pp. 51–3) of Benito Pereira, *De communibus omnium rerum naturalium principiis* (Venice, 1591), a work first published in 1562.

2

The changing fortunes of a traditional text: goals and strategies in sixteenth-century Latin editions of the *Canon* of Avicenna[1]

NANCY G. SIRAISI

Medical teaching in sixteenth-century universities inherited much from the medieval past. Textbooks and pedagogical methods that had proved their durability over several centuries continued to play a part in many university curricula. A copious late medieval Latin medical literature, the production of which had helped to establish the pre-eminent reputation of north Italian medical schools, continued – at any rate in the earlier part of the century – to be read. Aspects of practical instruction, notably anatomical demonstration on the human cadaver and clinical teaching at the bedside, although greatly developed and advanced in the sixteenth century, had much earlier medieval origins. And, of course, a fundamental reliance upon Greek, and especially Galenic, medical and physiological understanding characterized western medicine both in the middle ages and in the sixteenth century. Although the renaissance approach to Galen was marked by a fuller knowledge of and more attention to Galen's anatomy, and by a humanistic insistence upon the importance of direct knowledge of the Greek texts, a substantial body of Galen's works in Latin translation had been studied – along with various summaries and Arabized interpretations of Galenic thought – in western European universities since the late thirteenth century.

But while the heritage of the past survived in sixteenth-century medical teaching, it did not survive unaltered. Instead, the use of methods, materials, and concepts brought together in the Latin west in the middle ages continued in an environment profoundly affected by the humanist reverence for Greek medical texts and loudly proclaimed scorn for earlier Arab and Latin mediators of the Greek heritage, and by innovations in anatomy, in medical botany and pharmacology, and in the conceptualization of disease. Long-esteemed texts for teaching, including works of medieval Arabic origin, continued to be expounded, but by professors and to audiences whose priorities were not those of the past. Thus, even though a sixteenth-century medical student was likely to read some of the same books as his fourteenth-century predecessors, his intellectual experience was not the same as theirs. Nonetheless, so long as the system of medical education was to any significant extent based in substance upon Greek medicine and physiology and in form upon the exposition of texts, traditional materials retained their usefulness. Furthermore, apparently conservative aspects of teaching were in fact responsive to the changing intellectual environment, and were marked by efforts to adapt to the literary tastes, philological scholarship, and scientific needs of the age. The sixteenth- and seventeenth-century printing history of one highly 'traditional' text, the *Canon* of Avicenna, to which the present chapter is devoted, provides a case history of this process.

Between 1500 and 1674 at least sixty editions of the complete or partial text of the *Canon* were printed. Apart from one edition of the entire work in Arabic and two others of sections of the Arabic text with Latin translation, all these publications were in Latin.[2] In the great majority of cases, their context was the study of the *Canon* in western European, and especially Italian, university faculties of medicine. Hence, the content and chronology of these editions provide one measure of the changing fortunes of Avicenna, a leading representative of Arabic medicine and traditional authority, in sixteenth- and seventeenth-century medical schools. Far from simply perpetuating an unchanging and monolithic tradition, the various editions include a wide range of different material and display an equally wide range of apparent editorial objectives, attitudes to Avicenna as a medical author, and, in some methodologies of revision. Especially worthy of note are those publications which attempt to provide an improved Latin text or to accompany it with up to date apparatus of various kinds, an enterprise in which, collectively, a good deal of time and effort on the part of scholarly editors, revisers, and in a few instances translators, and of money on the part of publishers was evidently invested. Yet even routine reprintings of short excerpts from the *Canon* commonly prescribed as textbooks merit attention to the extent that such reprintings provide a clue to the call for copies of the work in the schools.

Among these editions, a handful were the products of a group of sixteenth-century Italian scholars, most of them associated with the university of Padua or with Venice, concerned to present the *Canon* in a form consonant with the tastes and scholarship of their environment. Of all the Latin editions of the work, this group of publications yields the most information about the ways in which the *Canon* was studied and expounded in sixteenth-century universities. From editions in this category, evidence may be gathered about the teaching of medical theory and medical practice in the Italian schools; about the latter stages of a regional tradition of scholastic medical learning that extended back to the thirteenth century; about the impact of renaissance Galenism; and about the arguments and assumptions of Avicenna's detractors as well as his defenders.

Accordingly, the present chapter will first survey broadly the entire output of *Canon* editions in an attempt to classify them by type and chronology, and then return to a somewhat more detailed but nevertheless necessarily brief discussion of the characteristics of the innovative Latin editions produced in Italy or with the participation of Italian professors of medicine that have just been alluded to. What follows is, however, very far from being a complete account of the career of the *Canon* as a Latin medical book in the renaissance and early modern period. Although valuable studies by Francesca Lucchetta and Marie-Thérèse d'Alverny have illuminated some attempts to revise the Latin text of the *Canon*, much remains to be learned about the textual history of the Latin versions of the work.[3] Furthermore, editions of the Latin *Canon* itself are only one variety of source for the history of the work's place in medical thought and education after 1500. Others, which cannot be examined within the confines of the present chapter, include the substantial body of formal commentary on various parts of the *Canon* written after 1500, renaissance printings of older commentaries, the literature of polemic over 'Arab' and scholastic medicine, and evidence regarding the actual and nominal place accorded to the *Canon* in different university curricula.

In content, the Latin editions of the *Canon* published after 1500 fall into six categories. These are: (1) the complete text in the translation produced in the circle of Gerard of Cremona before 1187, without commentary and with no recent 'modernization' of text or apparatus; (2) one or more of the five books into which the *Canon* is divided, accompanied by Latin commentary written between the thirteenth and the fifteenth centuries; (3) the complete *Canon* or a major portion of it with textual revisions and apparatus contributed by late fifteenth- or sixteenth-century medical scholars; (4) one or more of the short sections of the work used as university textbooks, either alone or in compilations of brief texts such as the articella; (5) compendia or collections of maxims based on the *Canon*; and, finally, (6) retranslations of portions of the work.

Broadly speaking, these publications may be divided into three chronological groups, each marked by a different distribution of the various kinds of content just indicated. However, the identification of these groups should not be allowed to obscure the extent of overlapping between them or the presence of elements of continuity through all three. With one exception, the first group of twenty two editions published between 1500 and 1525 essentially perpetuates approaches to and presentations of the *Canon* that had developed, most notably perhaps in the schools of northern Italy, but also in other western university centres, between the thirteenth and the fifteenth centuries. Among the twenty nine Latin editions published between 1526 and 1608 attempts to revise the text or presentation predominate. Most of the latter productions can, once again, be associated with the learning of the north Italian universities; moreover, this group, which includes the editions that are the focus of the present discussion, coincides chronologically with an active phase in the production and publication of commentaries on the *Canon* in the Italian schools.[4] Finally, a small group of nine editions was published between 1609 and 1674. They included efforts by northern European Arabists to provide a better Latin text of the *Canon* that were in some respects more far reaching than any earlier endeavours of that kind; but by the time these works appeared, neither the medical content of the *Canon* nor a pedagogical and investigative methodology based on the exposition of ancient scientific authorities aroused much further interest. Parts of the Latin *Canon* did indeed survive in various Italian university curricula until well into the eighteenth century;[5] but although this survival was not entirely nominal,[6] it was at any rate insufficient to stimulate demand for fresh Latin editions after the late seventeenth century.

The rapid sequence of editions in the first chronological group, like the appearance of the fourteen incunabular Latin editions that preceded them,[7] reflects the important place accorded to the *Canon* in medical teaching since the thirteenth century in the west. Many of these editions also demonstrate a high level of attachment to a major tradition of scholastic commentary that had developed in the fourteenth and fifteenth centuries. Although the *Canon* of Avicenna (d. 1037) in its twelfth-century Latin translation was well known to some Latin medical writers and natural philosophers before the mid-thirteenth century,[8] the earliest Latin commentaries on parts of the work – probably indicating their use as the topic of academic lectures or discussion – appear to date from the late 1200s.[9] It seems likely that sections of the *Canon* were incorporated as regular parts of the curriculum in Europe's leading medical schools about the middle of the thirteenth century.[10] Since Avicenna's work is in fact a collection of more or less self-contained treatises and reference works, portions of the *Canon* could easily be detached for study in various branches of a medical curriculum. Particularly appropriate for use as academic textbooks were the well crafted summaries of mainly Galenic teaching found in the opening two sections of book one on general physiology and principles of pathology, the fourth section of book one on general therapy, and the treatise on fevers that opens book four. No doubt the awareness of Aristotelian philosophy and Galen's differences with Aristotle displayed in the early part of book one, and the readiness with which that section of the work lent itself to the isolation and discussion of *quaestiones* regarding the nature of medical science, its relation to other branches of learning, and the fundamentals of physiology especially enhanced its appeal to scholastically trained learned physicians. Other parts of the *Canon* were a mine of information concerning simples (book two), the compounding of medicines (book five), and the various parts of the body with the ailments considered peculiar to each (book three, prescribed as the sole text for a four-year cycle of lectures on *practica* by the Bologna university medical statutes of 1405).[11] In addition, various compilations of excerpts from or compendia based on the *Canon* circulated no doubt chiefly among teachers and students, but perhaps also to some extent among literate practitioners.[12]

The authors who in the fourteenth and fifteenth centuries produced major commentaries on the portions of the *Canon* commonly used in teaching were most of them professors in the north Italian universities and included some of the most distinguished medical masters of their age – men such as Gentile da Foligno (d. 1348),[13] Giacomo da Forlì (d. 1414),[14] and Ugo Benzi (d. 1439),[15] whose accomplishments were a source of considerable regional and professional pride. Thus Avicenna, 'prince of physicians', came not only to hold a place alongside Hippocrates and Galen, but also to be closely linked with the major figures of Italian academic medicine of the fourteenth and fifteenth centuries.

Hence, in the period 1500–25, while two editions of the complete Gerard of Cremona text without commentary were published, both in the first decade of the century,[16] their appearance was overshadowed by a considerably larger number of publications of the text accompanied by the expositions of its principal thirteenth- to fifteenth-century commentators. Perhaps because he was apparently the only author to have written commentaries on all five books, Gentile da Foligno's expositions seem to have been especially favoured by the *Canon*'s early sixteenth-century editors. Even Gentile probably did not in fact quite accomplish the monumental task of commenting on the entire *Canon* since his exposition of book three is apparently incomplete.[17] However, his prolixity and that of other authors whose commentary was used to supplement his, was sufficient to preclude the presentation of the complete *Canon* with commentary in a single volume. Thus, to choose only one of several examples, books three and four with the commentaries of Gentile and the French physician Jacques Despars (d. 1458),[18] supplemented for parts of book four with those of Dinus Florentinus (probably Dino del Garbo, d. 1327),[19] and Giovanni Matteo Ferrari da Grado (d. 1472),[20] published at Venice about 1505, occupy three large folio volumes.[21] The culmination of this approach to the *Canon* came in 1523, with the appearance from the Junta press of Venice of a set of five massive tomes which announced itself as presenting the entire *Canon* along with the expositions of all its principal interpreters.[22] The round up of commentators included all those so far mentioned, as well as Taddeo Alderotti (d. 1295).[23] There seem to be no editions of the *Canon* subsequent to the Junta volumes of 1523 that are adorned with commentaries written before 1500; separate editions of such commentaries (some of which, as noted, include portions of the text), which were issued rather frequently between the introduction of printing and the mid 1520s, appeared much less often thereafter.[24]

If the goal of those responsible for the editions just described appears to have been to flank the *Canon* with the fullest possible scholastic commentary, others in the early years of the century followed another practice that also had earlier antecedents, and sought to make Avicenna's medical thought accessible by means of drastic abbreviations or rearrangements of the Latin text. Thus, the preface to a small volume of *Flores Avicennae* published at Lyons in 1508 refers to the importance in medicine of aphoristic works that can readily be committed to memory, and to the example of the Hippocratic writings.[25] The task of abbreviation was undertaken with such enthusiasm that Avicenna's chapter on the elements (*Canon* 1:1:2), for example, was compressed from about 550 words in the full Gerard of Cremona version into fifty three in the *Flores*. This compendium was twice reissued, in 1514 and again in 1528, in an expanded version that included similar treatment of other works by Avicenna.[26] A like emphasis upon the goal of easy memorization is found in the dedicatory letter that Antonio Rustico prefaced to his *Memoriale Medicorum Canonice Practicantium*, published in 1517 and intended to help students at the university of Pavia, where Rustico was a professor.[27] Rustico's first two sets of *canones* are based upon *Canon* 1:4 and 4:1, which he broke down into axioms grouped in numerous brief sections. A similar emphasis upon conciseness is present in the title of a 'very brief' so-called 'alphabetized' *Canon* published in 1520, although the contents of the work are actually a kind of index.[28]

In the early years of the century, too, excerpts from the *Canon* commonly used as university textbooks were several times printed as part of the *Articella*, the celebrated collection of brief medical textbooks first formed, probably in southern Italy, early in the twelfth century and subsequently expanded by the inclusion of additional works.[29] For example, *Canon* 1:1–2 and 4, and 4:1 are found in *Articella* published at Pavia in 1506 with a dedicatory letter by Antonio Rustico, and reissued at Venice in the following year.[30] Another version of the *Articella* printed at Lyons in 1515 subsequently several times reissued included the same portions of the *Canon* and, in addition, 4:3–4:5 (on surgery).[31] Although *Canon* 1:1 was in these collections printed, as since the early fourteenth century it had usually been taught, with the omission of a fairly substantial section on anatomy,[32] the texts printed in the *Articella* are excerpts from, not abbreviations or rearrangements of, the text of the Gerard of Cremona translation.

Thus, the salient features of the various types of *Canon* edition that appeared most frequently in the first twenty or more years of the sixteenth century – scholastic commentaries, aphoristic presentations, and the incorporation of sections of the *Canon* into the *Articella* – all testify to the continuing vitality of long-established forms of medical education.

But the presentation of the *Canon* did not long remain unaffected by newer developments. As is well known, the emphasis of medical humanists upon the study of Greek and especially Galenic medical texts was accompanied by a vein of denigration of Arab medicine and its Latin scholastic interpreters, as well as of medieval translators.[33] Nicolo Leoniceno had indeed published aspersions on the *Canon* as early as 1491; similar aspersions became a commonplace of advanced medical thought throughout Europe after the appearance of the first edition of the *Epistolae Medicinales* of Leoniceno's pupil Giovanni Manardi in 1521.[34] Controversies over the merits of the Arabs in general and Avicenna in particular broke out at Montpellier, Paris, and elsewhere in the 1520s and early 1530s.[35] The detractors of the *Canon* tended to focus upon Avicenna's supposed inadequacy as an interpreter of Greek medical thought, claiming either that he had distorted and misrepresented Galen or that he was merely Galen's ape who need no longer be read in an age in which the full range of Galen's work was becoming available,[36] and upon the confusion and inaccuracy of Arabo–Latin botanical and pharmacological nomenclature.[37] Meanwhile, the first efforts to improve the Latin rendering of the *Canon* in the light of a knowledge of Arabic had already been begun before 1500, efforts themselves apparently prompted by humanistic as well as more strictly practical medical motivations.[38] It seems unlikely that any scholarly reader of the *Canon* after the early 1520s could have remained unaware either that the work and its author had been subject to criticism or of the possibility of deflecting criticism onto the twelfth-century translator. At the same time, since the sections of the *Canon* most frequently assigned in university medical curricula in fact contained well organized summaries of a far more outmoded Galenic teaching, the work had by no means outlived its usefulness.[39] Hence there were good reasons for continuing to value the *Canon* in medical teaching, but many of those who did so could no longer be satisfied with traditional forms of presentation or established interpreters of the work. Thus a market for revised editions of the *Canon* was created which for more than a century editors, translators, and publishers worked to supply. While excerpts and abbreviations continued to be published for student use, scholars devoted themselves to various efforts – some of them parallel, overlapping or competing – to present the best possible Latin text of the *Canon*, to explore the relation of the *Canon* to Greek medicine, and to supply it with up to date apparatus and commentary.

Apparently the first edition to show awareness of some of the developments just sketched appeared at Lyons in 1522.[40] This was an edition of the complete Gerard of Cremona text which claimed in its title to be corrected 'from errors and every barbarism in all parts' by Antonio Rustico, and was preceded by a set of 'notes, errata, and castigations' by Symphorien Champier. Rustico, a professor at Pavia, had as already noted earlier compiled *canones* partially drawn from the *Canon* and contributed a prefatory epistle to an edition of the *Articella* containing excerpts from that work. Champier was, of course, one of the principal critics of the Arabs at Montpellier.[41]

Of considerably greater long term influence than the Champier–Rustico edition was the version of the entire *Canon* corrected and provided with a glossary of Arabic terms by Andrea Alpago (d. 1522), and prepared for publication by his nephew Paolo Alpago, that was first published at Venice in 1527.[42] The history of Alpago's long residence in the Middle East as a physician in the service of the Venetian republic, and of the formal endorsement of his version of the *Canon* by the Paduan College of Philosophers and Physicians has been well recounted by Francesca Lucchetta, and need not be repeated here.[43] Alpago's work was a basis of most subsequent major editions, and inspired several others produced in negative response to his efforts. Moreover, almost all later commentators on the *Canon* made use of the *versio bellunensis*, that is of Alpago whose family came from Belluno. Paolo Alpago's own awareness of the probability of large demand for the new version is doubtless reflected in his care to secure privileges from the pope, the king of France, and the Venetian republic granting him exclusive rights over the printing for a period of ten years.[44] This first edition of Alpago's work was published by the Junta press of Venice, which, the reader will recall, had only four years earlier issued the most majestic of the editions of the unrevised text with all its major thirteenth- to fifteenth-century commentators. In 1514, Paolo published a second edition, also with Junta, which included some further textual revisions, additions to Andrea's glossary of Arabic terms, a life of Avicenna translated by Nicolo Massa (d. 1569), and a set of illustrations showing an Arab physician manipulating dislocations.[45]

But dissatisfaction with the results of Alpago's efforts manifested itself almost immediately. In 1530 there appeared a new translation of *Canon* 1:4 by Jacob Mantino, a Jewish physician active in Venice.[46] In a letter of dedication to Doge Andrea Gritti, Mantino explained that owing to the difficulty of finding equivalents for Arabic idioms in Latin, the Gerard translation was marred by many major errors. Alpago, whom Mantino characterized as a distinguished physician equally learned in Latin and Arabic, had removed some of these, but many remained to cloud the true meaning of the work. Mantino claimed to have freed *Canon* 1:4 from these errors by translating it afresh not from the original Arabic but from Hebrew (an edition of the *Canon* in Hebrew, incorporating partial translations by Joseph Lorqi and others, was published at Naples in 1491.[47] Mantino announced his intention to go on to translate both the other parts of the *Canon* most frequently studied 'in the public schools,' namely 1:1 and 4:1, although he appears only to have completed the former. His versions of *Canon* 1:1 and 4 enjoyed considerable success.[48] The latter was printed at least four more times and disseminated across Europe (Ettlingen, 1531; Paris, 1532 and 1555; The Hague, 1533).[49] Although Mantino's translation of book one, part one, seems to have been printed only twice, both times in the Veneto (Venice, *c.* 1540, and Padua, 1547),[50] it was influential, judging by the rather numerous references to it by subsequent editors and commentators. Thus, for example, the sections of the commentary on *Canon* 1:1 by Oddo degli Oddi (d. 1558), a professor of medical theory at Padua, are headed by the passages commented on in both the '*translatio* (*sic*) *bellunensis*' and the '*translatio Mantini*,' and Oddo frequently weighed the relative merits of the two versions.[51] The success and importance of Mantino's translations of parts of the *Canon* from Hebrew perhaps serve as an indication of the limited role of Arabic studies in the approach to the *Canon* in sixteenth-century medical circles.

Three short excerpts from book three were also translated from the Hebrew by Jean Cinqarbres, regius professor of Hebrew at Paris, and published there in 1570, 1572, and 1586 respectively.[52] The first of these was dedicated to the dean of the college of physicians at Paris and described as a specimen of a larger future work. But the Cinqarbres' translations seem never to have achieved either the circulation or the influence of those of Mantino, no doubt largely because the portions selected for translation were not among those most frequently studied in the schools.

But whatever the merits of Mantino's claim to have provided better translations of two of the most widely used short sections of the *Canon*, Alpago's revision covered the entire work. It was the basis of yet another Junta edition published in 1555, with editorial additions by Benedetto Rinio of Venice.[53] The most important new features of the Alpago–Rinio version were the insertion of Alpago's emendations into the body of the text and the provision of innumerable cross-references keying the *Canon* to passages in Greek and other medical authors. Printed for the first time with the *Canon* in this edition were Alpago's translations of two other short medical works by Avicenna.[54] This first Alpago–Rinio version was reissued almost unchanged at Basel in 1556.[55] In 1562, however, Junta published a revised edition with the claim that it incorporated fresh emendations drawn by Rinio from manuscripts given him by Alpago's heirs.[56]

It might seem that the Alpago–Rinio presentation was destined to become the 'revised standard version' of the Latin *Canon*. But in 1564 a major rival appeared in the shape of a two-volume edition of the *Canon* and the four short medical works prepared by Giovanni Costeo and Giovanni Mongio and published, also at Venice, by Valgrisi.[57] It is, indeed, hard to avoid the impression that this edition was deliberately designed to compete with the revised Alpago–Rinio edition put out by Junta in 1562. Giovanni Costeo was a professor in the faculty of medicine at Bologna from 1581 until his death in 1603.[58] His best known work was a set of 'physiological disquisitions' (1589) which are in fact a commentary on *Canon* 1:1.[59] Mongio appears to have practised medicine in Venice and Padua.[60] Costeo and Mongio printed the text in the Gerard of Cremona translation and supplied variant readings from both Alpago and, where available, Mantino; they also appended substantial annotations to most sections of the text. In addition, they provided each of the first four books of the *Canon* with its own preface in the shape of a letter from either or both of them to a different medical personality. Two of the individuals thus honoured were professors of medical theory at Padua, and another held a similar position at Pavia; the fourth was the Paduan botanist Giacomo Antonio Cortusio. Book one was dedicated to Bernardino Paterno, first professor of medical theory at Padua from 1563 until his death in 1592, and himself the author of a commentary on *Canon* 1:1.[61] Paterno, at one time Costeo's teacher,[62] evidently had a more than nominal interest in the edition prepared by his former pupil; it was apparently on his advice that the editors decided to print the Gerard translation with emendations in the margin, rather than following Rinio's example and incorporating emendations into the body of the text.[63]

Nonetheless, in the eyes of Paterno himself and of other contemporaries, the Costeo and Mongio edition still left room for improvement. In 1580, yet another version of book one was produced by Andrew Graziolo, who had studied medicine under Oddo degli Oddi.[64] Graziolo worked with the assistance of a Jewish physician who knew the *Canon* in Hebrew and in the light of a manuscript left by Girolamo Ramusio (d. 1486).[65] Like Alpago, Ramusio had served the Venetian republic as a physician in the Middle East and had there learned Arabic; he apparently completed a translation from the Arabic of at least book one of the *Canon*, although this was never published. Graziolo's project acquired, as he informed his readers in his preface, the enthusiastic support not only of his own preceptor Oddo degli Oddi, but also of Paterno, of Nicolo Sanmichele and of Fracastoro. Since Graziolo's work had degli Oddi's support, it would appear that it was begun before the latter's death in 1558. It was thus presumably originally intended to improve upon the various Alpago and Alpago–Rinio editions, as Graziolo's emphasis upon his use of wholly different sources – the Hebrew *Canon* and Ramusio's manuscript – makes plain. However, the project was evidently completed after the edition of Costeo and Mongio first appeared in 1564, both because Graziolo asserted that he had only recently received the Ramusio manuscript, that is presumably shortly before the publication date of 1580, and because he identified the source of the manuscript as Sammichele, a recipient of one of Costeo and Mongio's dedicatory letters.[66] Presumably if the Ramusio manuscript had been in Sanmichele's possession when Costeo and Mongio were at work he would have made it available to them. It thus seems reasonable to assume that Graziolo's efforts were perceived by his backers as an advance not only over those of Alpago and Rinio, but also over those of Costeo and Mongio. Furthermore, the personal, institutional, and regional links between the scholars involved in one way or another in the Costeo and Mongio and Graziolo editions[67] suggest that the sense of the importance of an improved understanding of the *Canon*, manifested in the endorsement given to Andrew Alpago's work by the Paduan College of Philosophers and Physicians in 1521 (in which Oddo degli Oddi took part)[68] was still very much alive in some Paduan professorial circles in the 1550s, 1560s, and 1570s.

In the event, however, Graziolo's version of book one was never reprinted. Of the two competing major editions of the complete work, that of Costeo and Mongio seems ultimately to have been the more successful. Rinio's revised edition was reprinted once by Junta in 1582.[69] Thereafter, that press took over the edition of Costeo and Mongio, which subsequently appeared, revised and elaborated, in 1595 and again in 1608.[70] The 1595 edition was characterized by revisions by Costeo, by the participation of Fabio Paolino of Udine, and by the publisher's re-use of supplementary material from earlier editions of the *Canon* from the same press. Attention is drawn to Costeo's revisions both on the title page and in the latter's single preface (now addressed to his colleagues in the College of Philosophers and Physicians of Bologna); their presence is signalled throughout book one by references to his own 'physiological disquisitions', published as already noted in 1589, and by the expansion of some of the annotations. The multiple prefaces by Costeo and Mongio were dropped, presumably in the interests of modernization and in favour of the contributions of Fabio Paolino (1535–1604). The latter, who held a public lectureship in Greek at Venice, is perhaps best remembered as a Greek scholar, as the founder of the short-lived Accademia Uranica or degli Uranici at Venice, and as the author of a massive commentary on a single line of Virgil which, according to D. P. Walker, presents 'with remarkable completeness, not only the theory of Ficino's magic, but also the whole complex of theories of which it is a part'.[71] However, Paolino also obtained a medical degree at Bologna and wrote medical works. According to a late source he also learned Arabic, although on the basis of a statement made by himself in the edition under discussion, the extent of his study of that language by 1595 seems doubtful.[72] Paolino's acknowledged contributions to the 1595 edition of the *Canon* consisted of an ode on the merits of Avicenna addressed to Lorenzo Massa,[73] an essay in Avicenna's defence addressed to 'scholars of medicine' ('*studiosis medicinae*'), a complicated set of tables outlining the *Canon* and the medical *Isagoge* of Johannitius and intended to show that the plan of the two works was essentially the same, and a disquisition on the etymology and meanings of the word 'canon' designed to justify its use in the title of Avicenna's work. From the earlier Junta editions came Nicolo Massa's life of Avicenna, a poem on the *Canon* by I. M. Rota first included in the edition of 1562 (a few lines in praise of Rinio that had accompanied this in the 1562 edition being, not surprisingly, omitted), and the set of illustrations showing a turbanned physician reducing dislocations. The 1608 edition is a reprinting of that of 1595 with only minor changes.

So far as I have succeeded in determining, the two editions of the work of Costeo, Mongio, and Paolino were put together without reference to the most noteworthy event in the sixteenth-century history of the *Canon*, namely the printing of that work in Arabic in Rome in 1593. That publication was part of a project with goals that had nothing to do with medicine, was supervised by a scholar who was not a physician, and was intended for distribution in the Middle East; little is so far known about any European distribution. However, the editor, Giovan Battista Raimondi, had some medical contacts and it appears likely that a few copies may have found their way into the hands of European physicians.[74] Although it is certainly conceivable that the printed Arabic text was not available when Costeo was making his last revisions some time between 1589 and 1595, this could scarcely have been the case by 1608 (the Rome, 1593, edition was available to Peter Kirsten by 1609).[75] But by 1608 Costeo and Paolino (and probably also Mongio, who seems not to have taken part in the 1595 revision) were dead, and their work was simply reissued without significant alteration.

The prominent role played by the Junta press of Venice in the production of new Latin editions of the *Canon* deserves emphasis at this point. As we have just seen, Junta was responsible for the publication of the most lavish and comprehensive of the editions with older commentary (1523), for both the editions prepared by Paolo Alpago (1527, 1544), for the first edition of Mantino's translation of book one, part four (1530), for three of the four editions of Rinio's work (1555, revised 1562, 1582), and for the revised and expanded Costeo, Mongio and Paolino edition and its reprinting (1595, 1608). Given the reputation of the Venice branch of the Junta press for a certain pragmatism in the selection of titles for publication,[76] this output surely suggests the existence not merely of a market for copies of the *Canon*, but of a steady demand for continued revision and updating in the work's presentation from the 1520s to the end of the century. While such demand was not necessarily confined to the Italian schools, the programme of publication was presumably chiefly stimulated by local conditions.

Discussion of the small group of editions that appeared after 1608 carries us beyond the subject of this book, but they will be noted briefly both for the sake of completeness and to indicate the shift in goals and methodology that some of them represent. After 1608, no edition of the complete *Canon* in Latin seems to have been published until the Venice edition of 1507 was reproduced in facsimile in 1964.[77] The editions of sections of the work that appeared between 1609 and 1674 fall into two distinct categories. The first of these consists of small volumes produced to supply the market among students created by the continued survival of parts of the *Canon* in the Italian universities, notably Padua. Thus, editions of *Canon* 1:1 (general physiology) appeared at Vicenza in 1611, along with Galen's *Ars*;[78] at Padua 'for the use of the university of Padua' in 1636;[79] with the *Aphorisms* of Hippocrates and the *Ars* at Padua in 1648.[80] Both *Canon* 1:1 and *Canon* 4:1 (fevers) were included along with the *Aphorisms* and the *Ars* in a little book called *Schola Medica* published at Venice in 1647.[81] Book four, part one, was also published by itself at Padua in 1659.[82] All of these presumably cheap little books presented the Gerard translation without scholarly apparatus. Usually *Canon* 1:1 was printed without the anatomical chapters traditionally omitted in lecturing (although they are present in the edition published at Padua in 1648). As a result, the author of a preface included in two of these editions could without any apparent sense of incongruity refer to Avicenna's *opusculum*.[83] The author of the preface to the edition of book one, part one, issued at Padua in 1636 referred approvingly to the 'prudent institution of our ancestors' that had secured for Avicenna a place in the curriculum of the Italian schools.[84] The editors of the *Schola Medica* displayed a somewhat more realistic appraisal of the actual nature of their readers' interest in Avicenna by including a list of 'points for examination that are commonly propounded to degree candidates in the most famous schools' ('puncta quae laureandis proponi solent in celeberrimis collegiis').[85]

Of very different calibre were four publications that appeared in northern Europe during this period. Unlike the Italian editions, each of these contained a new Latin translation of a section of the *Canon* made directly from the Arabic; two of them also edited the corresponding portions of the Arabic text. The supplementary material provided by these editors and translators is also without precedent: in three of the four cases it includes, in addition to useful summaries of the history of textual scholarship on the *Canon*,[86] discussion of Arabic manuscripts used as well as scholia that deal with problems of Arabic philology or manuscript readings. Although the scholars responsible for these translations and editions had medical qualifications and medical interests, the context that made their work possible was the seventeenth-century flowering of Arabic studies rather than any developments in the world of medical learning.[87] Thus, Peter Kirsten (1575–1640), who published an edition and translation of book two in 1609, was trained in theology as well as medicine and had studied several other oriental languages besides Arabic.[88] While he believed book two of the *Canon* (on simples) to be highly useful for medical practice, and had learned from no less an advocate of the study of oriental languages than J. J. Scaliger that 'a true physician could better do without Latin than without Arabic or Greek',[89] Kirsten valued the knowledge of Arabic at least as much for religious purposes as for science and medicine. His version of book two of the *Canon* was one of a set of supplements to illustrate his Arabic grammar; others contained annotations on the four gospels and lives of the evangelists in Arabic.[90]

A project more exclusively medical in scope was undertaken by Vopiscus Fortunatus Plemp, a professor of medicine at Louvain who is remembered chiefly for his initial opposition to and subsequent acceptance of Harvey's teachings. For thirty years Plemp laboured over the preparation of an edition and translation of the complete *Canon*, which he planned to publish with Arabic and Latin on facing pages, accompanied by copious scholia. However, the volume finally issued in 1658 contained only his Latin translation of books one and two and book four, part one, along with relatively brief annotations on those sections. Plemp explained to his readers that he had resigned himself to the initial publication of only this portion of his work on account of the lack of locally available Arabic type, the small number of people in Christendom who knew Arabic (and the even smaller number who might be expected to know it in future) and, above all, the representations of his publisher.[91] No further volumes of Plemp's edition and translation ever appeared, but in the following year, 1659, Pierre Vattier, physician to the duke of Orleans and the author of treatises and translations, some of them in French, on various aspects of Middle Eastern or Moslem culture, published at Paris a Latin translation of some excerpts from book three, part one, having to do with mental disease.[92] In his preface, Vattier made a point of stressing that his translation from Arabic was completely his own, and that he had not followed the practice, so common even among great men in the past, of simply making interpolations in an older translation.[93] Finally, in 1674 Georg Welsch published his edition and translation of two chapters of book four, part three.[94] In Welsch's translation, the two chapters occupy four pages; they are accompanied by more than 450 pages of commentary and addenda which seem designed to appeal to Arabists, philologists, mythologers, and historians at least as much as to physicians.

Each of these four scholars presented his work as a 'specimen' or portion of a larger project, but none of them appears to have produced any more work on the *Canon*. Whether their editions aroused much interest in northern European medical schools or among scholars of oriental languages, I am not in a position to say, although the former seems improbable. Certainly, their efforts had little or no impact upon the practice of lecturing on the *Canon* in the medical faculties of the Italian universities. Alone among this group, Plemp chose to translate parts of the *Canon* still prescribed as textbooks, and, as G. B. Morgagni had occasion to remark,

Plemp's translation did not displace that of Gerard of Cremona in the Italian schools.[95] Conceivably the appearance of Plemp's work may have been a factor in discouraging further reprintings by Italian presses of any of the major editions of the *Canon* produced in the second half of the sixteenth century, but given other seventeenth-century developments it scarcely seems necessary to invoke this explanation.

Thus, the output of *Canon* editions after 1608 reflects on the one hand an outgrowth of a development of Arabic studies that doubtless came too late to have much impact on medical learning, and on the other the durability of sections of the oldest Latin translation of the work as introductory medical textbooks and as medical 'classics'. Quite different in character from either of these types is the series of publications of the complete *Canon* or a major part of it that began with the 1522 edition, which first showed awareness of humanist criticism of Avicenna and ended with the appearance of the last major edition to be published in Italy in 1608, to which we will now return. Most of the scholars involved in the production of this group of editions were primarily concerned with the *Canon* as a means of transmission of Galenic medical teaching, rather than with the study of Arabic. But they were equally far from commending the *Canon* solely as a book to be assigned to students because the tradition was bequeathed by 'the prudent institution of our ancestors'.

Instead, diverse though the editions they produced are, the Italian scholarly editors and revisers (and doubtless also their publishers) seem to have shared two common goals. The first was to present the *Canon* in a form that would be of practical use to the professors of medicine and graduate physicians who probably constituted the chief market for editions of the complete work or a major part of it. The second was to bring humanist medical learning to bear on the *Canon* itself, thus validating its continued study. The most obvious way to achieve both these goals was, of course, by the presentation of a Latin text that was 'improved' in any or all of several senses: truer to the original, truer to Galen, clearer, or stylistically more elegant. But the validation of the *Canon* depended not only upon the revision of the text but also on the provision of supplementary material – indices, glossaries, references, introductory essays, or explanatory notes – which would both facilitate consultation of the work and aid the reader in its interpretation. The editions under discussion reveal a succession of editorial strategies all designed to accomplish the goals just outlined. While, as we have seen, the successive textual revisions did not wholly satisfy contemporaries, some of the editors must be judged to have been rather successful in deploying their supplementary material to reinforce the position of the *Canon* in the medical learning of the second half of the sixteenth century.

Concerning the character of the revision of the text, only a few general observations can be made. As noted earlier, much remains to be learned about the textual history of the *Canon* in Latin; the fundamental need, namely investigation of the Gerard of Cremona version in the light of the original is only now being met by scholarly works in progress.[96] Moreover, except for the work of Alpago, none of the other sixteenth-century revisions or partial translations, whether from Arabic or Hebrew, seems to have been studied in detail by modern scholars. However, from what has already been noted it is apparent that no sixteenth- or early seventeenth-century edition of the *Canon* published in Italy contains an entirely new translation of any part of the *Canon* made directly from Arabic alone. Alpago's published work on the *Canon* consists of emendations to the Gerard of Cremona version, accompanied by a glossary of technical terms and an explanatory note. Graziolo's version of book one is different from that of Gerard, but not, as we shall see, translated directly from Arabic; the other partial translations published in Italy in the sixteenth century, those of Mantino, were made from Hebrew.

On the other hand, the claim that the text is revised, corrected, or improved is a prominent feature of all editions save one (that of 1523) of the complete *Canon* and of a number of the partial editions published between 1522 and 1608. I have not succeeded in determining whether this claim refers to actual textual emendations in the earliest of these editions (Champier and Rustico, 1522); comparison of a few selected passages shows only the Gerard translation, and there appear to be no typographical indications of textual emendation. It is possible that Rustico's 'castigations' are all incorporated into the front matter (see further below). The extent of Andrea Alpago's published revisions is made perfectly clear, both editorially and typographically in the first two editions of his work, those prepared for the press by his nephew Paolo. The title of the 1527 edition refers to 'correction' and 'restitution', the privileges accompanying the work refer to 'castigations and expositions' and the text itself is headed 'translated by master Gerard of Cremona' (*translatus a magistro Gerardo Cremonensis*). In both editions, Alpago's emendations are clearly indicated in the margin and keyed to the text with various typographical devices. The scope of Alpago's alterations was, however, obscured, advertently or inadvertently, by the editorial procedures of Benedetto Rinio. An advertized feature of the latter's editions was, as noted, the removal of Alpago's emendations from the margin and their insertion into the body of the text. This freed Rinio's margins for copious citations of Greek and other medical authors, but it also made it impossible to determine the extent of Alpago's corrections without comparison with another edition. Costeo and Mongio, by reverting to the Gerard translation with alternative readings from Alpago (and, where applicable, Mantino) in the margins, once again provided their readers with the opportunity to distinguish both the source and the extent of suggested changes. There is some justification, therefore, for the viewpoint of Johann Georg Schenk, who in his *Biblia Iatrica* (1609) expressed the opinion that the Costeo and Mongio edition was the best available.[97]

Both Rinio and Costeo and Mongio claimed to have added further emendations of their own.[98] In some cases these appear to have taken the form of supplying translations of Arabic words hitherto only transliterated, especially as regards the simples in book two. How new these contributions were, how accurate, and what level of linguistic knowledge they represented, I am not competent to determine. Costeo at any rate, indicated that in emending in this fashion he usually followed the judgement of 'more learned interpreters' who remain unidentified.[99] In the general theoretical treatise that opens book one, Costeo and Mongio offered very few suggestions for improvement of their own, relying almost entirely on Alpago and Mantino.[100] One gains the impression of a considerable interest in Arabic technical anatomical and botanical vocabulary that is not necessarily to be equated with substantial mastery of the language such as that attained by the elder Alpago. This conclusion seems to be reinforced by the intermittent development and chiefly religious focus of Arabic studies in sixteenth century Italy;[101] by even the younger Alpago's apparent inability in later life to translate a written narrative from Arabic, to which Francesca Lucchetta has drawn attention;[102] by the admitted ignorance of that language of Nicolo Massa, translator of the life of Avicenna first published in the 1544 edition of the *Canon*,[103] and of G. B. Da Monte (Montanus), one of the most distinguished of the sixteenth-century Italian commentators on that work.[104]

Graziolo not only made no secret of his own ignorance of Arabic, but also implied that he had no contact with anyone who did know it.[105] M. T. d'Alverny has drawn attention to Graziolo's own explanation of how in these circumstances he managed to produce a translation clearly different from that of Gerard of Cremona.[106] Graziolo stated that he had carefully studied all previous interpreters of the *Canon*, especially the annotations of Alpago, and had drawn on the assistance of the Jewish physician Jacobus Anselmus, who could read the *Canon* in Hebrew (as Graziolo himself therefore presumably could not). It was only when his work was already well advanced that he secured access to Ramusio's manuscript containing book one in Arabic with Ramusio's Latin translation. This explanation is doubtless true as far as it goes, but perhaps slightly disingenuous. Graziolo's version is not identical with that of Ramusio, as is shown by the notation of variant readings ascribed to the latter. However, a comparison of the opening of the chapter on humours in Graziolo's version and in the Latin translation of *Canon* 1:1 from the Hebrew by Jacob Mantino (Venice, c. 1540) suggests that for this part of Graziolo's work at least, Mantino was a major source.

If in their presentation of the text the Italian scholarly editors of the mid- and later sixteenth century were unable to go much beyond one or another combination of the work of Gerard of Cremona, Ramusio, Andrea Alpago, and Mantino, they displayed both learning and ingenuity in supplementing the text with other material. One variety of supplement that had earlier played an important role, namely commentary written before 1500, dropped out of *Canon* editions after the 1520s. Yet precedents for other forms of supplementary material which lent themselves to expansion and development were already in existence; for example the Venice edition of 1507, printed without commentary, contains a short life of Avicenna and a glossary of Arabic terms. Setting aside the purely complimentary dedications and the elaborate title pages that began to proliferate in printings of Avicenna as of other authors, and the textual apparatus indicating variant readings that has already been referred to, the expanded supplementary material found in the editions with which we are concerned can be broadly classified as follows: biography of Avicenna; indices and glossaries; evaluation of the worth of Avicenna and of the *Canon*; citations of other authors; explanatory annotations or scholia. It is from the last three categories that the priorities of the editors can most readily be determined, but the development of the first two deserves to be briefly mentioned.

Three different biographies of Avicenna appear in the various sixteenth-century Latin editions of the *Canon*. The short life included in the Venice, 1507, and other early editions may possibly be based on an Arabic source, but contains little specific information other than medical detail about the causes of Avicenna's death.[107] A slightly longer and purportedly more critical life was written by Franciscus Calphurnius of Vendôme, an associate of Symphorien Champier, for the Champier and Rustico edition of 1522. The author stressed the uncertainty and inconsistency of available information about Avicenna, and firmly repudiated the fiction of his correspondence with St Augustine. However, this biography retained the tradition that Avicenna had lived in Cordoba (where he flourished 'like a hyacinth among the nettles'), and also asserted that he was a contemporary of Averroës. A story that Avicenna's death was caused by poison administered by Averroës in a fit of jealousy was attributed to Champier.[108]

Avicenna's supposed association with Cordoba was laid to rest by a few biographical comments by Andrea Alpago, first published with the *Canon* in 1527.[109] However, much more, and more authentic information was provided in the well known life of Avicenna by Nicolo Massa which, as already twice noted, was printed for the first time in Paolo Alpago's second edition of 1544. This life was actually a free Latin rendering of the biography by Avicenna's pupil Abu Ubayd al-Juzjani, whose name was Latinized as Sorsanus.[110] It was reprinted in all the subsequent major editions of the complete *Canon*, with the exception of that published by

Valgrisi in 1564. In the editions of 1562 and thereafter, Massa's work, originally dedicated to the papal physician Tommaso Cademusto, was updated by a new dedication to Cardinal Carlo Borromeo.

A similar history of expansion, modernization of form, and greater precision can be told of the indexing of the various editions. In the Gerard of Cremona translation, the *Canon* itself incorporates a lengthy table of contents, adequate to locate the treatment of most topics in the bulky work, that is placed immediately after Avicenna's own preface. In addition, some early editions contain registers of the *quaestiones* discussed in the commentaries printed with the *Canon*.[111] Readers of the edition prepared by Rinio had the convenience of an alphabetically arranged subject index. In the Basel edition of 1556, this is relatively spare, occupying sixteen folios. In 1557, Junta published a much more comprehensive and complicated index, seventy-six folios long, with numerous subheadings and cross-references, compiled by the physician Giulio Palamede;[112] this was reissued in 1562, and replaced the former index in the revised edition of Rinio's work published in the same year.[113] The indexing of the Costeo and Mongio editions was even more elaborate. Not only did those scholars provide an index to the text of the *Canon* exceeding Palamede's in length, they also supplied a separate index to their own annotations. In addition, in their second, revised, edition Paolino's tables provided yet another guide to the whole work. In most editions, too, separate indices of the simples in book two were provided. That appearing in the Champier and Rustico edition of 1522 subsequently gave way to an index of Arabic names of substances compiled by Andrea Alpago (1527); in the editions prepared by Rinio, an index of Greco-Latin names for substances in book two compiled by Rinio himself was also added.[114] Both of these indices or lists were expanded in the Costeo–Mongio editions. The main change as far as glossaries were concerned was, of course, the introduction of the important and well known one compiled by Andrea Alpago.[115] Alpago's glossary, to which some additions were made by Rinio, appeared in all the major editions under discussion. However, the shorter, so-called 'old' glossary, sometimes ascribed to Gerard of Cremona, also survived and continued to be printed alongside that of Alpago.

The evaluations of Avicenna prefaced to the various editions are of course rhetorical, but nonetheless revealing of the goals and preoccupations of the different editors. The edition prepared by Champier and Rustico and published in 1522, just when bold criticism of the Arabs was becoming a shibboleth of modernism in medicine, includes prefatory material decidedly critical of Avicenna.[116] Champier set the tone of his 'castigations and errata' in a brief preface addressed to Robert Coleburn, Bishop of Ross, in which he explained Avicenna's importance for medicine as an interpreter of Galen, while deploring his membership in the 'filthy and wicked Mohammedan sect'. He then summarized the views on the soul of Avicenna, Algazel, and Averroës, condemning the last. Next follows discussion of seven supposed errors of Avicenna, all of them in the realm of philosophy, religion, and ethics, not medicine: among the errors repudiated are the legitimacy of divorce and the view that all supposed miracles are susceptible of a natural explanation. Then comes a set of *dubia* examining instances in which Avicenna appears to differ from Galen or other Greek medical authorities;[117] the topics relate to confusion or error in the names or attributes of medicinal plants and of diseases and in the prescription of treatment. Finally ten instances in which Avicenna appeared to disagree with Dioscorides are identified as errors and discussed. The issues of Avicenna's relationship to Greek medicine and of problems of pharmacological and botanical nomenclature, originally raised by critics of the Arabs, had now been introduced into an edition of the *Canon* itself. Subsequent Italian editors of the *Canon*, all of whom were principally concerned to defend, not attack, Avicenna were repeatedly to address these themes, although they usually avoided the religious issue also introduced by Champier. Overall, the Champier–Rustico edition seems something of an amalgam of conflicting intentions. The biography places Avicenna in a positive light; moreover, the claim that the text has been purified presumably indicates that the editors valued the work as a whole. Yet the message conveyed by the prefatory material seems to be that, on both religious and scientific grounds, the Christian physician should approach the *Canon* with a good deal of caution.

The brief dedication and preface placed by Paolo Alpago before his uncle's revision of the *Canon* are naturally chiefly concerned with Andrea Alpago's accomplishment, the circumstances that charged Paolo with responsibility for publication, and his editorial procedures. Of Avicenna, Paolo asserted only that he had drawn on earlier Arabic and Greek writers, above all Galen, so skilfully that physicians still regarded him as their prince and used the *Canon* as a standard work of reference for both theory and practice.[118] The substantial and carefully reasoned defence of Avicenna supplied by Benedetto Rinio was therefore a novelty in an edition of the *Canon*. In a prefatory letter to his four sons, whom he urged always to have Avicenna in their hands, he expressed his astonishment at the temerity of those who 'thirty years ago' (Rinio was presumably writing in 1555 or shortly before) attacked Avicenna.[119] He attributed these attacks to a rage for all things Greek, while asserting that a Greek, Latin, or barbarian origin should not prejudice a man. In defence of Avicenna, Rinio pointed out that none of the works of the major medical authors from Hippocrates to Haly Abbas was without some drawbacks. Avicenna's special merit was to have sifted the wheat from the chaff in the writings of his predecessors and to have presented the result aptly and harmoniously arranged. Consequently, reliance upon the *Canon* was both labour- and time-saving. Furthermore, those who condemned Avicenna for drawing upon the work of his predecessors should be aware that Aristotle and Galen had unquestionably done the same thing. Rinio admitted that Avicenna's dependence upon Arabic translations of Greek works meant that through the fault of the translators he had sometimes been misled or confused, especially about the names of plants and animals. These deficiencies had, however, largely been remedied by the work of Andrea Alpago. And in a few instances, Avicenna had supplied information about medicaments unknown to the Greeks.

Rinio called not only upon classical tradition and the modern work of Alpago, but also upon medieval sources in defending Avicenna. Possibly in indirect allusion to some of Champier's criticisms, he noted that Avicenna's merits as a philosopher had earned the approval of Albertus Magnus, Thomas Aquinas, and Duns Scotus, 'lights of the whole world'. Moreover, he pointed out that the long tradition of lecturing upon the *Canon* in the Italian medical schools had produced the commentaries of 'the great speculator Gentile, the clear expositor Giacomo, and the subtle disputator Dino'.

In the following decade, Costeo and Mongio echoed some of the same themes. They too deplored the prevalence of scorn for the Arabs, while pointing out that no-one had yet produced a work that surpassed the *Canon* in organization, comprehensiveness, generally accurate presentation of Greek medicine, and range of medicaments.[120] They took the war into the enemy's camp with the assertion that the Arabs were disliked by those who had entered medicine without any study of dialectic and philosophy and were themselves incapable of appreciating the weighty and recondite statements of Arab authors (by contrast 'the Greeks, indeed, with their suavity in words and copious effusion of speech are not difficult to understand').[121] And in Costeo's preface to book four the argument culminates in a diatribe against the 'Galenici' who act 'as if it were a sin to add anything to Galen's writings or as if it were a virtue to know nothing he did not know.[122] This was certainly quite unlike the behaviour of any men of real distinction in any branch of science, and certainly unlike Galen and Aristotle themselves, who had never hesitated to criticize their predecessors.

Around 1580, Graziolo elected to take a historical approach. His preface opens with a brisk summary of the transmission of knowledge from the Hebrews to the Egyptians to the Greeks to the Latins, of the devastating effects of the barbarian invasions, and of the rebirth of learning in Italy (dated by references to the flight of Greek scholars from Constantinople and the invention of printing.[123] Among the arts and sciences that were as a result 'recalled to their sources' and 'restored to light' was medicine. This conventional historiography was used to make the point that the arts, far from being confined to the Greeks, had arisen among barbarians (the ancient Egyptians!) and had been further developed by other peoples after

Greek ingenuity had grown old. Among the latter were the Arabs, who had not merely acquired but added to Greek learning, especially in mathematics (algebra), astronomy, astrology, and medicine. Graziolo also rehearsed some of the familiar themes: Avicenna's fidelity to Greek medical authors and skill in presenting their ideas, the outmoded character of disdain for Avicenna, and the faults of the *recentiores* 'who want to destroy medicine rather than teach and study it and who are ignorant not only of Avicenna but also of Hippocrates and Galen'. In hazarding the opinion that a man of such genius as Avicenna must have been a polished and elegant writer in his own language, Graziolo stressed the stylistic defects of Gerard of Cremona, Graziolo may here have been echoing G. B. Da Monte,[124] although he was doubtless also insinuating the merits on which he thought his own version should be judged.

Although it added little new in substance, the preface written by Fabio Paolino for the edition of 1595 was markedly more elegant in style than those of his predecessors.[125] Indeed, it may be that Paolino's principal contribution to the edition was to lend Avicenna's cause the support of a classical scholar of some reputation. Only a few points need be noted here. Paolino, like Costeo and unlike Rinio and Graziolo, admitted the existence of contemporaries, as well as of an earlier generation of medical teachers, who discouraged their students from reading the *Canon*. His account of the origins of hostility to Avicenna and the *Canon* among the medical humanists shows a fairly balanced historical perspective. Himself an ardent enthusiast for Greek letters, Paolino was unable to dismiss earlier critics of Avicenna as cavalierly as Costeo had done. Instead he asserted that although these critics had indeed included men of great erudition, their opinions were not based on close study of the *Canon* but were, rather, part of the polemic in which they engaged to foster the goals of a new medical sect that had arisen in their own time. This sect, called by its supporters the Galenic, had as its programme the union of sound medical teaching with elegance of expression. In the resultant polarization of the medical community, those who valued the substance of learning alone and were suspicious of rhetorical embellishments were stigmatized by the Galenic faction as 'Avicennan' or 'barbarous'. In reality, Paolino thought, the quarrel was more about translators than about medical content: since Arabic was much more linguistically distant from Latin than was Greek, it was scarcely surprising that translators from Arabic had committed barbarisms in Latin. In Paolino's view, it would have been preferable if Avicenna's critics instead of casting slurs on a great writer, had learned Arabic and translated him in good Latin style. This, Paolino had reason to think, would soon be done.

The provision of a systematic, precise, and comprehensive set of references to other, chiefly Greek, medical authors was an important, and in some respects novel, feature of all the major *Canon* editions produced in

Italy in the second half of the sixteenth century. Scholastic commentators had, of course, long since drawn attention to and discussed with a view to reconciliation both the echoes in the *Canon* of the differences between Aristotle and Galen, and various of Avicenna's own differences with ancient authors. In so doing, they frequently cited specific passages of the latter and compared them with passages in the *Canon*. But systematic identification of Avicenna's supposed sources or evaluation of his merits as an interpreter of Galen were, however, scarcely among the main goals of such commentators. In any case, the somewhat fragmented nature of scholastic inquiry by the question method, and the changing picture of Galenic scholarship itself in the late fifteenth and early sixteenth century, meant that for sixteenth-century readers of the *Canon* the older commentators were unlikely to prove a very helpful guide in this respect. Some of the critics of the *Canon* had, as we have seen, supported their arguments by pulling out instances in which Avicenna differed from Galen, Dioscorides, or other authorities, but such accounts were incomplete as well as biased. Benedetto Rinio, in his *Canon* edition of 1555, seems to have been the first to attempt to provide a comprehensive system of references which could be used not only to demonstrate the extent of Avicenna's dependence upon Greek authorities and the great number of instances in which he could be shown, even from the available Latin versions of the *Canon*, to have reported Galenic ideas accurately, but also the way in which Galen's teachings were re-ordered, abbreviated, and clarified (or oversimplified) in the *Canon*. Rinio did not confine himself to providing references to works of Galen, but also included other Greek authors (notably Dioscorides in book two), a few other Arabic authors, and cross-references within the *Canon*. Some indication of the scope of his endeavour and how much of his editorial effort it must have absorbed can perhaps be gained from the information that for the brief part one of book one alone (excluding the anatomical chapters), Rinio provided multiple citations of more than thirty separate works of Galen. Of these, the most frequently cited was the lengthy *De Usu Partium* to which Rinio referred over forty times. A check of the references to the three works most frequently cited in book one, part one, namely *De Usu Partium*, *De Temperamentis*, and *De Naturalibus Facultatibus* reveals Rinio as thorough and careful in seeking out parallels (and therefore presumed sources). He also noticed instances where Galen could be cited in opposition, but naturally in the physiological survey contained in *Canon* 1:1 instances of agreement are far more numerous.

Costeo and Mongio and Graziolo also gave considerable attention to the citation of ancient, and especially Galenic, sources, although they did not confine their own annotations to this in the way that Rinio had done. Instead, they wove the references into broader and more general *annotationes* and scholia to the text. Only the most salient features of the latter, illustrated by a few examples drawn from their treatment of *Canon* 1:1, can be indicated here. Costeo's own description of the objectives of his annotations seems to apply as well as Graziolo's scholia: the collection and citation of relevant passages from philosophers and physicians, the exposition of controversies, demonstration of the closeness of Avicenna's agreement with Hippocrates and Galen, and elimination of the objections of both ancients and *recentiores*. [26] Despite their relative brevity and somewhat episodic nature, the philosophical, medical, and bibliographical disquisitions in which these aims are realized have more in common with both the earlier and the contemporary tradition of Latin commentary on the *Canon* than with, say, the medical and philological scholia supplied by Plemp, let alone the mainly philological treatment by Kirsten. But although a good many of the issues discussed by sixteenth-century Italian editors ultimately derive from differences between the teaching of Aristotle and Galen that had been the topics of *quaestiones* discussed by Latin physicians since the thirteenth century (for example, the origin of the nerves, the existence and powers of the so-called female sperm, the identity or non-identity of *complexio* or *temperamentum* with substantial form), [127] little trace of dependence upon medieval treatments remains. Neither the form of the scholastic *quaestio* nor citations of Latin commentators on the *Canon* who wrote before 1500 can easily be found. Instead, in both form and content, the closest relationship is with the most recent commentaries on the *Canon*.

The tradition of Latin commentary on the *Canon* had been significantly modernized, in the sense of displaying the influence of renaissance Galenism, and abandoning the formal structure of scholastic debate a generation before the editions of Costeo and Mongio and Graziolo appeared. Some earlier sixteenth-century commentators had moreover approached Avicenna in a spirit of detached criticism mingled on occasion with outright hostility. The most notable Italian example is the commentary on *Canon* 1:1 by G. B. Da Monte, written at Padua probably in the early 1540s, in which Avicenna and the older Latin commentators are sharply attacked on a number of issues. [128] Certain subsequent Italian commentators on this section of the *Canon*, while equally or even more concerned with interpretation in the light of Greek medicine and current opinion, tended on the whole to explain rather than attack the work. It is to this latter group of commentaries – those of Graziolo's teacher Oddo degli Oddi, [129] Costeo's teacher Paterno, [130] and Costeo himself [131] – that the expositions in the editions by Costeo and Mongio and Graziolo can be most closely related. Their annotations and scholia are replete with allusions to controversy and bibliography dating from the middle years of the century. Thus, Graziolo's treatment of the nature of the mixture of elementary qualities in living bodies termed *complexio*, *temperamentum*, or *temperatura* is directed against the views of Jean Fernel and supported by arguments based on the *De Mixtione* of Alexander of Aphrodisias.[132] Fernel's attack on the definition of *complexio* used by Avicenna first appeared in 1542;[133] *De Mixtione* became available in an Aldine Greek edition in 1527 and was three times translated into Latin between about 1540 and 1553.[134] Similarly, it seems likely that Costeo's diatribe against those who identify *temperamentum* with substantial form is directed against G. B. Da Monte (who is not named), who had, from the philosophical although not the theological standpoint, endorsed that view in his commentary on *Canon* 1:1.[135] Costeo and Mongio introduced a paean of praise to sixteenth-century botanists into their annotations on book two, while simultaneously avowing Avicenna's work on this subject to be superior to that of earlier writers and disclaiming the intention to investigate it in detail.[136] In these and other instances, the evident goal was not the continuance of an older tradition of scholastic exposition, but the reactive defence of Avicenna against the adverse criticism of *recentiores* of the previous generation, and the demonstration that his work was indeed defensible in the light of Greek and some modern, that is mid sixteenth-century, medical learning.

To the seventeenth-century northern European Arabists who worked on the *Canon* the methods and goals of their Italian predecessors seemed worthy only of disdain. Of the efforts of 'the very learned Costeo' Peter Kirsten remarked drily 'he would have done better, in my opinion, if he had sought to restore this author from Arabic sources, rather than setting himself the task of restoring him from Galen.' Welsch simply noted that Costeo was 'extremely ignorant of all oriental languages.' Of Graziolo, Plemp commented: 'He called himself a translator . . . but he was utterly ignorant of the Arabic language; nor did he follow the words or content of the author, but took the sense from the commentators, often badly. Sometimes he inserted entire sentences from Galen.'[137]

Such procedures could scarcely fail to arouse indignation in men who had devoted themselves to the study of the *Canon* as an Arabic text. Yet it seems likely that Rinio, Graziolo, and Costeo and his partners in fact followed the approach most likely to secure the position of the *Canon* in the milieu in which they worked, where the influence of Galenism and medical humanism in general was still strong.[138] One may speculate that the display of Greek learning and awareness of recent concerns in their impressive editions helped to provide intellectual justification – if any were needed – for the assignment of sections of the bare Gerard of Cremona text to medical students for a good many years to come. In one sense, the study of Avicenna was thus at least in part perpetuated not by traditionalism but by efforts at modernization. The mid- and later sixteenth-century Italian editors of the *Canon* did not seek to preserve the traditions of medieval scholastic medicine unchanged; moreover, the drying up of the stream of printed editions of early commentaries on the *Canon* in the 1520s suggests that such an endeavour would have had little chance of success. But the form taken by their attempts to modernize the study of the *Canon* was in another sense backward looking, in that it was largely shaped by developments, progressive in their day, that had occurred between about 1490 and 1530.[139] In those years, the enthusiasm for Galen and the Greeks was at its height; attacks on the Arabs and scholastics were mainly on the grounds of their inadequacy in transmitting Greek medicine; and, also, the work of Alpago and Mantino on the text of the *Canon*, fundamental to the endeavours of subsequent sixteenth-century editors and revisers, appeared. The intellectual patrimony – even when they reacted against it – of the Italian scholars who devoted themselves to revising the *Canon* after 1550 was the medical humanism of the early part of the century.

The efforts of the *Canon*'s sixteenth-century editors, commentators, and partial translators were successful to the extent that they helped to secure the continued inclusion of parts of Avicenna's work in generally Galenic medical curricula. But although such formal curricula survived in some Italian universities until well into the eighteenth century, seventeenth-century developments in physiology relegated Galen, and with him Avicenna, to a position of marginal importance. In one sense, therefore, the effects of the labours of the scholars described in this chapter were short lived. In the context of sixteenth-century medicine, however, the re-assertion of Avicenna's usefulness as a summarizer and rearranger of Galen was a reasonable position, and the modernization of the presentation of the *Canon* a valid endeavour. Moreover, the endeavour was one that itself involved a loosening of established patterns of thought. The scholars who edited or revised the *Canon* accepted the need for a reasoned defence of Avicenna's work, did much to clarify Avicenna's relationship to Galen, and used improved editorial techniques to highlight inconsistencies and obscurities within the text. It seems likely that their editions facilitated a more detached evaluation than had hitherto been possible of the merits and defects of the one time 'prince of physicians'. Certainly, the story of the efforts to modernize the *Canon* makes it clear that the relation between tradition and innovation in sixteenth-century medicine was a highly complex one that allows for no easy delimitation of conservative and progressive areas.

The present chapter does not touch on humanist work on the *Canon* done in sixteenth-century Spain; on this important aspect of the topic, see Luis García-Ballester, *Los Moriscos y la medicina* (Barcelona, 1984), pp. 24–31.

3

Berengario da Carpi and the use of commentary in anatomical teaching

R. K. FRENCH

Introduction

The sixteenth century is widely held as a period of renaissance in medicine. Certainly there was a radical change in the style and content of teaching in the 1520s; and in anatomy this can be seen as the victory of the Hellenists over the men of the schools.

Some historical attention has been given to anatomy in the earlier sixteenth century, but much of it has been rather unbalanced. The principal reason for this is the historical eminence accorded to Vesalius, whose name is generally linked to humanism, renaissance, the beginnings of modern science and all the things that are good in common historical estimation.

In particular historians have attempted to group together the people who wrote anatomies before 1543 as 'preVesalians'. The implication is not merely that they were earlier than Vesalius, but that they were not so good as Vesalius. Thus Lind[1] speaks of the reasons (too much philosophy and not enough dissection) for their 'failure' (that is, their failure to be Vesalius). But the preVesalians were not striving towards a common goal, nor attempting to hit upon the proper method of proceeding. Some light can be thrown on what they were trying to achieve and what their conceptions of anatomy were by a closer look at Berengario da Carpi.

In fact a closer look at Berengario is long overdue. Historians have found it difficult,[2] because of its size, to tackle the *Commentary on Mondino*[3] of Berengario: this is the only major text omitted from Lind's collection of translations, yet it is almost a complete guide to the earlier anatomical literature,[4] is the first printed anatomy to be illustrated, and was the work identified by major figures like Fallopia[5] as that which initiated the revival of anatomy.

Many of Berengario's purposes in his teaching can be related to the commentary as a form. The commentary had been the vehicle of medical education for some two and a half centuries when Berengario produced his in 1521. The medieval commentary had a precise form, as is shown below, and differed in its structure both from its predecessors, like Galen's commentaries on Hippocratic works and those by the Alexandrian commentators on Galen, and from its successors, the humanist commentaries.[6] Broadly speaking, medieval medical education was based on a small group of short texts, the *Articella*, and increasingly upon the *Canon* of Avicenna. The substance of the teaching of different masters was commentary upon these texts.

The principal exception to this method of teaching was the anatomical demonstration. The essence of the dissection was that it was a *practical* affair. It was carefully controlled by regulations within the institutional arrangements of the university and formed a regular, if not frequent element of the curriculum. Probably dissections had been carried out since the Salernitan demonstrations[7] of the insides of pigs of the twelfth century. Human dissection seems to have begun in the late thirteenth century.

As a practical affair, dissection and the demonstration of the parts did not generate commentary. There was of course the necessary business of glossing anatomical terms as different authors became better known, and this extended to the establishing of sound texts and the correct attribution of works; but anatomical texts of the middle ages that had a direct bearing on dissection did not have the form of a commentary. Nor had there survived from antiquity any suitable text that might form the basis of a commentary. The only commentaries containing anatomical material were those upon book three of the *Canon*, which is much more than an anatomy text.

So Berengario was unique among his predecessors and contemporaries in producing a dissection-based anatomy in commentary form. Moreover, he was using the commentary – a device of the schools – at the time when the Hellenists were successfully making such great changes in medical education. A closer look at Berengario, then, should not only make available details of an unjustly ignored figure, but also illuminate the broader topic of the medical renaissance. We need to know details of Berengario that may help us understand his recorded actions; we should know what a commentary was, and why Berengario chose to use it; and we should try to understand how Berengario saw himself and his contemporaries.

Life

Berengario was born at Carpi in the early 1460s, for he was still a child, *satis puer*, in 1467. The records describe his father as a barber surgeon, but his practice indicates he had considerable skill in difficult cases and Berengario recalls two cases of badly fractured skulls[8] and a hysterectomy.[9] His father taught Berengario surgery as he grew up: while still a youth he helped to treat three serious wounds of the head, and later maintained that no one could learn to be a good surgeon unless he had spent his childhood at it. He seems not to have had a formal education in the early years and perhaps would never have been taught more than surgery had it not been for his friendship with the family of Lionello Pio, the *signore* of Carpi. Lionello's wife was Catherina, sister of Pico della Mirandola, and after Lionello's death, it was Pico's suggestion that his friend Aldo Manuzio should go to Carpi as tutor to the young Alberto and his brother.

The education of the future prince of Carpi then, was to be in the hands of a devoted Hellenist who had cut his intellectual teeth in a circle outside the universities. (The term 'Hellenist' has a particular significance in this chapter: see below.) The education of princes was of course a question much addressed by the Italian intelligentsia (and it was a question not only of teaching but of future reciprocal patronage). It was from such a network of personal contacts that the Hellenists waged their war against the academics. Aldo arrived in Carpi in about 1479, when Alberto was four and his brother two. Berengario in contrast, was about nineteen, and must have been a surgeon of some experience. By now he surely had mental habits that could not be entirely lost in the education he was to receive so (comparatively) late, and it seems likely that his later insistence on the importance of the senses of sight and touch in anatomy, his rejection of purely verbal demonstration of structure and his admiration for anatomists who were *artifices*, craftsmen, was owing to this.

We can gather something of Aldo's educational interests from his published 'letters' to Catherina Pio.[10] The favoured authors were Cicero, Horace and Quintilian, to be followed by the Greek studies so dear to him and to Pico. Alberto doubtless received great benefit from all this, but how rigorous Berengario's education was at the hands of Aldo is not clear. He says himself that his studies with Aldo were only of the 'rudiments of the gentler muses'. No doubt Berengario was later on pleased enough to be able to refer back to a period of instruction from a famous scholar, which, it has been suggested, he exaggerated, for critics like Haller have pointed out that Berengario's Latin style is not what we would expect from a pupil of Aldo. But as we shall see, Berengario's style was chosen for its purpose, and literary prose is restricted to his dedications.

We can assume that Berengario at least absorbed some Latin grammar from Aldo. This was characteristically humanist (for the particular use of the term, see below). The standard medieval authority was the two-thousand line versified *Doctrinale* of Alexander of Villedieu which, like the medieval lawyers' Code of Justinian, was treated as written reason and was committed wholly to memory. In contrast, Aldo *historicized* his subject by showing how language varies with time and by treating grammatical rules as codifications of practice, particularly that of the great classical texts. It was likewise a historical conception that 'everything that is worthy of praise' was first generated by the Greeks and subsequently passed into Latin.[11] The understanding of Greek became thus a matter of great importance, and it is easy to see that the Hellenists, with such a view, would come to see Latin as primarily the language of transmission, the language of the commentators.

We unfortunately do not know where Aldo placed medicine in his scheme of Hellenistic learning at this stage in his career. He was planning an edition of Galen at least as early as 1497 (the Greek *editio princeps* did not appear until after his death). However, Berengario says[12] that with Alberto and under Aldo's tutelage 'we had to dissect a pig', as if it were a considered part of Aldo's programme. Berengario was later asked to dissect a pig at the request of Ercole Gonzaga and in the presence of Pomponazzi and Bonamici,[13] but it is not clear that dissection and the knowledge it generated were parts of a humanistic or of a Hellenistic programme.

Whatever the details of Berengario's education at the hands of Aldo, by the mid 1480s (most likely) he was equipped to go to the university of Bologna, where he took the master's degree in arts and medicine in 1489. He was by now about twenty nine, unusually old for the degree, and again we may suppose he took from his surgical experience to the university and its systematic and largely theoretical medical courses, some firm ideas on the value of sense experience and manual operation. Probably too he had from Aldo an historical approach to his texts. His teachers probably included Manfredi (who taught astrology and was the *ordinarius* teacher of medicine) and Achillini (logic and philosophy). Manfredi's anatomy[14] is similar to Mondino's, is not cast in commentary form, and shows no evidence of Hellenistic tastes. Achillini shared anatomical experience with Berengario only later as a colleague, and Zerbi had left Bologna in 1483, almost certainly before Berengario arrived; but if Manfredi's was the only anatomical teaching Berengario received, it seems to have made very little impression on him for he never mentioned Manfredi's name in his published works.

By 1490 Berengario was back in his father's surgical practice. After 1494 when, it is said, the invading French army brought syphilis in its wake, Berengario began to use mercury in a – at least commercially – successful way in the treatment of the disease. It may well be that this treatment hastened both the beginning and ending of his teaching career: he must have been fairly notable as a successful surgeon to have been appointed in 1502 as the *ordinarius* to teach surgery at Bologna, and there is a persistent tradition (recorded by his biographer, Putti) that it was vivisection of syphilitic patients that led to his leaving the post in 1526.

He seems to have made surgical anatomy his prime interest and he based his teaching on the text of Mondino, his fourteenth-century predecessor at

Bologna. This, wrote Berengario, was the best text available, for it was short enough to be read in the necessarily short period of a dissection, and it covered all parts of the body. Above all, it was *practical* and *particular*. No other available text had all these characteristics: Galen's *Anatomical Procedures* was thought not to have survived and his *On the Use of the Parts* was not short nor particular, but general, teleological and lengthy. Galen's 'particular' books, like the *Anatomy of the Uterus* did not cover the whole body. The *Canon* of Avicenna was too unwieldy, said Berengario finally, and the commentators too diffuse and insufficiently practical. Berengario's first concern was to restore the text of Mondino to its pristine state, and then correct and amplify it for teaching purposes. These two stages are represented by his edition of Mondino in 1514 and the *Commentary* of 1521.

So in following Mondino and listing the shortcomings of the works of other authors, Berengario gives us some indication of what an anatomy text should be. Such a text should be practical in being closely linked to the manual operations of dissection, and should be particular in treating the parts of the body in turn, in terms of the particulars of sense perception rather than the universals of causality or general principles. Not every one had the same ideal, and we can usefully here look briefly at two anatomies published in 1502, the year of Berengario's appointment: as a new lecturer constructing a course, he probably read them. To historians who have read them they generally seem at either end of a scholastic–humanist spectrum.

These were the anatomies of Gabriele de Zerbi[15] and Alessandro Benedetti.[16] It is difficult to imagine two more different books. The difference is to be explained in the background of the authors and in their purposes in writing. Zerbi was a man of the schools: born in 1445, he had one intellectual foot in the manuscript age, and one of his tasks as a teacher was to bring together texts that were still expensive and hard to come by. He had taught medicine and logic at Bologna and had published his *Metaphysical Questions* before spending a period in Rome (when Berengario conceived an intense dislike for him). From 1494 he was teaching the theory of medicine in Padua. When he turned his attention to writing an anatomy, he was at least fifty five, and it is not surprising that the book is a thorough job by a professional teacher in a style of presentation that was not unique to anatomy. He declares that his purpose in publishing is to show that, properly understood, the principal authorities in anatomy do not disagree. The commentators are much quoted, and the whole work has the structure suggested by one of the earliest of them, John of Alexandria: each part of the body in turn is treated with the categorical–morphological *accessus* and the six observables.[17] Yet the book was intended to be a practical guide to dissection, as was Mondino's. The text is divided into alternate paragraphs of *textus*, 'to be read while the body is being dissected', and *additio*, to be considered at leisure between demonstrations. The book differs from Mondino's principally in the weight of authorities.

Benedetti's *Historia Corporis Humani, sive Anatomice* is very different. He too was a teacher (at Padua from 1490), but of practical medicine and anatomy. What makes his book so different from Zerbi's and Mondino's is his notion that anatomy is entirely a Greek affair. To have practised medicine for sixteen years in Greece, as he did, does not necessarily make a man a humanist, but it might well dispose him to become a Hellenist, with a knowledge of the language and a liking for the culture. As we look at figures like Benedetti and his circle of acquaintances we shall do better to call them Hellenists (rather than humanists) because this is how they saw themselves. Another Hellenist of this circle was Giorgio Valla, an important figure with a library of texts that was a magnet for other Hellenists like Leoniceno and Antiquarius. The members of the circle naturally supported each other's endeavours: Valla, discussing with Benedetti the latter's intention to write a history of the military campaigns of Charles VIII against Naples, urged him to model himself on the classical historians. Valla read the manuscript, and it was arranged that it should be printed by the humanist printer Aldo Manuzio. The arrangement not only gave Aldo the opportunity to print a work of which he approved, but it also gave him access *via* Valla and Benedetti to Venetian society.[18] In a similar way it was Antiquarius who urged Benedetti to publish his very Hellenistic anatomy.

Benedetti's dedication of the *Anatomice* makes his position very clear: he is to derive all his information from Greek sources, putting to one side the moderns who have tried to steal from the Greeks the honour of discovering medicine. Benedetti's terminology is studiously classical, and there is no mention of the commentators, their devices of exposition and their saving of the authors. His anatomy is certainly intended to be practical – he describes the construction and use of the anatomy theatre – but the message of the book is that anatomy is the *prisca anatomia* of the ancients which Benedetti is setting down in Latin for convenience of teaching. As a piece of Hellenistic propaganda, Benedetti realized the book would meet with the criticism of the great bulk of medical men brought up on Avicenna, and he loftily avoids the issue by declaring the book is intended not for them but only for the Emperor Maximilian, its dedicatee.

Turning back to Berengario, the scant evidence suggests that he was successful as a teacher. In an unidentified year between 1503 and 1512 he had ten or a dozen pupils, a number regarded by the university as satisfactory (his colleague, teaching surgery, had three, which was 'too few'). In the margin of these records, the university's 'reformers' noted that the teaching of surgery *non est multum honorabilis* but that it was popular with foreign students, those from across the Alps. (Other sources tell us that Bolognese medical education was popular among Poles and Germans. Berengario had at least one Spanish student, and perhaps the German Lange.) The same margin note says that student numbers would justify finding a temporary replacement for Berengario, but no one with his abilities could be found: *nemo practicus noscitur in hoc studio*. Perhaps these notes were written in 1512, for early the next year Leo X formally required the Bolognese authorities to release Berengario to go to Florence to treat one of Leo's relatives. Part of these arrangements was that Berengario was to have a replacement during his absence and that he was to be paid his normal salary. Before 1512 (when he died) Achillini could probably have replaced Berengario as a practical teacher, so almost certainly we are dealing with the year 1512–13.

What interests us especially about this episode is that surgical teaching was not highly regarded, not popular with the Italian students and perhaps only tolerated at the academic level of the *studium* because it brought foreign students into the town. Surgery clearly did not have the dignity of the other subjects of the arts and medical courses, and Berengario observed that physicians of his time disdained to be called surgeons. A professional teacher who had given courses on the natural philosophy common to the arts and medical courses could be naturally called up to teach medicine and anatomy, as an extension of the topics he was already teaching. In contrast, however, Berengario either could or would not teach other academic topics, and he must have felt himself in a somewhat isolated position in the *studium*: a confident and successful surgeon who was entrusted with the treatment of the pope's relations, a successful teacher, but not a member of the college of doctors and without the academic standing of his colleagues (at least in their eyes). This may well have combined with long-standing and firmly held convictions about the nature of anatomy formed in his early surgical experience to produce in him a suspicion of some of the sophistications and procedures of academic anatomy. Further evidence of this is perhaps found in his choice of Mondino as a teaching text. Although the traditional source of Italian anatomical teaching at least until the time of Curtius in the 1530s (a fact reflected in statutes), the text of Mondino was not an inevitable component of teaching, and neither Manfredi nor Achillini based their teaching on it. Zerbi disapproved of Mondino, and the Hellenists of course passed over him in a pained silence. But for Berengario (7v), Mondino was a craftsman like himself, for whom anatomy was to be conducted by hand: *secundum manualem operationem*, said Mondino. The edition of Mondino that Berengario brought out in 1514 and the *Commentary* itself seem to indicate a student-oriented[19] practicality that was neither purely academic nor Hellenist.

Whatever position Berengario chose to take up in relation to others who had an interest in medicine and anatomy, we must suppose that he saw the alternatives and rejected them for good reasons. To put him into a category of 'scholastic' or 'humanist' would be to impose a historical straight-jacket which would not explain anything. Although much of what Berengario wrote could be considered 'scholastic', we need not feel surprised, for example, that he shared the 'humanists' feel for classical culture. We know that in the year in which he published Mondino he bought an ancient stone torso, and two years later he bought a larger house in which to keep his collection of *objets d'art*. Five years after publishing the *Commentary on Mondino* he commissioned a pair of silver vases from Cellini in Rome, and when they were ready he shrewdly took away with them the drawings from which Cellini had worked. They therefore could not be copied and Berengario was able to pretend they were genuinely classical. In the circles in which he moved this was a compliment to his taste and, when the story got back to Cellini, his own stock in his circle of friends rose at once as the first man for a thousand years able to make such objects. There is no reason to suppose that such tastes came upon Berengario late in life, and no doubt he thought the same before the publication of the *Commentary*. He was approaching sixty when he began to write it, and he had long had the habit of accepting works of art in lieu of professional fees.

The Commentary on Mondino

The Venetian presses of Scotus and Junta continued through Berengario's lifetime to publish the commentaries on the *Articella* and *Canon* that formed the teaching material of the medical schools of Padua and Bologna. In publishing his own anatomical knowledge as a commentary Berengario was aiming at the same academic market. The form of the commentary encouraged a full and rigorous discussion of both morphology and procedure, and Berengario seems to have chosen the form as the one that first, did justice to the questions and which second, would most effectively convince the reader. His commentary was unusual in that its subject was an author comparatively recent and homely, in the non-academic typographical appearance of the book and in some of its purposes (all of which are discussed below). Nevertheless, the *Commentary on Mondino* has a structure that had been common to commentaries for two hundred years.

A medical commentary in Bologna would normally take such a form as follows. It would begin with a proemium praising God and the book under review. Berengario does so in the dedication and at the opening of the text. The first commentary would seek to place the subject matter of the book in its context in natural philosophy as a whole, perhaps through a device like the *accessus*. Here Berengario discusses the status of anatomy as a *scientia* and its relation to natural philosophy. The traditional commentary then began with an analysis of the book as a whole; for example the Bolognese commentators Taddeo Alderotti[20] and Gentile da Foligno[21] preferred to see the whole work in terms of a fourfold Aristotelian causality. In this place Berengario has some parallel general remarks on the necessity and use of anatomy, its 'final' cause. After the first, subsequent commentaries were invariably devoted to each section of the work, so that those standing at the head of a book, fen, doctrine or chapter would analyse the flow and stages of argument of the text, indicating to the reader the subdivisions of the text. The ultimate subdivisions of the text were perhaps only a sentence or two long, and each is identified within the preceding commentary by a quotation (within some typographical device serving the purpose of inverted commas) of its *incipit*.[22]

Thus the reader knew in advance which would be the fragments of text to be found embedded in the commentary and the whole exercise was designed to make clear the sequence of events in the text. Up to this point the exercise was an *expositio* designed to throw light on a difficult text (Taddeo says[23] picturesquely that the *expositio* is a light that brings out the colours of the text), and those whom we call commentators called themselves *expositors*.[24] Berengario and his predecessors as expositors characteristically subdivide the text in a hierarchically ordered way, so that the first level of division may reveal, say, six parts, the description of which by the expositor always begins at the second part, followed by the third and so on. The expositor then returns to the first part for a further level of subdivision, again with the second part receiving the first analysis. The purpose of this is that the expositor can preserve a continuity of analysis through the hierarchy, and so that by the time he has reached the end of his first *expositio* he has fully analysed the *beginning* of the text and can move on in subsequent expositions to the subsequent and already identified fragments of text.

Because Mondino's text was readily understood, Berengario allows it to stand in chapters without fragmenting it. He does however move through the stages of the *expositio* as outlined here, frequently concluding abruptly with the remark that Mondino's words are clear and should be read.

Having made his *expositio* in this form, the commentator would then bring forward a number of other aids to understanding the text, generally drawn from external sources. This would normally include an examination of the way in which the author used his terms. Just as the medieval disputation proceeded by the opponent (among other things) 'distinguishing' the terms of the proposition – that is, showing that the terms can have meanings inconsistent with the subsequent reasoning – so here the commentator explains in what specialized sense the author is using a term and how other authors may be using it in a different sense without necessarily contradicting each other. Where the *expositio* as described above has broken the text down into fragments of about a sentence in size, these can be treated as propositions and the whole text can thus be exposed to the rules of logic.

The commentator has now proceeded as far as he can in elucidating the text; the *expositio* is at an end. But the newly lucid text can now be seen, perhaps, to contrast with some other authority, and perhaps there are inconsistencies within it that cannot be resolved by the techniques of distinction. The next stage in the commentary form is thus the introduction of *quaestiones* or *dubia*. (The older commentators or their copyists or editors listed these *dubia* separately. Berengario does not do so, allowing the text of Mondino to be the guide to the contents of the commentary.) Here, then, Berengario brings forward the opinions of the authors for comparison and (generally) resolution. He, as a commentator, is reporting to the reader what the major issues in the field are. Sometimes, when the topic is a large one such as the formation of the foetus, the sheer bulk of Berengario's treatment is such that the commentary form is lost. He calls these *digressiones* (518r) – that on generation is about a hundred pages in length.

But more often the commentary form is retained and Berengario completes his review of the opinions of the authors before announcing any major discovery of his own, such as the structure of the vertebrate (490r) the existence of voluntary muscles within the nasal cavity (466r) the structure of the ventricles of the brain (444r) and the absence of the Galenic *rete mirabile* (459r). The novelty of these assertions necessarily meant that Berengario was in conflict with the authorities; it also meant that such bald and unsubstantiated assertions were unlikely to convince the reader. For these reasons Berengario generally introduced his assertion, or proposition, as something that would have to stand the examination of the learned and be seen separately by other skilled anatomists.

Berengario is not merely inviting his readers to 'see for themselves'. Rather, he is putting forward his anatomical discoveries as *propositions*, not because he is not convinced of their truth, but because the only way to convince others of that truth was through the stringent requirements of academic procedures. The formal structure of his commentary would have been perfectly clear to Berengario's readers, and they would have been perfectly familiar with the logical procedures of commentary, disputation, rhetoric and dialectic. Above all at the two points where Berengario could introduce his own interpretation of structure – in resolving a conflict of authority, and at the end of each comment – his readers would have felt the need of some form of *proof*.

But what kind of proof could be applied to morphological *structure*? The commentator was on traditional ground in dealing with the writings of the authorities, which could be treated as 'opinion', the premisses of the dialectical syllogism. Dialectic logic then has the business of demonstrating the falsity or truth of 'opinion' and the validity of related arguments. The process was akin to that of the disputation, with its technique of 'distinction'. Berengario is 'distinguishing' when he draws out of a single term, for example *siphac*, several meanings, not all of which fit the context and argument. Taken very strictly, *strictissime*, (50v) *siphac* means *peritoneon* (95v), but it means something else when taken merely *stricte* or *communiter*. Likewise *mirach* is used *large* and *stricte* to mean the whole abdominal wall, or simply the skin, fat and muscles (50v).

But all these are purely verbal techniques, and offer no 'proof' of structure. Certainly they could be very useful, particularly in association with detailed scholarship, to clarify the authors' texts, resolve their conflicts and so 'save' them. Berengario often calls his resolution of a conflict of authority a 'determination', the term used when at the end of a disputation the master decided in favour of one or the other disputing students; at other times he uses technical terms of rhetoric, and in both cases he seems to be invoking academic procedures to lend support to his conclusion. Now, his conclusions could be of three kinds: an assertion that an organ or part was this or that shape; an assertion that a part was *not* there, despite authority (like the Galenic *rete mirabile*) or an assertion that a part was there, but could not be seen. As we shall see below, Berengario expressly excluded the last kind of assertion as improper for anatomy. Among other things, this meant that he could not 'prove' the existence of a part from the existence of a function assigned to it.

In order to find some kind of 'proof' for the first two anatomical assertions, Berengario turned to the practical side of medicine. The commentators he had read had argued since the late thirteenth century that there were some areas of medicine where only sense-experience could lead to knowledge.[25] While it might be possible to treat the text of the *Aphorisms* in a completely syllogistic way, the only way to *know* the action of a medicine upon an individual was by experience. Berengario as a surgeon was above all a practical man, and as he many times announced his intention of writing a book on surgery, we might even see the commentary on Mondino as a 'theoretical' work, preliminary to the real business of medicine. But it would be quite wrong to think that Berengario's practical instincts led him out of scholastic anatomy and into a new methodology based on sense perception. He had chosen the commentary form and was addressing the academics in their terms, and any contributions he thought he was making were to their science. In seeking to substantiate his conclusions he used what we might call 'practical logic'.

This practical logic was *demonstration*. Derived from the simple physical *demonstratio* or *ostensio* (479v; 438; 351r) of the school anatomy, the term carries over some of the force of logical or even geometrical demonstration (450r). In general terms it meant for Berengario 'conclusion': in dealing with an insoluble problem in the field of generation, Berengario gives almost a complete bibliography of authorities and cries 'Oh! that I could demonstrate which of the foregoing opinions is true!' (139v). In this sense the word is close to *determinatio* of a disputation. Thus Berengario cannot 'determine' another conflict of authority on generation (227r) or another on the action of the heart (355r).

But the main force of the word *demonstratio* to Berengario is that it speaks directly to the senses. 'Proof' in anatomy is to expose the structure to the sight and touch, ideally to a number of observers, and at least in such a way that the reader can perform the dissection and employ his own senses (216r, 254r, 494r, 259v). Many eyes make proof; and when, in its proper place, Berengario introduces a new discovery, he puts it up as a proposition to be examined in the usual academic way and to be given a final *determinatio* or *demonstratio* by repetition (466r, 444r).

The image of the disputation provided by Berengario's commentary is strengthened by the place given to *sensus* in his method. Sense, he says, will always be his master, *magister* (that is, in providing a *determinatio*) and his guide, *dux* (that is, in investigation: 4r, 434v). More often sense is the ultimate arbiter, the *judex* (443r, 259v, 83v). Where sense has been unable to provide a final *determinatio* the question remains *sub judice* (239v, 227r). The legal analogy is present too in the very frequent use of *teste sensu* (and the occasional *necessarius est visus testificatio*: 75r). *Ad sensum* is used several hundred times.

In short, what is demonstrated to the senses is also proved to them (73v, 74v). In contrast, Zerbi uses *rationabiliter* as Berengario uses *ad sensum*, and 'proves' the warmth of the spleen syllogistically (Zerbi 22v). For Berengario the ultimate use of demonstration as proof was in the form of sensory experience that we call experiment. In the school anatomies hollow organs were often inflated to demonstrate their shape. The same technique could also prove that the organs had, or did not have, channels communicating to other organs. A major use of the proof by experiment for Berengario was the resolution of conflicts of authority. An example will make this clear: one such dispute concerned the sequence of appearance of organs during the development of the foetus, and was the result of the very different accounts of generation given by Galen and Aristotle. By Berengario's time it was also important to know at what period in its development the foetus received its soul and its animal virtues. Inspection of the early stages of the foetus could go some way to answering these problems by showing what organs had not yet developed: was the liver the first to develop, as Galen said, or was it, with Aristotle, the heart? Secondly, did the foetus, which received ready-made faculties and nourishment from the mother, need the organs responsible for these faculties while still *in utero*? For example, receiving pure concocted blood from the mother did the foetus need kidneys? Did it urinate?

Berengario realized that the only way to settle these old questions was through sense experience, the teacher or *magistra cui credendum est* (248r). But such experience was very difficult to obtain because it could only be gained from aborted foetuses 'which we see only on the rarest occasions, and with difficulty, because of the practice of our women, who refuse to show anything except secretly and with difficulty' (248r). At length and by means of furtive payments to midwives, Berengario gained the experience he desired about the early appearance of organs. Pursuing the question of development to the point where the foetus may be thought to urinate, and considering the possible role of the foetal membranes in collecting the urine, Berengario found himself in flat opposition to Galen. The only way to 'save' Galen was to assume that the relevant text was corrupt, but Berengario did not really believe that this was the case (253r, 254r). Berengario proves his case in the way outlined above:

. . . what I have said agrees with true sense; I have seen it many times and shown it to many scholars. Today, that is, 17th May, 1520, I have shown in a single anatomy (of a woman who died in the eighth month of her pregnancy, unable to give birth) and before many trustworthy doctors and scholars, that everything I have said above is very true (254r).

Pursuing the matter still further, Berengario asserts that the foetus does eject waste material in the *later* months (257v) and in particular that it expels urine through the same route as the adult, and not through the umbilicus as Avicenna has it (259v). That this is true only of the later foetus Berengario demonstrated by forcing water from a syringe into the bladder of a foetal dog, whence it passed to the umbilicus. He found this always to be the case with the early canine foetus, but the bulk of his human foetal material was at a late stage of development, and the pathway could not be found. Again Berengario resorted to *experientia*, compressing the bladder of a nine-month foetus and finding no transfer of fluid to the umbilical region. Thinking that there might have been no urine in the bladder, Berengario injected a 'notable quality' of water from a syringe into the bladder through the penis and repeated the experiment, with the result that the water emerged only along the route by which it had entered. There still remained the possibility that the water had merely chosen the most obvious of alternative pathways, and so Berengario repeated the experiment, this time tying a ligature round the penis after the water was injected to prevent reflux. The same result was obtained. Finally Berengario injected the ureter within a kidney to demonstrate the normal flow of urine, and explored all possible pathways with a small silver probe (260v). He offers similar experimental proof of his analysis of kidney function (178v) and the connections of the gall bladder (153r).

Anatomia sensibilis

We have now looked at a number of reasons why Berengario might have chosen the commentary form, chief amongst them the need to adduce a proof to convince the academics – *scolastici, scolares* – to whom the book is addressed. As a commentary in form it goes far beyond the brief text on which it is based, and we can distinguish between the form and the content of Berengario's book. The content is his idea of what anatomy should be: the purpose of anatomy is, simply, the possession of anatomical knowledge, but the acquisition of knowledge, through the procedures of anatomy, is far from simple.

In discussing anatomical knowledge and its acquisition, Berengario draws upon the tradition of commentary that contained anatomical material, that upon book three of the *Canon*. Broadly speaking, the *Canon* came to be the biggest single authority in the two centuries before Berengario, and although, as in other fields, the logical and physical works of Aristotle provided the principal tools for academic business, in medicine the substance of the topic was provided by the non-Aristotelian *Canon*. Aristotelian natural science could in principle extend to medicine as well as to the rest of the natural world. Yet there were no Aristotelian works on medicine itself, and medical men took the substance of their discipline from elsewhere. This substance did not extend to other parts of the natural world, and the natural result was that the medical commentators of the *Canon* felt that medicine was a province with clearly marked boundaries, outside which it should not tread, but within which the writ of the philosophers did not necessarily run. In particular, book three of the *Canon*, providing a complete conspectus of medicine from anatomy to treatment, became the *via medicorum*, the path to be trodden by the medical man.

This is illustrated by one of the earlier commentators, whom Berengario quotes extensively, Gentile da Foligno.[26] The first part of his commentary on book three of the *Canon* is the common exercise on the wisdom and goodness of God. It is God the Creator who is presented to us, *artifex istius mundi*: God the practical craftsman. The advantages of this presentation to the medical man are clear, for the *medicus* can fit into his world picture the western theological tradition, the church fathers and, from within his own profession, the divine and creative Nature of Galen and the creating and protective Allah of the Arabs and Avicenna himself. Nowhere is the hand of God more evident than in the microcosm, which is the body of man and the special concern of the physician. God presented in this way is very different from the abstract ultimate Good of Aristotle, presiding over an eternal (not created) world. Gentile's views allow for God to have created the world through the mechanisms of Aristotelian causality and categories, and so an Aristotelian natural science is still possible in the world at large. But in the *via medicorum*, the professional preserve of the medical men, physical reasoning was not the most appropriate. Book three of the *Canon* was vocational and practical; it was the *only* text specified in the Bologna statutes of 1405 for the *practica* course.[27] Gentile's commentary develops the theme of the skilful doctor never stepping aside from the *via* and reaching medical virtuosity by treading the path from the practical business of anatomy to the equally practical application of remedies. Gentile's remarks refer to the educational training of the physician: the implication is that while the philosophers may have a satisfactory account of the *causes* of the parts of the body, or of the mode of action of medicines, the only way to acquire knowledge of the shape of a part or the actual action of a particular medicine is by experience.

These practical features of the *via medicorum* as outlined in Gentile's commentary clearly appealed to Berengario, and he picked them out of Gentile's largely non-practical context. He then greatly developed the doctrine within anatomy. He used the term *anatomia sensibilis* to indicate a method of teaching *and discovery* that yielded a body of knowledge enclosing in its boundaries only those structures perceptible in practice to the senses. By definition other *kinds* of questions, in themselves legitimate (like those concerned with the 'origin' of parts) were excluded. For example invisibly small parts are *imaginabiles* (for example 344r): not 'imaginary' but perceptible to the mental faculty that perceives *images*. This is the faculty of reason, which Berengario identifies with imagination because of its power of handling images. This power he says, distinguishes the *sensata*, brought in by way of the *sensus communis* from the external senses, from the *non sensata*, which are composed images partly drawn from the memory and seen, then, by the internal sense or 'eye of reason' (426v, 444r, 446r) which has no place in anatomy: *anatomia non notat insensibilia* (427v). Berengario energetically denies the existence of Galen's *rete mirabile*, which had played so important a part in these functions in traditional psychology: he claims to have opened hundreds of heads in search of it and claims Galen *imaginatum fuisse*, misled by reason, not wishful thinking (459v. Compare the misled Aristotle, 64v).

There were a number of other questions which now fell outside the boundaries of anatomy: perfectly proper questions, but not to be asked of the anatomist. If much-disputed questions as that of the origin of the nerves (brain or heart?) were pressed upon the *artifex sensibilis*, they had to be answered by him – indeed by all *medici* – 'at the brain' where they can be observed (346v). Nevertheless, the 'physical' (philosophical) reasons for supposing the heart to be sentient, says Berengario, are strong, and can even overcome the medical reasons. It remains the duty of anatomists to 'speak medically', and it is quite outside the bounds of anatomy to save both opinions and declare that sentience is *virtualiter* in the heart and *actualiter* in the brain, as the commentators had done. Almost as an act of faith Berengario declares himself to be a medical man and therefore incapable of leaving the *via medicorum*, which is a pathway across the 'whole ocean' of such disputes (68v): it is the job of the theorizing physicians and philosophers to deal with these questions (475r). The tone of Berengario's words closely recalls Gentile's 'Peritum medicum non decet transgredi hanc viam'.[28] A related question concerned the origin of the veins. Both Galen and Aristotle had argued for an 'origin' of the veins (in the liver and heart respectively) on the functional basis of a faculty flowing out from a central organ. Berengario is thinking in morphological terms (and not in functional or embryological ones) and he argues that there can be no 'origin' of the veins *nisi improprie et metaphoriae*, 'unless speaking metaphorically' (161v).

So at its simplest and most fundamental level *anatomia sensibilis* was the anatomy of what could be seen. But the acquisition of such knowledge was far from simple. No one dissector could by his own unaided efforts come to a knowledge of the whole body, and necessarily had to derive some information from elsewhere. The 'science of the nature and function of the parts' says Berengario (6r) grows co-operatively, by the addition of new knowledge to old, so that we are like boys on the shoulders of giants, able to see further than they. Berengario was aware that even Galen had said that others would come after him to add to the stock of knowledge (7r).

The necessity of deriving some information from sources other than the body, combined with his insistence of sense perception, led Berengario to examine very carefully the roles of observation and reason in anatomy: how can we *evaluate* information from other sources? On their own, even the senses can be deceived, and many anatomists mistake one part for another (7r). Simply to identify and put a name to the parts of the body, the anatomist must be a master of the literature and of the problem of historical terminology; he must also discuss the problem with other learned anatomists. Where sense and authority agree, all is well, but where it can be seen that sense cannot be made to agree with the authorities, they must be rejected. Berengario constantly refers to the practitioner of *anatomia sensibilis* as an *artifex* (for example 346v), the craftsman working with eye and hand. This craftsman can learn from others: the dispute over the alleged opening of the pubic bones at birth could be settled if anatomists would visit carpenters and see how doors and windows are made so that they will open (493r). The sutures of the cranial bones is best understood by examining the carpenters' dovetail joints (417r). The entire body has been put together by God, the *primus artifex* (367r) and so can be understood by lesser *artifices*. Because of its divine origin, nothing in the body, says Berengario, is made in vain (219v–210v). It also follows from this that the body has not changed substantially since its Creation and although aware of variation of the body (14r) (for example, the gluttony of modern man has reduced the size of the caecum (115r) to a mere appendage), Berengario had good reason to believe there was an unchanged normality of bodily structure common to ancients and moderns.[29]

The role of sense observation in *anatomia sensibilis*, said Berengario, was to be extended in a number of ways. A knowledge of comparative anatomy should be gained by the dissection of different animals and of both sexes in each case. The females should be dissected at different stages of pregnancy, and much attention was to be given to the structure of the foetus, in which many things were clearer than in the adult (46v, 53v). Animals should also be vivisected (6v). Dissections should be repeated, for one organ is necessarily destroyed in revealing another. Hollow organs can be inflated, and bones and fibrous parts dried for leisurely inspection (484v, 489r). Berengario while writing to refute the earlier commentators sat with a dried specimen of the vertebrae in front of him (484r). These are largely teaching devices; the research aspect of the use of the senses is discussed next.

Berengario often distinguishes public from private dissections. Public anatomies were the customary university dissections, attended sometimes by citizens (222v) and always by students, for whom Berengario says he is writing the *Commentaria* (192v, 287v, 305v). These were the inexperienced *scolares* who can be often led 'into the pit' by the blindness of teachers, and the school dissections they attended (*in gimnasiis publicis* 479v) were concerned with the traditional 'three venters' and their contents, and were necessarily brief affairs. Their function was to reinforce in the memory the words of the accompanying text with visual images, or to make clear the shape of organs that could not be adequately explained in words (the *clarificatio eorum qui in occulta sunt* of John of Alexandria[30]). Berengario adds that such 'common' anatomies cannot show a large number of things, firstly, the bones, muscles, nerves, blood vessels and fibrous parts, all of which need special techniques for their demonstration: boiling, maceration in running water, drying. The common anatomies were generally limited to a single body, and many organs were imperfectly demonstrated in being destroyed in order to reach another organ (119v); for example the top of the cranium was generally sawn off, making it difficult to see how the dura mater is attached to it (422v). The observing students were very often misled in such a complex dissection as that of the brain. When Berengario talks of private dissections, in contrast (424r), he implies that he was dissecting to decide a particular point, like the presence of water in the torcular of Herophilus, or the existence of the Galenic *rete mirabile*. Many bodies were to be secured in private dissections for the sake of a single organ (438r) and Berengario's vivisections of animals, undertaken to decide on such points as the presence of water in the pericardium (439r), must also have been private affairs.

In other words *anatomia sensibilis* was also a set of practical precepts for anatomical *research*, the generation of new knowledge about the body. In contradicting the major authors it provoked the students of the school anatomies into reading the texts of the authors and performing dissections and vivisections in order to discover the truth (398r). *In anatomia* stated Berengario, *locus ab auctoritate contra sensum non habet veritatem* (413r), and sense observation, gained in the cemetery and by boiling the skulls left over from ordinary anatomies, will free the student from the confusion induced by reading the authorities. If the new discoveries of *anatomia sensibilis* are provocative, so much the better in stimulating intellectual activity of the *scolares* (494r).

New medical knowledge was also to be gained in another area: some diseases were reckoned to be new, because modern man, it was often thought, either by degeneration or from the effects of an undisciplined regimen of life, was less hardy than the ancients. Doctors in northern Europe found for example that there was no classical description of scurvy or scrophula, and in the Italy of Berengario's time syphilis, believed to have been brought in by French troops in 1494, had no classical precedent. The dissecting surgeon or anatomist was therefore on his own, and was necessarily making pathological discoveries. In 1521, the year of the *Commentaria*, Berengario reissued Hutten's book on the guaiac treatment, and Benvenuto Cellini records that Berengario made a great deal of money while in Rome in 1526 by the mercury treatment. Berengario intended to discuss the disease in the book on surgery (308v). As a surgeon and as an anatomist he must have wondered about the internal pathological changes: here was an *aegritudo* without classical precedent, the last of the routine observables in a dissection (according to Guy), and a category best observed in vivisection (according to Mondino). Berengario was well aware of the changes in pathological appearance brought about by death (5r, 118v), and the consequent advantages of vivisection. Fallopia records the persistent rumour that after his stay in Rome, it was a charge of having practised vivisection on a syphilitic patient that cost Berengario his post in Bologna. A man with apparently homicidal tendencies in respect of his colleagues and political enemies (as noted by Putti)[31] may indeed have been too prompt in bringing to the dissection table a body in which life still lingered.

But what of 'reason' in *anatomia sensibilis*? When Berengario says at the outset in the *Commentary* that he will be guided by 'sense [observation], the authority of the divine Galen, and various reasonings' (4r) what did he have in mind? So far we have seen that he attempted to limit the part played by reason in anatomy; and to this we can add that he rejected the idea of the 'eye of reason'. This was a technique sometimes used to argue for the existence of invisibly small or subtle parts, like the veins or humours that nourish the transparent cornea, or the invisible superfluities of the spine (497v) on the grounds of the manifest nature of their *function*. This could easily be related to the Aristotelian principle that true knowledge of a part was not generated by the particulars of sense observation or morphology, but included the more general principles that lay behind the particulars, of which the most important was function. All university-trained physicians, we may suppose, were familiar enough with 'reason' of this sort, and the argument from function was much more widely used in anatomy than inductive and observational techniques that could equally have been derived from Aristotle. A model of a deductive argument from function had been provided by Galen, who had argued that nature did nothing in vain and that therefore the apparently blind pits on the surface of the cardiac septum are not useless. Their only conceivable function was to communicate with invisibly small pores from one ventricle to another: therefore this must be their function. We may recall that it was his attention to morphology and rejection of the argument from function that led Berengario to dismiss as inappropriate to anatomy any discussion of the 'origin' of the veins.

The answer to the question of Berengario's 'reasons' is probably to be found early in the text of the *Commentary* where he spends what at first sight seems a surprising amount of space on the 'similar' parts and their qualities. The similar parts were the homogeneous and fundamental parts of the body, described by Aristotle and constituting the first step of any synthetic treatment of anatomy. The qualities of the similar parts were similarly Aristotelian and fundamental. Yet some of the commentators and Berengario himself held that in the body no similar part as such was perceptible because each was inextricably bound up with others in the construction of the parts. It would seem that the similar parts constituted just such a part of theoretical anatomy that Berengario the *artifex*, the surgeon, would reject as improper to *anatomia sensibilis*. And how far were the theoretical qualities perceptible to the senses? In the pages where Berengario discusses the similar parts and qualities we do not see these as so much medieval mud sticking to the shoes of a traveller striving valiantly for the dry ground of the renaissance. Berengario goes deep into the question of the perceptibility of the qualities and similar parts because this was anatomy's principle link to theoretical medicine. All disease at root was a qualitative imbalance and so the complexion and temperament of the parts was of great importance. If anatomy was to be of help to physicians as well as to surgeons, it must deal with the qualities. Berengario concludes that the similar parts do in fact predominate in actual organs to the extent that their elementary qualities are perceptible to the touch (but that the commentators' seven degrees of comparison were absurd).

In seeking in this way to link anatomy with theoretical medicine, Berengario is not of course trying to make anatomy theoretical, but to demonstrate that it is the observational basis for the understanding of health and disease. And just as importantly it was necessary in an institutional and academic setting to show that anatomy was not just a manual art, but related to a *scientia*. Medical commentaries since the thirteenth century (at least) had argued in a similar way that medicine itself had the dignity of natural philosophy: these were at least partly professional arguments used in defence of young faculties of medicine. In short then, these 'reasons' of Berengario were part of *anatomia sensibilis* not in telling him more about the body but in making clear anatomy's external relations.

Part of *anatomia sensibilis*, in addition to establishing a relationship between the body, text, sensory experience, reason and authority, was the establishment of a sound text. A good anatomy text, of whatever age, was one that agreed with the body; and a text was bad either from the fault of its author (or his circumstances) or because it had suffered in transmission and translation. It followed that corrupt passages in otherwise good texts

could be identified and *corrected* by the use of dissection. Practical anatomy
was also an answer to the interminable disputes of the authorities and a
guide to the correct attribution of texts to their authors. An example of
Berengario using dissection to establish the correct reading of a text occurs
in the case of the abdominal wall: Berengario has three authorities, the
printed works of Haly Abbas, a manuscript version, and a version quoted
by Nicholas, all of which differed and which Berengario decides between
on the basis of dissection, providing a woodcut to illustrate the sensible
anatomy of the part (85r). Berengario's first duty as a commentator, of
course, was to restore the text of Mondino to its *pristinum sensum* (102v),
for he says parts of the original are missing, other parts are expanded and
the sequence of others has been changed (103r). Berengario's technique is
to establish Mondino's mode of exposition as a whole, the *totus processus*,
and to argue back to the opinion behind the suspect passage, avoiding a
literal translation. Thus where Mondino appears to say there are ten
contained organs in the abdomen, Berengario argues that it is a corruption
introduced by the commentators who have been misled by Mondino
treating thirteen organs under only ten textual headings.

Illustration. The *Commentary on Mondino* is one of the first illustrated
printed anatomy texts. The modern mind so naturally seizes upon the idea
that an anatomy text should be illustrated that it is difficult not to see
Berengario as taking the first essential step. But for Berengario, of course,
it was not in the least natural that an anatomy text should be illustrated,
since no treatment of any length of the body before him had been
illustrated, and in particular the structure of the commentary form did not
admit of non-verbal elements.

Rather than taking a first step towards an ideal, Berengario's use of
illustration was an answer to his own problem of presenting anatomy.
Anatomia sensibilis was the anatomy of visible things, and visible things can
be drawn, and engraved on to a wood block. The essence of his emphasis
on sensory experience in teaching and discovery within *anatomia sensibilis*
was that sense would reveal and commit to the memory shapes that could
not be described adequately in words: illustration was a printed *anatomia
sensibilis*. Thus the complex shape of the vertebral processes, or that of the
ventricles of the brain (494r) defy full verbal description. We have seen that
within the commentary form Berengario attempted to bring forward a
mode of *demonstratio* that would convince his readers, and in the *Commentary on Mondino* in 'proving' that (for example) the uterus does not have
seven cells, he provides not only a description of its actual shape but also a
printed *praesentalis ostensio* – a woodcut – of the demonstration he would
have made to his students in life.

Another reason for providing woodcuts was that the *Commentary on
Mondino* described parts of the body that were not reached in the school

dissections. Thus the bones were not normally boiled free from flesh in the public anatomies, and were not seen by the students: Berengario provides woodcuts of the articulated skeleton and detailed illustrations of the bones of the hands. As a surgeon he is aware of the greater medical usefulness of such a presentation, in comparison with the older anatomists' concern with the total number of bones (he is thinking of Achillini: 517v). Other woodcuts are designed to show where to let blood, and how to avoid cutting muscle when excising tumours, both better seen than described. (The limitations of the technique were the skill of the artist and more particularly of the block cutter, and the woodcuts in Berengario's *Commentaria* and *Isagoge* are somewhat crude, and he remarks that the print of the vertebrae does not represent the reality of structure.)[32] Other of his illustrations were intended also for the use of artists who, like the surgeons, would have been thought of by Berengario as *artifices*. Again we see Berengario, as a *practicus*, relating himself more closely to the medieval surgeons who had illustrated their works (Guy de Chauliac and Henri de Mondeville) than to his contemporaries, whether Hellenists or 'aggregators' (see below).

Berengario first used illustration in his book on cranial fractures to illustrate the trephine. He tells us he used the instrument on Lorenzo Medici and part of the message of the book is the need for a full armoury of instruments and a skilled hand. But Berengario's trephine was a *cranked* instrument very similar to a carpenter's brace, and quite distinct from that of the prime surgical authority of the time, Albucasis, which was straight rod rolled between the open hands. It is very much easier for a reader to grasp the idea of a crank and of the complex shape of its cutting tools, from an illustration than from a verbal description, and this is one of Berengario's reasons for including the woodcut. Characteristically, he is concerned with the variety of names and of the structures they represent: *terebrum, terebellum* and *trepanum* are all 'trephine' but all differ structurally. To avoid creating confusion in the surgical reader – *ne operatores ambulant in tenebris* (90v) – Berengario publishes, in the book on cranial fractures, a *catalogue* of names *with illustrations*.

Another reason for Berengario to use illustrations was that Albucasis himself had illustrated his text on surgery and instruments and so Berengario's own library provided a model (from his will we know that Berengario not only owned a copy of Albucasis but that he considered the book fundamental to medicine).

Scholasticism and humanism. So far in this chapter we have seen Berengario as an individual presenting his own view of anatomy in accordance with his aspirations and circumstances. Can we fit him into the usual picture of humanists and scholastics? What do these terms mean in the context of medicine and particularly anatomy? To attempt to answer the question we must first look briefly at the nature of medical scholasticism.

The Italian universities before the early thirteenth century enjoyed a prescholastic period during which they supplied largely vocational training in the skills of government, trade and the professions (the *ars dictaminis*, mathematics, law and medicine).[33] Scholastic techniques were introduced from the north (principally Paris) and by student demand. These techniques were probably most closely associated with the growth of the study of the *libri naturales* of Aristotle, which gave a natural–philosophical or 'physical' content of the vocational training.

The 'physical' subjects were closely associated with medicine and were generally taught by medical men. Aristotelian natural philosophy could be made to underpin the whole of medicine, but only after some problems had been solved. The first was that these works of Aristotle did not always agree with extant medical knowledge, partly derived from Galen. Second, the largest single authority in medical education quickly came to be the *Canon* of Avicenna and this too had to be reconciled with Aristotle and Galen. In particular (from our point of view) while the general principles of anatomy were tackled by Avicenna in book one, its topographical detail was dispersed through book three and the anatomical commentator had to re-assemble it (the topographical anatomical *summae* of book one were omitted from the medieval curriculum).

So medical scholasticism was at least in part a technique of dealing with texts. These were products of alien and sophisticated culture, and they naturally created problems in the medieval Latin west. To understand these texts, and to teach them, medieval scholars devised systematic methods of enquiry and presentation. The simplest was perhaps the topical question and answer of, for example, the Salernitan questions.[34] A more complex question–doubt–resolution routine is exemplified by Peter of Abano's *Conciliator*, also arranged on the basis of topic. An elaborate approach to individual texts was the *accessus ad auctores*, a set of formal questions asked of the text by the commentator in his introduction. Designed to explain the works of Aristotle and relate them to the rest of knowledge, the *accessus* came to be used in many areas of the school curriculum including, as has recently been shown, medicine. For our purpose it is important to note that a form of the *accessus* that is closely related to the Aristotelian categories was used by John of Alexandria in commenting on Galen's *De Sectis*. This gave rise to a *physical* 'accessus' – the observables in the body – when human dissection began in the middle ages (see note 17).

The overall purpose of the scholastics was to present knowledge in an ordered whole which could accommodate new knowledge and which was structured for ready teaching and learning. The world picture became largely Aristotelian, medicine and physics having a common substrate. The agreement between the related divisions of knowledge was ensured by drawing out the 'true' meaning of the texts. In such an ordered scheme ancient authors apparently differing in their opinions were 'saved', that is, shown to agree by revealing their 'true' opinions. Close logical analysis of the texts was one means of doing this. This scholasticism varied from subject to subject. The *accessus* ranged from the anatomical to the legal. In the study of the Bible, the question of saving the authors, so important in medicine, could not arise in the same way, and scholastic study was a question of drawing out essential meanings and moral parables by close application to the text. Legal scholasticism centred on the Code of Justinian, which was treated as 'written reason',[35] and again close study of the text was necessary in order to apply it as closely as possible to society. Given the importance of this one author and text, the lawyer did not have to save his authors as the physician did. The last of the traditional higher faculties was canon law, which developed as an assemblage and codification of papal decrees: in this case the given text was fragmentary and the scholar worked from internal evidence to build up a wider scheme. The role of the commentator, then, was different in all these branches of study. The medical commentator had not only his important texts (the *Aphorisms* of Hippocrates had been used in medical education from antiquity and approached in weight of authority the fundamental texts of the other major disciplines) but was obliged to reconcile his important authors. Moreover, the physician had to carry his precepts into practice, and the anatomist had the dissected body to place in his overall scheme.

Correspondingly, the humanism which replaced these forms of scholasticism differed as much as they. Perhaps the only feature we can identify with confidence as common to them all is a sense of historical distance the humanists felt between themselves and the ancients. The associated desire to recapture classical culture led to the use of classical models in rhetoric, and the pattern of arguments used by Cicero was opposed to the formality of the rules of the *ars dictaminis*. The legal humanists came to see the Code of Justinian as the product of an ancient imperial culture that was quite different from the cities of Italy and therefore inapplicable to their society. The scriptural humanists now saw that Paul's letters to the Romans had to be understood also in the circumstances of Roman political power. In the 1440s Lorenzo Valla showed that the church's 'Donation of Constantine' was a forgery: he did so on historical grounds, by pointing to anachronisms. A related weapon of the humanists was philology, or more precisely, historical terminology, the establishment of the meaning of a word at the time it was written. This concern with language was linked to the humanists' cultivation of a purely classical prose style, from arts–course rhetoric to technical exposition in the higher disciplines.

Armed with this historical awareness, the humanists began to see that the commentators, seeking to apply the Code of Justinian to contemporary society or seeking the real religious message of the words alone of the scriptures, were engaged upon an enterprise that looked increasingly foreign to the humanists' own aims. They attempted not only to show that the commentators had misconceived the nature of their sources, but that their techniques were mistaken. The humanists naturally objected to the fine logical distinctions made by the scholastics in penetrating the 'real' meaning of the text, and to their readiness to construct neologisms to explain these distinctions. These neologisms often included ugly indeclinable words from Arabic sources, and the humanists were tempted to step right over the Arabs and commentators back to the Greek and Roman sources.

These changes were spread over a long period of time, but some important ones occurred in the period when Berengario was reading and teaching. Thus the legal humanism of Valla and his followers crossed the Alps to France only in the first decade of the sixteenth century, in the hands of Budé. Valla's denunciation of the Donation of Constantine became known to a visiting German, Ulrich von Hutten, while he was in Bologna in 1512 or 1517.[36] When he returned home von Hutten published this *exposé* with 'explosive' results in reformist thinking.[37] von Hutten seems to have met Berengario in Bologna, and when he had gone, Berengario reissued Hutten's book on the guaiac treatment of syphilis, a disease that interested them both. We have seen that Berengario was acquainted with other important figures and their techniques in the intellectual battles of the day, and the fifteen years of his productive lifetime was a crucial period for the humanists' battle.

It seems that the extent to which medicine could be 'humanized' was limited. A 'humanist' physician would be aware of himself as being historically severed from the classical world and certainly to place his authors in a time scale suggested by this would be of value, but he could not historicize his texts in the same way as the legal humanists were doing. Taking the aphorisms of Hippocrates as an example again, however much they were seen to be the products of an alien society, they applied to physical and unchanged individual people, not to a changed set of relationships between people. The same applied *a fortiore* to anatomy: a good anatomical text carried the same message as the body itself. For the same reason it was not easy to dismiss the commentators, whether their subject was the anatomy of the *Canon* or the densely aphoristic Hippocratic writings. In other words these commentators were engaged in the *same kind* of activity (despite the uncouthness of their language) as the 'humanist' physician, because the ultimate object of enquiry was the truth about the physical human body. Moreover, the *Canon* seemed more complete than any Galenic work available[38] and study of it was indispensable. The 'humanist' physician might do what he could to avoid barbarity of language, but the Ciceronian style that suited rhetoric so admirably was not easily suitable for dissection guides and descriptive anatomy (Vesalius was to lose a number of readers for this reason). The humanists' tool of historical terminology was of great importance in a descriptive science like anatomy, but it had to be based upon Arabic as well as Greek terms; in using it the humanist physician found not only that he was engaged upon the same kind of enterprise as the scholastic commentator, but that the commentators had been doing it for about two centuries.

Hellenists. These general remarks may serve to locate Berengario and his contemporaries, but when we come to try to force them more tightly into this background, we find we cannot. We are obliged to suspend our historical categories. Berengario saw himself as an *academic*: he calls his colleagues and pupils *scholastici* and *scholares*.[39] But we cannot call him and them 'scholastics' because the term still has the pejorative sense attached to it by the later humanists, implying that such people were characterized by a want of practicality in an excess of dry and sterile argument. On the contrary, Berengario saw himself as extremely practical, devoted to the principle of the superiority of sense observation over reason, and at the same time heir both to a rigorous academic tradition that had established rules for the evaluation of knowledge, and to the best medieval surgeons.

Nor does Berengario use a term that we can translate as 'humanist'. Instead he contrasts the academics with the Hellenists, one of the principal spokesman of whom was, for Berengario, Leoniceno. It was argued above that Aldo Manuzio may have been responsible for some of Berengario's 'humanist' traits; and we should recall here that these Hellenists formed a circle of acquaintanceship with widespread influence. When Berengario pursued Demetrius Chalcondylas for the text of Galen's *Anatomical Procedures* he was mixing with members of this circle: Bonamici was a pupil of Musurus, who followed Aldo as Alberto Pio's tutor. Chalcondylas himself and his teacher, Theodore Gaza, were not merely Hellenists, but were *Greeks*. This serves to remind us why northern Italians of Berengario's generation saw Hellenists rather than humanists amongst them. In short, while for a long time elegant and classical pieces of the Latin authors had been used by some university teachers the Greek interests of the Hellenists have quite a different origin. Behind this was the Council of Florence of 1439 when a Byzantine delegation spent some eighteen months in Italy. Hard pressed by the Turks, the Byzantines sent the group in an attempt to unite the Greek and Italian churches, and so secure Italian military help in the East.[40] In thus negotiating with the Latin west the Byzantines were putting to one side a political antagonism that dated back from the Crusaders' capture of Constantinople: it was simply that the Turks were a more present danger. But many of the Byzantines were impressed enough with Florence to return later; and in turn the Florentines were not only equally impressed with the unfamiliar philosophies of their visitors, but also continued to be aware of the advantages of friendly relations with the Byzantine East. There were thus also political and economic reasons why the sons of north Italian nobles, who had been previously trained in the arts of seamanship and commerce, should be taught Greek.

So both before and after the advancing Turks captured Constantinople, Byzantine emigrés were a feature of life in northern Italy. Where they contributed to a growing Hellenism, their cultural interest lay primarily in the Greek language. To the Hellenists Latin was simply the language in which Greek ideas were to be expressed for convenience, without a great cultural inheritance of its own. It was also the language of the commentators. Thus fifteenth century Hellenism was very different from the humanism of the previous century.

Berengario's charge against the Hellenists, as far as their activities touched medicine, was that they had chosen the elegance of the study of antique letters and had abandoned the wide reading, thorough scholarship and rigorous standards of argument of the academics. We have seen that Benedetti anticipates some of such criticism in his little Greek anatomy, and it is certainly true that to regard anatomy as purely Greek reduced the necessary reading to Galen and fragments from Hippocrates and Soranus. In contrast Berengario argued that the good anatomist must above all be a master of the literature. His own commentary assesses the work of nearly a hundred authors; of these Galen was clearly the most important for Berengario, for his name appears in the commentary more than fifteen hundred times, three times on every folio. Avicenna, whom the Hellenists resented as stealing Greek glory, is quoted over a thousand times by Berengario (and Aristotle about six hundred times, Zerbi two hundred and the commentators and lesser Arabs each between one and two hundred times).

Berengario's attitude to the Hellenists is illustrated by his dispute with Leoniceno, one of the *periti Eleni* (skilled Hellenists) in the phrase of Berengario and Zerbi (49r and Zerbi, 7v). Berengario approved in principle of Leoniceno's attempt to establish a sound Greek terminology (40v, 42r, 480r, 486v, 495v) but argued that to ignore the Arabic authors would lead to error. Thus Leoniceno uses the term *epigastrion* for the entire abdominal wall, evading the vigorous academic debate about the identity of the Arabic *siphac* and *mirach* and the Galenic *panniculus carnosus*, all of which seemed to academic anatomists to be parts of the abdominal wall. Consequently *epigrastrion* was unsatisfactory to Berengario.

Again as a Hellenist striving to write in pure Latin, Leoniceno translated the *peritoneon* of Galen's *Commentary on the Aphorisms* as *membrana abdominis interior* because there was no single-word Latin equivalent to the Greek and because he did not wish to use the 'barbaric' Arabic term *siphac*. Berengario insisted not only that *siphac* was a perfectly proper anatomical term that precisely expressed the meaning of 'peritoneon' but that Leoniceno was unjustified in inserting additional words into the text, words moreover that introduced confusion by restricting the meaning to an *inner* membrane. The argument (104ff) had a very real surgical importance, for Galen's text asserts that if the omentum penetrates the abdominal wall, it necessarily putrefies, and Berengario as a practical surgeon understands this to mean if the omentum reaches the air: to penetrate merely an interior membrane (as occurs in the zirbal rupture) is not necessarily to putrefy. Arguing from observation and due consideration of the Arabs, Berengario feels himself to be in a stronger position than Leoniceno, who is concerned primarily with 'good letters' (*viri profecto omnium bonarum litterarum con-sumatissimi* (105v)). Leoniceno's reply[41] is textual, without reference to observation or Arabic authors. However elegant Leoniceno's 'good letters', it seemed to Berengario that they constituted mere unverified *authority* and that Leoniceno's method was therefore at fault. In particular he objected to Leoniceno attacking Mondino (the *artifex sensibilis*) *per auctoritates et non per sensum* (154v).

Berengario's position is that, given a knowledge of the literature, both in terms of its content and its *historical* sequence, we can understand how errors have arisen and give due weight to the important authors: there is no need to short-cut the Arabs, for we can sift their contribution to anatomy if we use the critical aspects of *anatomia sensibilis*. In particular although Galen's *On the Use of the Parts* had been known in Greek and a good Latin translation from the early fourteenth century, and was a natural focus for the attention of medical humanists with an interest in anatomy, yet more popular and easier to read was an abbreviated and corrupt form of the work that had reached the West through Arabic.[42] This must have seemed very different to the Hellenists of the renaissance, and Leoniceno denied that the two had the same origin (89v). But Berengario had read both works thoroughly and could see that the sequence of argument was the same, despite the battered state of the text of *De Juvamentis Membrorum*. That is, he considered that he had recovered the *via Galeni*, the essential Galenic doctrine (akin to the *totus processus* of Mondino: compare 34r) which was the criterion against which the shortcomings of the corrupt text (which he realized were acquired at the Greek–Arabic stage of transmission (89v)), could be judged.

In anatomy at least, the Hellenists did not have that historical approach to their texts which has been seen as such a feature of humanist scholarship. What inspired the Hellenists was the belief that they were recovering a true *prisca anatomia*; true, because Greek. In contrast Berengario did historicize his texts, realizing that their content must be understood in terms of the circumstances of their composition. Aristotle, said Berengario, lived in an age when anatomy was not highly developed and so was ignorant of a great deal; Galen too was often wrong in little things (for example in his description of the veins: 162r) as in big, notably in his description of the *rete mirabile*: 'I too' cried Berengario confidently 'have a keen eye and hand and suitable tools' (459r). Other authors in Berengario's view had suffered the accidents of history as their texts have been lost or corrupted (166r). Berengario had perhaps in mind Galen's *Anatomical Procedures*, for he had read in Galen's *On the Use of Parts* of Galen's first, short version of the text and his plans for a fuller version. Perhaps Berengario had not yet realized that the fuller version was represented partly in the Greek text with the medieval name of *De Anatomicis Aggressionibus* for he often bewails the loss of Galen's particular and practical anatomy (that is, in the style of Mondino) and he spent the years between 1521 and 1529 tracking down the Greek version and improving Chalcondylas' Latin version of it for publication.

Berengario continues by placing the Arabic authors in their historical context. The first of the *cardines* of medicine after Galen, he says, was Rhasis, followed by Haly Abbas and Avicenna (162v), and their different historical contexts including their different purposes in writing, for Rhasis was much more practical than Avicenna and Haly, who were less inclined to use observation than theory, and so repeated many errors (165r, 168v). Moreover, adds Berengario, although Avicenna depended heavily on Rhasis, it was Avicenna who became known first in the West, and the *Canon* was widely accepted without its derivative nature being understood. Its status ensured that subsequent anatomists simply 'made books from books' without recourse to observation.

An important part of the techniques of establishing sound texts was the study of historical terminology. seen throughout the *Commentary* and particularly in the anatomical 'catalogue' or glossary, which occupies some forty pages in the earlier part of the work. Berengario's statement that the purpose of listing anatomical terms accurately is to establish their meaning *as used historically by the authors* could hardly be bettered as a 'humanist' programme, but of course much of Berengario's philological enquiry is directed at the important Arabic authors. The reader, says Berengario, must make every effort, *ultimo conatu*, to discover which authors have used a term, and what it can mean in different contexts, in order to understand the 'mind of the author' who uses the term (15v, 29v). The essence of the technique is to grasp the idea in the author's mind, and not to be over-concerned with the literal appearance of words, over which some scholars waste their lives (61r). Having done so, terminology can be simplified in two ways: first, a good Latin word from an approved author will replace all synonyms, as *adeps* indicates 'fat' well enough to render all the synonyms unnecessary (54v, 55r), and second, barbarisms and corruptions will be avoided. But, says Berengario, it is in the end only by means of observation that we decide which is the better of two texts. Again Berengario points to the difference between *Du Usu Partium* and *De Juvamentis Membrorum* as an example (153v). In the larger work, Galen compares the insertion of the ureters into the bladder to that of the bile duct into the intestine (so that a flap acts as a valve) but the corrupt version makes the comparison with the insertion of the bile duct into the *gall bladder*.[43] Berengario accepts from observation that *De Usu Partium* is correct, and that the error of the corrupt version is one of translation, probably at the Greek–Arabic stage (89v). Moreover, since similar errors occur in *De Juvamentis Membrorum*, Haly Abbas and Avicenna, it must be assumed either that all three texts have suffered corruption in the same direction, or, more likely, that Haly and Avicenna depended upon *De Juvamentis Membrorum*, and did not have available either *De Usu Partium* or the opportunity of sensory observation. Since all the moderns, adds Berengario, 'walk with Avicenna', they are all in error. Many of the elements of *anatomia sensibilis* are involved in Berengario's examination of the question of the insertion of vessels into the gall bladder: Berengario wonders, *miror, ac longe miror*, how Nicholas, Zerbi and all the modern *cardines* of medicine have been deceived by *authority*, since to *observation* it is clear that the insertion is perpendicular, not diagonal; *reason* would suggest a diagonal entry (on the analogy of the ureters) because such an insertion provides a valve that prevents reflux, but this must be denied in the face of observation. There is no middle way to 'save the authors' except by saying their texts are corrupt; and the good anatomist will see by *dissection* that Berengario is correct, and can confirm his opinion by *experiment*: squeeze the gall bladder and the bile moves easily into the bile duct and intestine (there is no valve) (152–3).

Similar considerations persuaded Berengario that the text of Avicenna then common, that of Gerard of Cremona (91v) was corrupt in places, in particular where concerned with the structure of the abdominal wall. The result is that Mondino and all the modern authors are in error (49v), deceived by authority. However, the text available to some of the early commentators, particularly Nicholas, was superior, and Berengario concludes (92v) that it was possible to restore the text of the Gerardine translation by adopting Nicholas' report of certain passages *and by dissection*. More generally, the older commentators, says Berengario, had inferior texts, often from the Arabic. Thus Dino, Gentile, Ugo and Nicholas had only the old, ex-Arabic translation of Aristotle's '*De Animalibus*' (232v) which has *zirbus* and *mirach* interchanged in sense as the components of the abdominal wall, while the new translation (by Theordore Gaza (232v)) more correctly identified as *De Partibus Animalium*, had 'membrane' (103r–v) in a correct usage.

This *historical* evaluation of texts, translations and technical terms was, far from being a 'humanist' activity, the very substance of what the commentators had been doing since the translations had been made. The commentators had always been critical of the translations. Taddeo called Constantine the African a 'mad monk' incapable of good translation. Taddeo preferred the translations of Burgundio of Pisa, but was obliged to base his commentary on Constantine's text because it was so widely used in teaching. As better translations were made they were ofted added to the older, so that, for example, some of the printed commentaries include three translations, the latest being perhaps that of Leoniceno. As Berengario observes, Jacobus de Partibus was aware of the identity of *De Juvamentis Membrorum* and *De Usu Partium* and of the reasons for their different appearance (388v); Gentile recognized corruptions in the text of Avicenna (111) and considered whether or not *De Juvamentis Anhelitus* was correctly attributed to Galen (137v–138v). Peter of Abano questioned the Galenic attribution of *De Spermate* (220v); Jacobus de Partibus saw *siphac* as a good modern Arabic term, replacing the antique Arabic 'superscripts' (glosses) *berbentinem, alberiteron* which are clearly Arabic attempts to handle the Greek *peritoneon* (and which were *auditu horrenda* to Berengario). This improvement within Arabic terminology was seen by Berengario as a process parallel to the later coining of neologisms by the Latins to generate concise technical terms. We can see from Berengario's text that such terms could be Latinate in form or adoptions from the Arabic, and we have also seen what Berengario considered the advantages of a precise terminology of this form. The Hellenists, needless to say, considered both adopted Arabic and new Latin terms as barbaric, and translated from their Greek in circumlocutions when there was no Latin counterpart.

We can now see more clearly Berengario's view of the Hellenists. He was aware of a great amount of scholarship and a shrewd historical awareness of anatomical texts that had begun at least as soon as the early fourteenth century. The fruit of this scholarship was still to be reaped in Berengario's time, especially with his own critical techniques, which in their practical nature were not necessarily sympathetic to the Hellenists. This scholarship was academic, comprehensive and businesslike, but without the elegance of 'good letters'; but to avoid it, at least in anatomy, was a failure to grasp the nettle: without such scholarship it was all too easy to fall into elementary errors such as supposing that Galen did not make mistakes (and all that was needed for truth was a sound text) or being unable correctly to attribute works of Galen that had suffered in transmission (like Leoniceno and *De Juvamentis Membrorum*).

Aggregators and barbarians. Having looked at how Berengario saw himself in relation to the Hellenists, we must examine his opinion of other identifiable groups among his contemporaries. As suggested above, Berengario saw himself as an academic. Some of the outward signs of academic medical teaching were the heavy folios of double-column, black-letter printed commentaries and text of the *Articella* and *Canon*. This format identified them as academic; Zerbi was not 'unfortunate'[44] in his printers, but undoubtedly chose the format to suit his readership. The sheer bulk of these Venetian folios represents a considerable publishing investment, that could only be recouped by steady sales to a large educational market. The disappearance of these folios from the publishing programme of the houses of Scotus and others from the 1520s was the victory of the Hellenists.

But although an academic Berengario did not identify himself with the bulk of school anatomical authors. His admiration was reserved for the practical texts of Mondino and Guy de Chauliac, who, he said, like himself had practised *anatomia sensualis* (464r) while no-one else among the moderns did so. Guy, Berengario further explained, was the *maximus anatomes* whose work was read in the public anatomies of Montpellier as that of Mondino was read in those of Italy (171r). Like Mondino, Berengario addresses his text to the practical *operatores* (for example 78r).

Berengario particularly objected to those modern anatomists who undervalued sensory experience and dissection. Those who compiled their anatomies from books alone Berengario called *aggregatores*, a term that indicated most of the commentators and which was derived from the literary habit of collecting simple recipes. Zerbi in Berengario's eyes was the *magnus aggregator* (307v) who had in Bologna a following of 'Zerbists'. These often clashed with the 'Partists', the followers of the fifteenth-century commentator Jacobus de Partibus (310r); clearly Berengario felt as distant from them as from the Hellenists.

Lastly, since Berengario, the Hellenists, the aggregators and the commentators all had their different views on what anatomy was and what an anatomy text should be like, we may usefully enquire into what at first sight seems to be their common enemy, the 'barbarians'.

Zerbi, the academic aggregator, is clear enough on the point: Guy de Chauliac, the medieval surgeon, and his kind. Although Zerbi regarded him as a useful author (for he quotes him often enough) yet he observes that Guy is barbaric in his language, using medieval terms like *pincherium* (Zerbi 47v) to express the capacity of the bladder. Probably Zerbi was also aware that Guy used his native French. Zerbi himself did not cultivate a high style of prose, and was not above using neologisms (like *cerebri factiva*, 'brain-making' 38r) but he did his best to keep his language as Latinate as possible. Thus where Berengario invariably uses 'Haly' for the Arabic author, Zerbi uses the compound 'Haliabbas' which he can decline: it has the ablative form 'Haliabbate'. Even 'Averroys' is given the ablative 'Averroy' by Zerbi (30v, 33v) while 'Rasis' (for Rhasis) becomes 'Rasi' (32r). The normally indeclinable 'siphac' becomes 'siphacia' in the nominative plural (12v).

Zerbi's attitude to Guy was not shared by Berengario, who admired him as one of the few practical authorities. Like Mondino, Berengario consciously avoided an elevated prose style as unsuited for practical descriptions and where possible tried to 'walk like Celsus among the Latins' (393v). His own view of barbarisms differs from that of Zerbi and from that of the Hellenists. He defends his own usage in telling us that Arabic terms rendered into Latin characters (like siphac and mirach) although undeclinable are not in themselves barbaric, and that barbarisms are *corruptions* of a pure original introduced by the errors of copyists, translators and printers (45r, 46r). 'God preserve me' he pleaded 'from the translators' use of unknown names for known structures' (78v). Some of the *horrida nomina* that have found their way into Averroës' *Colliget* are so fearful in sound that Berengario cannot bring himself to use them (30r). As examples of corrupt terms we may take Berengario's list of variants produced by the Greek *peritoneon* passing through Arabic into Latin: *beriteron, berbetinem, berterin, alberiteron* and *albentirion*. The proper forms in the three languages says Berengario are *peritoneum, siphac* and *membrana*, and good scholarly anatomy reveals the identity of the *idea* behind the three different words by relating it to structure.

All such names derived from the Arabic, whether corrupt or not, were regarded by the Hellenists in their search for the pure Greek form as barbaric. Their barbarians were the academics and medieval surgeons. Berengario, who felt sympathy with both these groups, naturally felt that the barbarians were some other group. Yet when he was urged (he says)[45] by Bonamici, Pomponazzi and Ercole Gonzaga to publish his edition of Chalcondylas' translation of the *Anatomical Procedures* he seemed to share the Hellenists' views on barbarisms. In giving the book 'a true birth into Latin' he spoke with a characteristic Hellenistic rhetoric of the 'pure fountains of the Greeks' and of the 'very turbid streams' of the barbarians. This rhetoric was addressed to Ercole who, we may suppose, understood and approved of it. These barbarians were not Arabs, however. Berengario's barbarians are some of his contemporaries, those who draw their *remedies* (even though the context is the *Anatomical Procedures*) from the turbid streams. For the 'lack of skill' of these barbarians, Berengario uses *imperitia*, a word he elsewhere seems to relate to *empiricus*, 'an empiric'. In either case what is implied is a lack of thorough training, particularly anatomical; the training provides skill, and the anatomical knowledge provides the basis for a *rational* practice of surgery. This lies behind his attack, in the dedication of the *Commentary*, on the *cardines* of the medical faculty, ignorant of anatomy. Much more revealing is the text of his book on fractures of the cranium. He supposes that one of the most reliable surgical authors, because one of the oldest, was Celsus. He accepts the Arabs' historical judgement that by their day most of the old surgery had been lost, so that (by implication) both Arabs and the commentators were at a disadvantage. Nevertheless, *magnus* Guy de Chauliac (12v) was an ideal practitioner combining surgery, medicine and natural philosophy (30r). But since Guy's time, says Berengario, things have deteriorated, and physicians are not willing to undertake a long period of surgical training (ideally from childhood), and surgeons with good manipulative skills are rarely well-read. Learned physicians, he explains (29v) disdained to be called surgeons, but were very conscious of the money to be made in surgery; in this perplexity they pretended to be surgically knowledgeable, and covered their ignorance by pretending also to be too faint-hearted to operate: they attended patients, taking with them stout-hearted if ignorant *chirurguli* who performed the operation and shared the fee, 'the blind leading the blind', as Berengario observed.

These *chirurguli* in Berengario's eyes were empirical, ill trained and mostly Jewish. Most of the ancient authors had sought cause and effect (60v) (that is, they were rationalists) but the ancient sect of Empirics (who held that a knowledge of anatomy was neither useful nor decently gained) flourished principally among the Jews (58r), and although Berengario says some of them have not been negligible, yet none of them have become famous. Berengario has in mind his father's great friend Jacob the Jew, who treated Ercole, Duke of Ferrara; he also has in mind Master Abraam, to whom he resented playing second string in the case of Lorenzo Medici. Although he was not above obtaining the receipt for his own cranial ointment from Jacob by deception (Jacob imagined him to be of the ducal family), Berengario became most indignant over the claim of the empirical Jewish surgeons who believed that a depressed fragment of the cranium could be raised by the use of ointment alone. These ignorant empirical idiots (64r) are Berengario's barbarians, so different from the anatomically learned *scholastici* (103v).

4

Humanist surgery

V. NUTTON

The modern historiography of renaissance surgery resembles a moral fable concocted out of ignorance and tralatician prejudice. The story has its heroes, principally Paré and Fabry von Hilden; as well as its villains, the London College of Physicians and sundry Frenchmen; it has its great stage settings, the deaths of rulers and the prosecutions of surgeons; and it has its intellectual shibboleths, the proper treatment of gunshot wounds and the correct site for bloodletting. In this gory tale of vice and virtue, the surgeon emerges triumphant over the follies of the physicians and the prejudices of the fastidious, and his availability and the effectiveness of his treatments have been contrasted with the small numbers and useless therapies of the physicians.[1] It would be foolish to deny that there is a good deal to be said in favour of the the traditional account. It is not easy to minimize the force of the observations by a man as wise and as sceptical as Montaigne, who saw around him the physicians 'bastelant et baguenaudant à nos despens en tous leurs discours' and who preferred surgery which 'me semble beaucoup plus certaine, par ce qu'elle voit et manie ce qu'elle fait; il y a moins à conjecturer et à deviner'.[2] Nor can the career of Paré be disregarded as an example of the workings of professional prejudice against a less well-educated but technically superb practitioner. But neither example proves all that champions of surgery have wished it – after all, Montaigne preferred self-medication to being cut for the stone by a surgeon – and a review of other, less well-known texts offers scope for a rather different interpretation. In this chapter I want to suggest that the gulf between surgeon and physician was not as wide as has been thought; that, particularly when contrasted with the barbers and barber-surgeons, the two groups had much in common; and that there was a strand of humanism that was as important in the development of surgery as in that of medicine.

I begin with one obvious point in the surgeon's favour. Montaigne's support for the surgeons was based on their greater certainty in their treatment. Unlike the doctor, whose diagnosis, no matter how circumscribed it might be, still depended upon a doctor's hunch, and whose possible therapies in any given case might be almost unlimited, the surgeon was often faced with conditions that were at once obvious and curable by only a restricted variety of techniques. A broken leg, with a simple fracture, does not require great sophistication of diagnosis or more than competence to set it satisfactorily. Similarly, the link between healer and cure was more immediate. Since most diseases would have cured themselves, given time, it is often hard to see whether the doctor's intervention actually hastened the cure or, maybe, did little to hinder it. Yet in many cases treated by a surgeon, his expertise would be obvious to all who watched him perform. He also had the advantage over the physician of treating fewer chronic cases, and even in acute cases, his intervention was frequently seen as a last resort, where failure was not to be imputed largely to his bad treatment. This impression of the certainty of the surgeon might also be enhanced by the guild craft traditions in which he was trained. At Bordeaux, whereas the graduate physician publicly disputed with others before the mayor and council, the corresponding act for the surgeon was to be presented by the guild of surgeons as a well-trained and competent member of their craft. No arguing over doubtful cases here; merely a show of solidarity by all surgeons over the essentials of their craft.[3]

Yet if one turns to another area in which surgeons played a major role in diagnosis and treatment, but where the condition was less amenable to cutting and burning, namely skin diseases and syphilis, a different picture emerges. A glance at the pages of Proksch's *Geschichte der venereischen Krankheiten* or at its sixteenth-century predecessor, Luisini's *De Morbo Gallico*, reveals a melancholy story that only confirms the fortitude of the syphilitic patients. There is little to choose between doctor and surgeon; both use the same arguments (largely borrowed directly or indirectly from Leoniceno), and the same examples and classical texts to prove their case. The noble art of plagiarism is as much likely to be practised by a surgeon on a physician as the reverse, and both sides express their pride in difficult cases successfully cured. But it is not until the middle of the seventeenth century, with Richard Wiseman, that we get an exaltation of surgical technique as a means to alleviate, if not cure, venereal diseases, for both surgeon and physician accepted the validity of remedies using guaiac, mercury or sarsaparilla. It is well also to remember that when dealing with a condition whose cause was as obscure as sciatica or whose course was as difficult to follow as that of syphilis, the surgeon fared neither better nor worse than the physician. The surgeon's apparent certainty depended at least as much on the conditions he generally treated as on his own ability. But, as traditional historians of surgery have stressed, the new developments in warfare in the sixteenth century led to a consequent re-examination of surgical techniques, the invention of new instruments and artificial limbs, and the discovery of new techniques for managing wounds. In these situations, the obvious relationship between treatment and cure (or amelioration) gave the surgeon a benchmark against which to test any novelty. He could then adopt whatever seemed most effective and jettison what seemed to him useless or outmoded. Not that one should immediately equate the outmoded with the classical texts of Greece and Rome; for as well as bringing to light again writings on medical philosophy and on anatomy that had been hidden for centuries, the renaissance saw the restoration of classical surgery.

The surgical treatises in the Hippocratic Corpus, which have deservedly received praise from a distinguished line of surgeons from Vidus Vidius to Owen Wangensteen, were unknown to the middle ages. Pearl Kibre lists only a couple of Munich MSS., CLM 161 and 614, which are said to contain Latin versions of *On Head Wounds* and *On Cancer and Fistulae*, but their connection with the actual Hippocratic treatises seems to me to be slight. The so-called Hippocratic *Surgery* is equally little more than the shadow of a great name.[4] One can find traces of Greek manuscripts of the ancient Hippocratic surgical texts owned by or accessible to physicians before 1520 – Cornarius used MSS. once in the possession of Johann von Dalberg, bishop of Worms, and of Adolphus Occo, *Stadtarzt* at Augsburg[5] – but it was not until the Aldine Greek edition of 1526 and, still more, the Latin versions that followed from it, that knowledge of these texts became in any way widespread. Only in the third quarter of the century did Hippocratic surgery make any major impact on academic medicine. Leaving aside as a curiosity the 1556 statutes of the University of Ingolstadt, which prescribed as anatomical texts *On Glands, On Fleshes* and *On Places in Man*, I,[6] only *On Wounds in the Head* became a standard set text in a university course on anatomy and surgery.[7]

Two other Greek sources for ancient surgery, Aëtius and Oribasius, have a similar *fortuna*. The main surgical sections in Aëtius, Books XV and XVI, were in fact never printed in Greek until this century, and were not available in Latin until Cornarius' translation of the whole sixteen books, Lyons, 1549. The section on eye diseases and head wounds had appeared in Greek at Venice in 1534, but little account seems to have been taken of this author by renaissance scholars.[8] As for Oribasius, the later surgical books of his great medical encyclopaedia were never printed in Greek until the edition of Daremberg and Bussemaker, Paris 1851–76, and were not included in the sections translated by Giovanni Battista Rasario into Latin, Paris 1555, and in subsequent reprints.[9] However, some sections, Book forty-eight, 1–18, and Book forty-nine, took on a life of their own in the translation of Vidus Vidius, Paris, 1544, as part of his surgical collection. As *De Fasciis* and *De Machinamentis* they were included by Gesner in his 1555 collection of surgical texts, and appeared in a French translation at Lyons in the same year.[10]

Three other major medical authors remain to be discussed, Celsus, Paul and Galen. Celsus presents a great problem. His works, in their elegant Latin, were first published in 1478, and were frequently edited and reprinted. Yet it is hard to discover them playing any major role in university teaching, either of physic or of surgery, and the fact that their last two books contain a very detailed exposition of graeco–roman surgery seems rarely to have been mentioned by publishers on their introductory title pages or prefaces, with the exception of the edition produced by Lucantonio Giunta at Venice in 1524. Whether this was the text from which Johansen Khüffner made his German version, published in 1531, I cannot say, but his title *Die Acht Bücher von beyderley Medicine: das ist von Leib und Wund Artznei* at least suggests that he was aiming to attract readers among the surgeons. I leave it to others to pursue the influence of Celsus on the medical world of the sixteenth century, on Paré, for example, but it is worth noting that if Celsus was among the favourite authors of medical humanists, Guenther's complaints, in his 1542 edition of Paul, about the difficulty of creating a new surgical vocabulary in Latin, are not easy to interpret.[11]

Book six of Paul of Aegina's *Compendium of medicine* is the best short account of ancient surgery, and comes from an author whose merits as a textbook writer were well known to the Greeks. The early medical humanists made good use of him, even though his works did not appear in print until the Aldine edition of 1528. Leoniceno quotes him often in his treatise on syphilis,[12] and other manuscripts were owned by Guillaume Cop, Jean Ruel and Thomas Linacre.[13] Like the Aldine Galen, the Aldine Paul stimulated a flurry of Latin translations.[14] Of the vernacular versions of book six I shall speak later, as they form part of a deliberate, and, I would argue, Galenist attempt to influence surgeons.

Galen's surgical works, like his anatomical texts, had remained in obscurity in the middle ages. No translations had been made of his commentaries on the Hippocratic surgical texts, and his book on tumours, the surgical sections of the *Method of Healing* and the spurious *Introduction* were available only in bad translations or in the accurate, but not always accessible, versions by Niccolò.[15] The *Method of Healing* had the honour of being the first genuine Galenic work to be printed in the original Greek, at Venice in 1500, with the support and encouragement of Leoniceno, who supplied the editors with manuscripts on the express condition that they publish them.[16] This text also had the privilege of an extremely competent translator, Thomas Linacre, whose Latin version successfully cornered the market and was printed almost thirty times between 1519 and 1598.[17] This was a major achievement, and one that might have been expected to bear fruit. But there is one *caveat*: several of the copies I have seen of this large work seem to have been opened with enthusiasm, but as interest waned, particularly in the middle books, seven to twelve, on humoral disorders, the pages bear fewer annotations, and often remain uncut for the last two books, which describe some complicated surgical techniques.

On 15 July 1524 the first renaissance translation of the *Introduction* was dedicated to Pope Clement VII. Its author was Euphrosynus Boninus, a Florentine, who had qualified in medicine, and who from 1522 held the post of *praeceptor* in oratory and poetry at Pisa. He admitted that he might be less imbued than some with the precepts of rhetoric, grammar and poetry, but offered as an excuse his medical experience in curing fevers and in cauterizing and in cutting sores and ulcers. The translation formed part of an ambitious project, suggested to Boninus by Clement before his elevation to the papacy in 1523, to put into Latin hitherto untranslated Greek works. The first fruits were his versions of Philoponus' commentary on the *Posterior Analytics*, Galen's *Medical Definitions*, the *Introduction* and, in about 1525, a version of Paul. Unfortunately, these versions were never printed and, although the version of Paul claims to be complete, its two surviving MSS. are both defective, and there is no trace yet of Books four to six and the later chapters of Book seven. His version of the *Introduction* remained similarly forgotten and exercised no influence on subsequent authors.[18]

It was left to the young and impecunious Guenther of Andernacht to produce the first printed translation, for Simon de Colines in 1528. Its association with Guenther's version of *De Sectis*, its small format, and the substantial number of surviving copies, all suggest that it was deliberately aimed at a student audience (or one which needed a basic grounding in Galenic medicine). Like Linacre's version of the *Method of Healing*, it held the field unchallenged for the rest of the century. Two months later appeared Guenther's version of *On Tumours*, which enjoyed a similar *fortuna*, although the subsequent compilers of the big *Galeni Opera Omnia* from 1541 onwards preferred the translation of the otherwise obscure Horatius Limanus.

The other surgical works had to wait until the 1540s before being turned into Latin. Feliciano, 1543, Trincavella, 1545 and Vidius, 1544, all completed their rival translations of Galen's commentaries on the Hippocratic surgical texts, and Vidius added in 1544 a translation of the little tract *On Bandaging*.[19]

The rediscovery of these Galenic tracts provided all those who could read Latin with two things, new information on surgical technique, and, secondly, a model for the integration of medicine. Throughout his writings, Galen constantly stressed the unity of medicine, a unity of head and hand, of logic and experience. There is a constant emphasis on *ascesis*, practice, and on the need for the doctor to experience the workings of the body for himself. It was not enough simply to read a book on the subject – or even to attend an occasional demonstration of anatomy. It was essential for the true physician to keep practising, to repeat anatomies, in order, at the very least, to keep his abilities well honed. It was precisely for this reason that Galen continued his private dissections long after he had been forced to abandon them in public.

Although Galen never completed his own book of surgery, he constantly referred to his own surgical successes – excising a suppurating breastbone, bandaging and healing the suppurating finger, half-amputated accidentally, of a careless vine-dresser, and removing foreign bodies from eyes, heads and stomachs. The pseudo-Galenic *Introduction* apparently confirmed his expertise by providing details of a complicated series of internal operations, of methods of suturing, and of restoring damaged limbs, which have excited the praise of a modern surgeon, albeit under the impression that they were genuinely Galenic.[20] In this context, Galen's insistence on the importance of anatomy takes on a dual function. At one level, it is a *Forschungsinstrument*, essential for anyone who wishes to understand how the body works, at the other, it provides essential practical training in surgical technique. It also carries with it the implication that, even for the surgeon, there must be some approximation to the Galenic ideal of a medical man who not only can carry out complicated and difficult tasks, be they in physic, surgery or pharmacology, but also knows why and how he is doing them. At its best, this ideal of the unity of medical knowledge is an inspiring one, even today, and it would be unjust to see those who championed it against less-intellectual practitioners, like the Paracelsians, simply as motivated by narrow professional jealousy or a desire to maintain the status quo in their favour. Such cynicism underestimates the force of an ideal which led to so much ink being spilled, so many words written, and so many proposals uttered.

It is the believers in this ideal that can best be characterized as 'humanists', scholars convinced of the practical utility of linking the present with a classical past, and prepared to be guided by the precepts and the example of the ancients. It was more than mere philology. The violent polemic of 1578 of the Parisians Duret and Martin against the comments on Hippocrates' *On Wounds in the Head* prepared by the young J. J. Scaliger and his surgeon friend St Vertunien, was intended to show that textual criticism by itself was not enough.[21] Many of its adherents also took the liberal humanistic view that their surgery could bridge the ever-widening gap between physician and barber surgeon. The surgeons could be educated up to a proper understanding of what they were doing, while the physicians, who might otherwise remain aloof from the body and thereby condemn their patients to the tortures of the illiterate and incompetent, could be encouraged to take up again therapies they had long neglected.

This humanistic programme might further strengthen the position of surgery (and, incidentally, of anatomy) within the university.[22] Particularly in southern Europe, it was possible for a student to attend a limited course on medicine – usually only the first year courses on medicine – and graduate with a degree in surgery. Such a graduate would have a great deal in common with the learned physician. He too might obtain a civic post as a result of an examination by an official appointing body, although his salary was generally lower. His lecturers might be the same, and the set texts similar to those of the medical student proper. The professor of surgery, if there was one, could happily lecture on Galenic or Hippocratic texts and might attract medical students eager to hear in simple language theories whose import was not easily grasped when dressed up in the philosophical rhetoric of a senior professor. The *Aphorisms* were a mine of information for the surgeon, and the Spaniard, Juan Fragoso, whose *Surgery* depended largely on them, found himself with a best-seller. First published in 1586, his book was still being reprinted a century later.[23] The Hippocratic Corpus and the voluminous works of Galen provided ample weapons for almost any conflict, whether it was for Matteo Corti in the debate on bloodletting that rocked the 1530s or for Laurent Joubert and his friends in the 1580s, who compared with equanimity the varying defective approaches to the treatment of gunshot wounds advocated by Hippocrates, Galen and Paracelsus.[24]

By an alliance with the humanism of some physicians, the academic surgeon could further strengthen his own position within the academic hierarchy, which was by no means assured. When in 1550 the German Gryllus, on his sponsored tour of European medical schools, visited Rondelet at Montpellier, his delight at finding there 'as frequent a practice of surgery as of the rest of medicine', together with the rarity of his other references to surgery, emphasizes the special position of Montpellier and Rondelet in this regard.[25] At Pisa the University authorities had made great efforts to secure distinguished teachers of surgery in 1488, yet from 1496 for the next half-century our knowledge of surgical teaching there is almost nil.[26] At Bologna, where a continuous tradition of surgical instruction is easy to trace in the sixteenth century, Roger French has pointed to the feelings of academic inferiority of even a Berengario da Carpi.[27] A graphic illustration of this can be found in the letters of Johannes Lange. Of his medical teachers at Bologna, he mentions only the obscure Ludovicus de Leonibus: his admiration for Berengario is an invention of a modern savant for whom it was inconceivable that a visitor from Germany would not rush to hear the great anatomist.[28] A similar argument over the status of surgery has been revealed in fifteenth-century Padua,[29] and here it may not have been until the middle of the sixteenth century, with the triumph of anatomists like Vesalius, Falloppia and Fabricius, that the professor of surgery and anatomy gained appropriate recognition. But at a price, for here anatomy, which was usually and rightly seen as the handmaid of surgery and as possessing merely propaedeutic value, began to oust surgery and to gain a certain degree of autonomy. But this was Padua, and it should not be forgotten that in many universities, anatomy in the sixteenth century was by no means a separate research discipline. It was taught with a deliberately practical aim, to produce better doctors and surgeons. Anatomical dissection was rare and, in terms of time, took a distant second place to the discussions of the treatment of wounds, ulcers and dislocations.

It was perhaps in France that this new humanist surgery had its greatest impact, as can be seen from the list of sixteenth-century medical writings in French drawn up by Howard Stone.[30] Before 1537 Stone records only ten translations, none from the Greek, and only three directly relating to surgery, including two editions of Guy de Chauliac. The picture is drastically altered for the years between 1537 and 1546. There are some twenty works on surgery, as compared with seven that are not, and the figure rises even higher if it is allowed that several of the Hippocratic and Galenic texts, particularly on drugs, were avowedly intended for the instruction of surgeons or composed at their insistence. The proportion of strictly surgical translations diminishes after 1546, but is regularly around a half to a third of all French medical texts until the end of the century. Before 1557 Stone lists some forty editions of works translated from the Greek, including not only Hippocrates and Galen, but also Paul's book six (1540), Dioscorides (1553), Adamantius on physiognomy (1556) and the fragments of Oribasius published by Vidus Vidius (1555).

To explain this sudden burgeoning of classical versions is not the simple task it once appeared. Both Stone and Durling take the phenomenon almost for granted, and seek to explain its delayed arrival either on the grounds of a paucity of French *belles lettres* or of professional jealousy. True, there was a reluctance on the part of the doctors to impart the secrets of their sacred art to those who had a lesser education and no Greek or Latin. They might also, like Jean Canappe, fear the anger of distinguished colleagues for trying to impart physiology and medical theory to non-physicians.[31] Indeed, Guillaume Cop had been asked to suspend his lectures on Guy de Chauliac in 1498 because he had read the text in French to the surgeons. This was over and beyond his duty to lecture to them in French as part of the Paris faculty's undertaking to teach them the rudiments of anatomy and surgery.[32] One might add also the feeling that what should be said in Latin and what in the vernacular were two different things. This was certainly true for the Englishman John Caius, whose two treatises on the English sweat, in English (1552) and in Latin (1555) show considerable variations of style and even of content. But with the late exception of Daléchamps' textual notes on Paul, which were ready in both Latin and French by 1566, I know of no parallel in French.[33] All this would provide a reason for the late introduction of vernacular versions of classical texts, for relative rarity and for a somewhat sketchy quality, but the sheer quantity of French versions, as compared with those in English, German, Spanish and Italian, and the high level of scholarship at times displayed in them call for a different explanation.

Part of the answer lies in the somewhat ambiguous relation between Paris and provincial medical centres. Paris was acknowledged even by

Montpellier doctors as being the place that attracted the highest talent. Its doctors were learned, its professors eloquent, and the linguistic skills of its orators, particularly in Parlement, unsurpassed.[34] Medical discourse could, indeed should, be carried on at a high level in appropriate language. But when a medical graduate of Paris, like Jean Canappe, or of Montpellier, like Pierre Tolet or Jacques Daléchamps, obtained a teaching post in the provinces, he found himself confronted by surgeons and surgeon-apothecaries who were not 'nurtured on Greek and Latin' and who had only their native French.[35] Guillaume Chrestien, teaching at Orléans, found his audience of young apprentice-surgeons unable to muster Latin between them, while the barbers could not even read or write French, let alone Latin.[36] These young surgeons were not without native wit; they lacked but one thing, a good education, *bonas literas in scholis*, and if they had had that, they would have become doctors, not surgeons.[37] The vernacular translators, being perhaps closer to the actual situation of average medical practice than the Parisian élite, were in a position to see the problems and to act upon their findings.

It is no coincidence that the centre of this new movement was Lyons, a major city yet without a university, or that the two most important of the early surgical translators were both men of talent and ability there. Jean Canappe, a Paris graduate, was an MD, and a lecturer in surgery at Lyons, while Pierre Tolet, a pupil of Rondelet at Montpellier, and doctor at the Hôtel-Dieu alongside Rabelais, was equally involved in surgical education. He was dean of the Lyons College of Physicians (an institution whose qualifications for membership were stiffer than those of a Montpellier MD), and in 1574, towards the end of his long life, he drew up a programme for the proper academic study of surgery.[38] These were no provincial backwoodsmen, but important figures in a city whose leading medical institutions were the College and the Hospital. The fact that there was apparently close collaboration between the two institutions (unlike at Paris) may also have helped to push surgery to the fore. Finally, Lyons was the centre of the publishing trade, and in the Lyons publishers were to be found backers willing to exploit any market that could be opened. These humanist versions, printed in small octavo or duodecimo format, were clearly aimed at students or apprentices of surgery, who could not afford massive folios.

According to Durling's catalogue, the series begins with Canappe's translation of the books of Galen's *Method of Healing* that concerns ulcers and sores: book four, 1537; books three, five and six, 1539; and surgery proper: books thirteen and fourteen, 1538. The second book of the shorter *Method of Healing*, also for surgeons, followed in 1539. The year 1540 saw three important versions by Tolet, Galen, *On Bloodletting*, Galen, *On Unnatural Tumours*, and Paul, book six, on surgery, while in Paris Guillaume Chrestien produced a translation of a 1534 Latin epitome of the first half of the *Method of Healing*. Canappe continued his translations for surgeons in 1541 with Galen's *Anatomy of Bones* and *On the Movement of Muscles*, while the next year he published versions of two books of Galen's *On Simples* and Vassaeus' *Anatomical Plates*. It is an impressive achievement, particularly since in the process he and his collaborators were having to forge a new French surgical vocabulary in order to be understood.

The motive of these translators was Galenic and educational. Canappe's prayer was for greater learning for the surgeons, in order for them to carry out the duties demanded of them. The physicians had no wish to go in for bleeding, burning, cutting, cauterizing and other manual operations, but even here the surgeon required help from a man like Canappe. He needed up-to-date anatomical knowledge, which in the 1530s meant Galenic, not Arabic, anatomy, and with this he would be better able to carry out his traditional functions; he would be less the author of death than of health. Yet the role of the surgeon was gradually broadening; it was going beyond the limits of the older surgery in order to fill the gaps that were appearing in medical care. Surgeons, who needed to know about drugs in order to treat skin diseases and prepare dressings, were now being asked to prescribe diets and all types of drugs. But, if the aid of the physician was lacking, who could blame those who involved the surgeon, or even the surgeon himself for trying, perhaps unsuccessfully and ignorantly, to do his best? Better any help than none.

But how were the surgeons and even barbers to gain 'everything necessary to reach perfection in their art'? How were they to rise above the crowd of 'erratiques et coureurs' with their placards promising instant and universal cures, above the empirics, 'circulateurs, basteleurs, theriacopoles, vulgairement triacleurs, ou imposteurs et abuseurs', without doctrine or method, who became like dumb brutes the moment they were asked for an explanation of their cures or who, if once they lost their precious recipes, were totally useless, unable to do anything. The answer was simple; by adopting Galenic method. Surgeons and apothecaries, by knowing the *Aphorisms* and their Galen, would be better prepared. If their profession demanded it, even they must be 'methodiques et dogmatiques'. They needed experience, practice and learning (a prescription recommended by Galen, Quintilian and Hippocrates), and thereby they would be able to show, by swift, sound and unshatterable reasoning, how best to proceed in any situation. Manual dexterity was not enough; they needed 'chirurgie theoretique', a touch of Galen.[39] Without Galen's doctrines of the causes and symptoms of disease, one could easily err and thereby bring into disrepute a noble art: the example of the Greek surgeon Archagathus, nicknamed 'the hangman', figures frequently as a warning to the present.[40]

Admittedly there is little here that could not have been said by any learned surgeon from the fourteenth century onwards, and these pious hopes and exhortations are so traditionally Galenic as to be but a pale reflection of their source, and very stale beer indeed. But the proof that the new humanist Galenism could give renewed 'fizz' to an older brew and that the result is qualitatively different is given by Canappe's exposition of the prologue to the *Surgery* of Guy de Chauliac, first published at Lyons by Etienne Dolet in 1542, and republished there in 1552 by Jean de Tournes in his *Opuscules de Divers Autheurs Médecins. Redigez ensemble pour le Proufit et Utilité des Chirurgiens.* Although Canappe faithfully follows Guy's praise of the high estate and noble calling of the surgeon, he adorns it with much classical learning, with many references to Galen and the new learning, and to the true type of physician. The surgeon needs philosophical training as well as practical expertise; he needs to understand the future course of disease, to prognosticate. Indeed, he can show himself superior to the physicians by adopting an appropriate morality. Like Montaigne, Canappe describes the contentiousness of contemporary physicians. They fight like gryphons, horses or dogs. They are constantly at each others' throats. If one prescribes sleep, another orders waking; one wine, another water; one fasting, one eating. They deliberately contradict each other, and try to gain profit for themselves; they are worse than animals, for snakes or fish do not attack others of the same species. By contrast, the surgeon, possessed of a proper morality, reinforced by Galenic precept, will be led towards kindness and charity to his colleagues; he will preserve a decent semblance of order, as well as being right in his judgements and advice. Traditional craft loyalty is here being strengthened by classical precept, and Guy's heroic surgeon becomes a sort of Galenic saint.[41]

It should not be forgotten in all this that the classical texts were providing new practical material for the would-be surgeon. The celebrated letter of Giovanni Manardi (Ep. VII. 2), written to a Parisian surgeon in 1530 and first published by Rabelais at Lyons in 1532, clarified and categorized the nomenclature of skin diseases, and was provided in 1555 with an independent existence in a French translation by a 'friend of the surgeons'.[42] The message of humanist surgery found its greatest expression in the work of Jacques Daléchamps on Paul of Aegina. Jacques Daléchamps was another provincial, born at Caen in 1513. He took his medical degrees at Montpellier with Rondelet, graduating MD in 1547. He taught and practised medicine for a while at Grenoble and Valence before becoming the physician at the Hotel-Dieu at Lyons in 1552. The rest of his life was spent there, and until his death in 1588, he was at the centre of the thriving cultural and medical life of that great city. He conducted a correspondence with distinguished humanists and medical men in France, Spain, Italy and Germany, and enjoyed a European reputation for his writings on botany. He also was a skilled translator, of Athenaeus and Theophrastus into Latin, and, significantly, of Greek anatomical and surgical texts into French. His version of Galen's *Anatomical Procedures* 'traduictes fidelement . . . par M. Jacques Daléchamps, docteur en

Médecine & lecteur ordinaire de Chirurgie à Lyon' appeared in 1572 and again in the next year: it was the only renaissance version in the vernacular. More important than this was his work on Paul of Aegina, book six. To the 1567 edition of Guenther's Latin translation, Daléchamps contributed a series of marginal notes, explaining various changes and amendments in the text. The editor, Jean de Moulins, in his preface invited the learned reader to admire the erudition and perspicacity of such a scholar, who had done more than any other for the understanding of this difficult author. The accolade is justified; Daléchamps alone can compare with Francis Adams in the nineteenth century, but the praise should be less for his help with the Latin edition than for his French translation and commentary.[43]

His *Chirurgie Françoise*, for this is its title, received its *privilège du roi* on the same day, 20 February, 1566/7, but it was not in fact published until 1569, with reimpressions in 1570, 1573 and 1610. Its table of contents is misleading, for it suggests that it includes translations of Hippocrates, *On Bones, Fractures and Joints*, parts of Celsus and Aëtius, as well as sundry other ancient surgical texts.[44] What Daléchamps in fact does is to provide an immensely learned and valuable commentary, incorporating sections from these texts, abbreviating and summarizing them, and referring to the whole range of surgery down to his own day. His commentary has an avowed proselytizing intent. Although directed to the 'compagnons et maistres Chirurgiens', without Greek and Latin, it is also intended to rectify 'the infelicity of an age when so few physicians give themselves to learning, practising and enriching the divine science of surgery', which is the most important part of medicine; to remind the world of the distinguished work of contemporary surgeons; and to enable the surgeons to fill with greater confidence and skill the gap that has been left by the withdrawal of the physicians. He does this in two ways. First, by stressing the agreement between the greatest surgeons of antiquity and his own day, even when this has been unwitting, and by illustrating this concord with pictures of ancient and modern surgical instruments, some provided for him by Paré and by another royal surgeon, Jacques Roy, he takes pains to emphasize the friendship between physicians and surgeons, and their unity in a classical frame of surgery. Secondly, Daléchamps goes out of his way to emphasize that ancient surgery can indeed teach something new. Yet there are many reasons why Daléchamps' contemporaries should not be criticized too harshly for their ignorance of their predecessors. Much of what survives is badly preserved, badly transcribed or badly understood. Operations recorded in Paul or Galen may have been replaced by something simpler, or the condition calling for such treatment has become rarer. Maybe, it is the fault of the doctors and surgeons who are no longer of 'si vif et prompt esprit' as to be able to follow the complex operations set down before them. Or the blame could lie with the patients, possessed of a 'si mignarde et délicate complexion' that they (like Montaigne) refuse to submit to drastic surgical treatment.[45] Whatever the cause, Daléchamps insists that he is providing new and effective techniques to help both doctor and surgeon. His commentary, a masterpiece of compressed learning even in its more than nine hundred pages, shows what humanist surgery could contribute. It sets the work of the Greeks, the Arabs and Daléchamps' own friends and contemporaries into context, explains what is happening and what is to be done, and provides a manual of surgery for the expert. Like contemporary work in botany, this book shows that there was a place for the humanist tradition in late sixteenth-century surgery, and that the union of past and present, even if outside the four walls of the university, could lead to practical as well as intellectual benefits.

This claim of the humanist surgeons that their rediscoveries were of practical utility was by no means new. It had been made twenty five years earlier, although with a different emphasis, by Vidus Vidius, in the introductions to the various texts contained in his *Chirurgia e Graeco in Latinum Conversa*, published at Paris in 1544. No-one, he says, should blame him for his abundant annotations and commentary (themselves based largely on classical authors), for they were intended merely to clarify the text of Hippocrates. One had only to look at the elegance and accuracy of Hippocrates' treatment of headwounds and then at the work of modern surgeons, and a vast gulf would be instantly visible (p. 61). A book like his was a necessity; witness those

who are incapacitated for some time by ulcers, and who by reason of broken or dislocated limbs have become lame or less capable of their usual activities, and who think that they are receiving excellent treatment when they do not actually die; and those who, after a head injury, suffer torture at the hands of their doctors and still die. Not to mention any individual cases, is there a single one of our surgeons who can use his hands as the case demands, apply bandages properly, use the right machines for setting broken bones, replace them when dislocated or cure head injuries? But they have a good excuse, for they have not until now possessed the Greek authors with the greatest reputation for this practice of this branch of medicine (sig. aa. iii r.)

Thus, by authorizing the publication of this book, Francis I would be a public benefactor.

The researches of C. E. Kellett, W. Brockbank and M. D. Grmek have done much to set Vidius' book into its personal and medical context.[46] They have shown how the young Vidius (b. 1509) attached himself in Rome to the household of Cardinal Ridolfi, grandson of Lorenzo Medici, where he met many noted humanists and artists. With occasional interruptions to visit his native Florence, he remained in Rome until the end of 1541 or slightly later. His book of surgery was based largely on a copy done for Ridolfi of a ninth- or tenth-century Greek codex of ancient surgery which incorporated drawings going back to Hellenistic Alexandria. A Greek copy and Vidius' Latin translation were brought by him as gifts to Francis I, when he made his way to Paris in 1542, and they were gladly received into the royal library. Vidius' reward was swift. 'Vidius venit, Vidius vidit, Vidius vicit'. He was appointed royal physician and the first *lecteur* in medicine at the new Collège de France, although the Paris Faculty would have preferred Sylvius; he added anatomical demonstrations to his lectures, and students from the Faculty attended in large numbers. The death of Francis I in 1547 and the consequent uncertainty allowed him to accept an offer to return to his native Tuscany. Cosimo I, in his munificent restoration of the intellectual organization of Florence and Tuscany, invited him to become his personal physician, as well as professor of philosophy, and later of medicine, at Pisa, where he died in 1569.

But it is not just his commentary, redolent of humanist philological medicine, or even the illustrations by Santorinus of Rhodes and, in the printed book, artists associated with Salutati and Primaticcio, that demand our attention here, but Vidius' attempt to bring to the notice of his contemporaries the instruments used by his classical predecessors. The tract *'On Wounds'* ends, pp. 113–30, with a detailed and illustrated description of the saws, trepans, scalpels, forceps and scissors that were described by Celsus, Galen and Paul, and the later tracts of Galen and Oribasius on bandaging and Oribasius on mechanical devices contain many practical illustrations. For the last tract, which in the original Greek lacked any illustration whatever, Vidius sought the help of model-makers: 'I was keen to depict and make models in wood in order to give a better idea of them than by description and set them before the eyes of men.' The result was an improvement on the illustrations to Apollonius found in the Greek original, and Vidius' reconstruction of the Hippocratic bench (p. 519) and the uses to which he claims it can be put go far beyond the work of his own contemporaries. Not always for the better, however. Although his machines might be technically superior to their ancient models, the cases in which they were to be employed were not always appropriate. Whether a dislocated jaw could be put back by the procedure depicted on p. 521 is an open question; at best, it would have been extremely painful. But it would have had more chance of success than the attempt by similar means to reset a broken humerus (p. 524), but, as Brockbank points out, Vidius was not alone in confusing the treatments of dislocations and fractures or in assuming that traction was the manoeuvre necessary to reduce most fractures.[47]

Vidius' handsome folio, with its magnificent illustrations and copious commentary, was intended for an audience of quality, and it exploited the art of the designer and typographer to this end. But if all humanist surgeons had been published so lavishly, their impact on their fellow professionals would not have been great. Vidius' illustrations, important and necessary as they were for suggesting new instruments and new techniques, were also expensive, and his erudite discourses somewhat above the heads of the average student and surgeon. But there were others, equally imbued with the classics, who aimed at a wider audience, and who saw in the ancient surgical texts the essential theoretical foundations for modern practice. One such was Giulio Cesare Aranzi, whose tiny commentary on Hippocrates' *On Wounds in the Head* stands in marked contrast to Vidius' folio. The distillation of years of lecturing on surgery at Bologna, this book is avowedly practical. It seeks to resolve a limited problem, the proper treatment for head wounds, on which each doctor seems to have his own opinion, with possibly fatal consequences. Aranzi's editor, his pupil Claude Porral, recalls how, when he was with the army at Turin, a doctor from Rome killed a young man by his botched treatment of a minor head wound.[48] Aranzi suggests two reasons for this unhappy state of affairs: doctors have simply distanced themselves from surgical practice or they have neglected the golden book of the divine physician, Hippocrates. For Dr Porral, the claims of his master to expound the truth need little support from him, for they are obvious: Aranzi's twenty-two years as lecturer and professor of surgery at Bologna, and his close adherence to the precepts of Hippocrates.[49] He might also have added family tradition, for Aranzi was the nephew of another distinguished Bolognese surgeon and lecturer, Bartolommeo Maggi.

Two things above all distinguish Aranzi's commentary from what has gone before, its severe practicality and its Hippocratism. Unlike Daléchamps and even Vidius, Aranzi is highly selective in his commentary, an impression heightened by Porral's editorial labours. There is only the occasional reference to classical authors, and little of the orotundity of the earlier medical philologists. Instead Aranzi concentrates on practicalities, on the medical problems to be tackled, in an endeavour to render the words of Hippocrates both intelligible and memorable. With these precepts firmly in his mind, the student could approach any head wound with confidence. Secondly, the hero of the book is Hippocrates alone. Galen and Paul are adduced from time to time, but only as confirmation of the 'dogmata sacra Senis' (p. 8) and the 'doctrina bonorum omnium Parentis' (p. 11). Hippocrates thus provides the general guidelines for the true understanding of the treatment of head wounds. He can thus speak, through Aranzi, directly to the doctors and surgeons, because he is telling the truth, and there is little need of a mass of complicated erudition to explicate it.[50] This surgical Hippocrates is a far cry from the Galen of the physicians, yet we are still dealing, I would argue, with a humanist surgery. This is a surgery based on classical texts, but freed from any suggestion of antiquarianism. Hippocrates, the author of truth, can be confirmed, not from books, but in everyday practice.

But it is one thing to record as a historian one's own impressions of the merits of the works of Vidius and Aranzi, and another to attempt to estimate their effect. A glance at the publication dates of Aranzi's lectures suggests a brief burst of popularity (two editions, Lyons and Geneva, in 1579, with two similar editions the next year) followed by oblivion, broken only by a Leyden edition two generations later in 1639.[51] A slightly different history can be written for Vidius' collection, although it too had a solitary republication after a very long gap (in French, Paris 1634).[52] With the exception of a few small reprints of individual Hippocratic texts, all the publishing activity after 1544 is concentrated into a single year, 1555. The *Surgery*'s later sections from Galen and Oribasius were included, along with their illustrations, in a collection *De Chirurgia*, edited at Zurich by Conrad Gesner and intended to show the best (and the most literate) of modern surgery. The significance of this collection I shall explore in a moment; all that is here necessary is to note that Vidius' tastes and style coincided well with Gesner's philological interests. In the same year, 1555, there appeared two different French versions. F. le Fevre, a doctor from Bourges, translated the Hippocratic texts along with Vidius' commentaries on them, while the whole volume was translated anew by an anonymous doctor of medicine and re-published with much inferior plates.[53]

The *Surgery* had a considerable success; according to Lehoux, it appears, in French, or usually, Latin, in ten or so inventories of doctors in the sixteenth and early seventeenth centuries, more than any other surgical text save for the writings of Paré.[54] It was cited in 1560, interestingly from the French, by Leonardo Botalli of Asti, a doctor in medicine and surgery from Pavia, who was equally a supporter of Galen and Hippocrates as the true guides to surgery.[55] Five years later, in 1565, he revised his tract and incorporated in it a long discussion of the various instruments unearthed by Vidius from his classical sources. This time his quotations from Vidius, 'vir quidem de medicina optime meritus', are taken from the 1544 Latin edition, and there is much greater evidence of Botalli's humanist leanings, including untransliterated Greek.[56] But by now Botalli was a star, doctor to Charles IX, king of France.

The merits of Vidius and his book were sung at length by another contributor to Gesner's collection, Jean Tagault, whose *Institutiones Chirurgicae*, with its supplement on drugs by Houillier, opens the volume. Tagault was a stylist as well as a surgeon, and his prefaces are filled with references to the barbaric Latin of Guy de Chauliac and other medieval authors. He himself has purified the old surgical compendia by an admixture of the purest founts of Greek and Roman learning, Hippocrates, Galen, Paul, Aëtius and Celsus. He has taken from the new Galenic anatomy what is most relevant to the surgeon, and has clothed it in splendour (*nitidius*) and elegance. He rejects a pure Ciceronianism as not always appropriate to a technical text, but there is still a place for the flowers and ornaments of eloquence.[57]

Gesner's choice of authors for inclusion in his collection is motivated by precisely similar reasons. His aim is to print in Germany and to make accessible there works on surgery by distinguished authors. He himself is not a surgeon – indeed, his list of surgical authors at the end of the book devotes the greatest amount of space to a discussion of the origins of surgery in mythological Greece – but he knows what will last. Large composite volumes are better looked after, and they are produced and, significantly, sold with greater ease and delight than single texts. Besides, students keep them in better condition. Yet Gesner confesses to have encountered a problem which exemplifies some of the difficulties that humanist surgery had to face in Germany. Some of the books he wanted to include were unobtainable in Zurich, others were too long, and many were written in a 'filthy and scarcely Latin style'.[58] The result is a curious blend of the up-to-date and the old-fashioned. On the one hand, Vidius, Bartolommeo Maggi of Bologna on gunshot wounds 'according to the doctrine of Hippocrates, Galen and other Greeks', Alfonso Ferri of Naples on the same topic (but with a greater mixture of Arabic doctrine), Tagault and Lange; on the other Jacopo dei Dondi's *Remedies* of about 1350, Bolognini on unguents, of about 1520, and the surgical compendium of Mariano Santi, 'who attended with care to the precepts of great Galen'. This large work, which begins with the legends of Marcus Scaevola and Decius, was started while Santi was a doctor and surgeon in Rome in about 1517. Its value is not great. Even the charitable Gurlt finds little to praise in it, but it had one thing that appealed to the humanist in Gesner.[59] It was written in the remarkable form of a Ciceronian dialogue between Santi and his teachers, and ends with a wondrous *Liber Quidditatiuus de Modo Examinandi Medicos Chirurgos* designed to help others in their choice of (probably) state doctors and surgeons.

Although this collection was intended for the German market, it contained only one section written by a German, Johannes Lange's *Themata Chirurgica*, eleven letters taken from his *Epistolae Medicinales*. Lange's singularity demands explanation. One can point at once to the long and distinguished series of writings in German on medicine and surgery. Perhaps more than any other vernacular, German by the renaissance had already established for itself a broad and detailed vocabulary for all aspects of medicine. The fact that relatively few lengthy tracts have survived is less significant than the sheer variety and number of the medical texts that we now possess. University doctors were equally prepared to write down their thoughts or notes in German or Latin, and a court as cultivated as that of Herzog Sigmund of Tyrol, with Italian-trained doctors as well as experienced local men to hand, was not divided among itself linguistically.[60] In particular, there was a flourishing learned craft-tradition of surgery that owed little or nothing to the universities. The so-called surgical school of Strassburg, with Hieronymus Brunschwig,

Hans von Geyersdorf and Otto Brunfels among its representatives, produced around the turn of the century an impressive series of medical and
surgical writings in the vernacular, that far surpassed anything the
humanists could provide. Not surprisingly, none of these authors entered
Gesner's pantheon of surgery.[61]

The German universities could offer little to the surgeon. Only
Tübingen, from 1497, offered lectures on surgery and the possibility of
obtaining a surgical degree in addition to, or instead of, a medical one.
Here the would-be surgeon either spent an extra year at lectures and
gaining practical experiences or could study for two years, including
practical anatomy and accompanying his professor on his rounds for a
year, before making his formal disputation on a surgical theme.[62] But
statutes by themselves cannot bring about a revolution, and the early years
of the Tübingen faculty were not easy. The religious and political crises
affecting Wurttemberg, the vacillations of its rulers towards education in
general, led to a general decline in the numbers of those attending the
university and by 1525 the students were fewer than they had been in
1500.[63] The next decade was one of chaos and confusion, and only the
return of duke Ulrich in 1535 brought about a revival and filled the vacuum
of university teaching with new and ambitious men.

Like almost all the German professors of medicine in the sixteenth
century, the Tübingen faculty had spent some time in Italy and had sat at
the feet of distinguished humanist physicians in Padua, Bologna and
Ferrara. Yet these men rarely brought back with them the practical results
of humanist enquiry.[64] One can point to Fuchs' teaching of botany at
Tübingen from 1535, to the introduction of botanical field trips for
medical students at Frankfurt-an-der-Oder by 1550, and to the occasional
requirement of viewing a formal annual anatomy, but these are isolated
examples.[65] Far more typical was Jacob Schegk, Fuchs' colleague and
successor, a walking embodiment of Aristotle, or the Ingolstadt professors
of 1556 whose curriculum was based entirely on the books of Galen and
Hippocrates.[66] At the new University of Jena, although its professors, like
Cornarius, had a great reputation for humanist learning or as poets and
mathematicians, their practical abilities (and even interests) were severely
limited.[67] These were not the men to interest students in the new Vesalian
anatomy, let alone in surgery. But there was one exception to this picture
of peaceful philological medicine, of a medical humanism remote from the
body, and that was Heidelberg in the late 1550s, partly under the influence
of Lange.

Johannes Lange (1485–1565) was born at Löwenberg in Silesia, to a
wealthy and well-connected family. He studied first at Leipzig, graduating
in philosophy in 1514, and he remained there for some time lecturing to
large audiences on a variety of classical topics, including Pliny's *Natural
History*. But the lure of Italy was already proving too strong. He went first

to Bologna, where he learned the rudiments of Greek from Petrus de Aegina, who was lecturing on Aristophanic comedy (p. 523).[68] Whether Lange also began to study medicine at Bologna under Ludovico de Leonibus at this time (p. 231) or a few months later after his return from Venice is uncertain. He implies that it was to gain a knowledge of medicine and the true method that led him to Ferrara (and he was also bored with Bologna) (pp. 523, 312). At Ferrara he met Leoniceno. He then visited Padua, where he found the medical professors all attending cases in Venice (p. 523), to where he turned his steps. His visit to Venice does not appear to have lasted long, and he may have returned to Bologna and then to Pisa, where he took his medical degree in 1522 or 1523. He also spent a short while in Rome, where he made the acquaintance of John de Vigo, the Papal surgeon and doctor (p. 32). On his return to Germany he was soon appointed to the post of doctor to the Elector Palatine at Heidelberg, in whose service he remained until his death. In the company of Elector Friedrich, he travelled round Europe, to Spain (pp. 683, 248), perhaps again to Italy between 1526 and 1536[69] and on campaign against the Turks (p. 22). Lange, then, was a man who had been everywhere, and met everyone of note among the humanists. He had talked with the leading men of Venice, and the Papal court; and, so he claims (p. 419), he had been the first to tell Giovanni Francesco Pico della Mirandola of the death of Reuchlin in 1522, and to commiserate with him on 'the great loss to Hebrew studies', 'but one which the learning of Melanchthon will be able to repair'. Here is a man made out of finer stuff than the average surgeon.

It thus comes as something of a surprise to find that Gesner could count him among the most important writers on surgery and include eleven of his letters in his collection when they were almost hot off the press (*Ep. Med.* I.3–10, 32, 77, 82; Basel 1554). The later books of letters, particularly II.4, and the case histories of III.3–5, confirm an interest in surgical questions – and also that Lange was not a man for the knife. He preferred plasters, bandages and the removal (by internal means) of swellings and tumours. But at least in his young days (p. 32), he had shown an interest in surgical instruments, for he intervened in a debate between 'empirics, each boasting of the superiority of his own instruments from Augsburg or Nuremberg', to ask whether they had ever heard of the trepan called 'abaptiston' in Galen. They laughed at him, saying that in Germany only bells and children were baptized, not surgical instruments. When he replied that he had not only seen this trepan but also been shown by John de Vigo, the Papal surgeon, how it should be made, they accepted his story for, since the Pope was in Rome, it was only too easy for him to baptize instruments if he wanted to.

This amusing confrontation exemplifies Lange's relationship with the surgeons. He associates with them, wishes to help them, and is totally convinced of the superiority of his classical authorities, even going so far as to christen guns with Greek descriptions (p. 562). He was, in my opinion, the widest read of the humanist physicians, and used his classical texts expertly to provide himself with solutions to difficult medical problems. His range of knowledge was vast, and he clearly had up-to-date information on medical debates and events going on round Europe. Yet at times, it seems that, like Cornarius trying to browbeat the wife of Riquinus,[70] he was endeavouring to get his way by sheer bulk, and with as little success. Learned reference after learned reference pours out, sometimes to the point, sometimes not, and his arguments at times almost disappear under a mountain of classical precedent.

Yet his stay in Italy had awoken him to the needs of Germany, and implanted in him a desire to bring there the best of the new humanist knowledge. It was not native wit that was lacking, it was knowledge and good instruction. Around him Lange could see a mass of what he would term half-trained empirics – doctors pronouncing solemnly on the fate of the patient simply from an examination of urine (pp. 2 ff.), surgeons entirely without education, even totally illiterate, lacking knowledge of how to cure dislocations and fractures, not using the Hippocratic bench, gladly accepting the continuous oozing of pus from a swollen wound as a good sign of the *Gliedwasser*, the humour from within the joints. They tried to cure *Causo* by applying dung to the tongue; their cures of skull fractures, gunshot wounds, or erysipelas caused wholesale murder. Their treatments were more deadly than war; their victims more numerous than the population of Paris. Lange's whole life can be seen as a crusade against these 'threepenny doctors', ignorant boors, Jews, renegade monks, and conniving magistrates.

The surgical letters offer some detailed guidance to surgeons from the works of Hippocrates and Galen, showing particularly how a general theory can be modified in individual cases, and parading a few of Lange's successful cures, but they take second place to his crusade for better education for doctors and surgeons. Lange does not despise surgeons as such, witness his courteous refutation of the Strassburg surgeon whose argument on the treatment of wounds 'smelled not of the barber's shop, but of the Roman school of surgeons'.[71] But he wishes them to become men of learning ('*docti*').

How this was to be brought about was further summarized in a separate work, *Medicum de Republica Symposium*, which appeared in 1554 and which was later included as the final letter in the entire collection, *Ep.* III.6.[72] The same examples and the same scapegoats recur (not surprisingly if Lange had been harping on the same topic for almost twenty years (p. 998)), rustic surgeons, superstitious old women, particularly the Jews, who bribe magistrates to let them murder Christians by their drugs (pp. 1001, 1018, 1045), greedy ecclesiastics, eager to supplement their income by promoting the sale of relics and organizing healing shrines (pp. 1051 ff.).

The denunciation by Lange and his friends of the dreadful state of contemporary medicine extends for almost sixty pages, and it is only the imagined onset of night that puts an end to their symposium. Before they depart, their chairman, Count Auerbach, presents their recommendations for the revival of medicine in the Palatinate: the expulsion of the Jews, the legal banning of superstition and the *pseudomedici*, with their corrupt advisers, and the declaration by Lange of errors that should be punished by law or should be generally avoided. Above all, too, the state should provide money for better education (maybe even including grants for students, p. 1056, cf. p. 1054), and better pay for experienced and good doctors, who will be the anchors for a sick community. There should be a reform of the university. Not only should the Count Palatine summon lawyers, teachers, theologians and doctors from all over the world to revive the university (p. 558), he should also create a great library. If the popes, the kings of France, and even the count of Mirandola (p. 558), could do this, then it was certainly possible for him to do the same, and provide the books with a dignified home, where neither moths nor worms could destroy them. National pride suggested that there should be a library in Germany, the home of printing, at least equivalent to those elsewhere, and where better and more fruitful than Heidelberg (p. 560 f.)? At the university also doctors could be taught philosophy (pp. 16, 654) and up-to-date medicine instead of the false opinions of the 'barbari' (p. 13), and they could be given proper instruction in anatomy. Only if one knew the make-up of the human body could one resolve a dislocation or set a fracture properly. Anatomy must be human anatomy. One reason for the incompetence of surgeons was because, like unspeakable tyrants, they assaulted the bodies of the sick after once having seen a butcher gut a calf or piglet (p. 17).

It would be easy to dismiss all this as empty rhetoric from a man who never mentioned Vesalius (although he praised Maggi and Belon (p. 565)), were it not for the fact that when the statutes of the university were changed in 1558 under Count Otto Henrich, Lange submitted his own proposals, several of which were incorporated almost word for word in the final statutes.[73] A law was passed against Jews, parsons, and old women, without university education, practising medicine. Control of the physicians rested with the professors, who also were not only to examine the apothecaries' wares but also to advise on drugs to be bought at the Frankfurter Messe.[74] Surgeons were to be allowed to cure certain conditions, provided that they were sufficiently trained or experienced – cutting for stones, restoring limbs, setting fractures, treating wounds, couching for cataract and so on. The surgeons were thus second-class citizens, but, compared with the others, citizens none the less.

Surgery had a prominent place in Lange's ideal university. He proposed four professors of medicine, one for the *lectio Galeni*, one for the *lectio medicinae Arabicae*, one for the *lectio Hippocratica*, and one for the *lectio Chirurgica* 'because in Germany very few surgeons experienced or properly learned in medicine are to be found'.[75] But the statutes themselves did not go so far as Lange wished. There were only three professors, who lectured entirely on Greek texts (although the faculty had the power to supplement them with whatever they found 'most useful'), and there was no provision either for a professor of Arabic medicine or of surgery. But practical medicine was not entirely left out. Although attendance at hospital visits does not seem to have been allowed before 1595,[76] the students were to go on a botanical field trip at least once a year, and were encouraged to look at plants for themselves. Anatomy and surgery were particularly encouraged. 'Since it is impossible to examine, recognise and treat human disease without a knowledge of the internal parts, organs and bones of the human body, or to understand and learn properly all that pertains to surgery', and since this knowledge was not to be obtained solely by ocular inspection and external demonstration, the medical faculty in its formal anatomy was to use also anatomical plates, a skeleton, and, oddest of all in a sixteenth century context, Copho's anatomy of the pig, an early Salernitan text. The bodies of executed criminals and those who died suddenly or without cause, were, with the relatives' permission, to be handed over for dissection and inspection by those who were to practise surgery and wound management, so that this needful and health-giving art could lack nothing for its propagation.[77]

These statutes with their emphasis on practical surgery, go beyond anything elsewhere in Germany in stressing the importance of the visual. To what extent they were put into practice is another question. Not until 1574 do we have a record of a public anatomy at Heidelberg, although this may be the fault of our evidence, not of Lange's contemporaries. Perhaps significantly, it was then performed by an Italian exile on the fringes of the university, Antonio Francesco Pigafetta,[78] doctor to the hospital, whom his opponent and successor in the anatomies, Thomas Erastus, disparagingly called 'surgeon', an obvious insult to a well-trained academic.

Lange's crusade, to improve the instruction of the surgeon by a massive dose of humanist theory and by the introduction of proper anatomical training, has its exact counterpart in England in the work of John Caius. Caius, an editor and translator of Galenic texts and the reinvigorator of the College of Physicians, had an interest in anatomy that was much more than merely linguistic. No one who had lived with Vesalius for eight months while he wrote the *Fabrica* could fail to be impressed by his passion, even if he did not always agree with his conclusions. Caius had also sat at the feet of another distinguished anatomist, Matteo Corti. This interest was translated into action. By 1546, at the wish of King Henry VIII, he was giving a course of lectures on anatomy to the Barber-surgeons, 'which gave enlightenment and great solace to the surgeons, that they might know your parts, O Anatomy', as the verse inscription on his portrait at Caius says. He was also instrumental in securing permission for the College of Physicians, and also for Cambridge, to obtain bodies for public dissection. In these anatomies he himself took the leading part: he talks of lecturing for almost twenty years before the Barber-surgeons, and attracting some devoted hearers.[79]

In all this, as Sir Walter Langdon-Brown emphasized, Caius was maintaining the Galenic unity of doctor and surgeon, and continuing the Linacre tradition.[80] That too was how he was seen by his contemporary, William Bullein, whose praise of his learned lectures and secret anatomies, 'revealing the hidden jewels and precious treasures of Galen' and showing himself to be the second Linacre, is well known.[81] Bullein, a country clergyman turned doctor, waxed enthusiastic for surgery.[82] His ideal was the learned surgeon, not 'vagabounde beggars; robbinge the people; and more hurtfull than private murders in kyllyng men, for lacke of knowledge', who kill soldiers far more than bullets (5v–6r).

> Yet neyther reede, Tagaltus, Marianus, Guido nor Galen,
> Olde Hippocrates, Dioscorides, Rasis nor Auicen.
> Latine nor Englishe, little or none, do they reede,
> Small is their knowledge, much lesse is their speede.
> Yet lacke they no Brimstone, Quicksilver or Litharge,
> Oyles grosse and lothsome, to beare out the charge.
> They haue Palmestry and Charmes, at eche wights desire,
> Good store of Blessinges, for toothache, and saynct Antoines
>   fire . . .
> Worse then the valiaunt beggars and mendicant Fryers.
> Murderers of mankind in know of no arte.
> Banish them from Chirurgi, commende them to the Carte. . . .

Bullein's message is clear and vigorous. It is a direct counterpart of Lange's trumpetings, both in language and in example. But, it might be argued, Bullein, who is presumably a university man, although not an MD, represents the views of the humanists, and his remarkable list of those interested in surgery, from Achilles to Vicary, could be dismissed as propaganda, for the College of Physicians.[83] Certainly Drs Bunn, Butts, Bartlet, Carr, Clement, Caldwell, Chambers, Edwards, Geynes, Hatcher, Huyck, Freer, Linacre, Langton, Lorkyn, Corembeck, Masters, Ludford and Wendy, all leading members of the London College of Physicians or of the Cambridge academic hierarchy, are strange bedfellows with Otto Brunfels, Albertus Magnus and (an unidentifiable) Thomas Colphus, *pharmacopulus Ang.* The explanation lies partly in Bullein's source, Gesner's list of surgeons at the back of the 1555 *Chirurgia*, and partly in Bullein's acceptance of the Galenic or Linacre tradition of the learned surgeon. I suggest that Bullein is including the physicians both for their remedies for surgical conditions and because, in some way, they seemed to him, by example, precept or some other means, to foster the art of surgery.

But this view could also be upheld by many of the leading surgeons in London. The complaints of William Clowes of a 'rude rabble of obscure and unperfect experimenters' 'bungling botchers, ignorant makeshifts, caterpillars in a commonwealth'[84] echo Bullein, Caius and Lange. From the 1560s, leading members of the College of Surgeons, like Roger Coplande, George Baker, Thomas Gale, and, at the end of the century, Peter Lowe, were actively involved in translating humanist surgery into English.[85] As well as the older Guy de Chauliac and Giovanni da Vigo, their texts included Galen, Hippocrates, the more modern Almenar, Botalli and Tagault. It is as though English-learned surgery was being dragged forcibly into the European world. But before one could argue that the torch of humanist surgery had passed from Knightrider Street to Monkwell Street, one important qualification must be made. This tradition of humanist surgery was not acceptable in Latin, still less in Greek; it reached England in French dress. Baker, Coplande and Gale did not feast on Caius' Greek Galen, but on Canappe's.

In this chapter I have endeavoured to show that there were, in the sixteenth century, practical men as well as theoreticians who believed that the newly revived medicine of Galen and Hippocrates might contribute a great deal to surgery. For some, it might offer a theoretical basis for diagnosis and treatment, for others it gave new instruments and techniques; it could be seen as an attempt by physicians to impose their views on surgeons (and this presumption called forth bitter rebukes from surgeons and apothecaries) or as a well-intentioned and well-thought out plan to make the surgeons better able to carry out tasks that, *faute de mieux*, were falling to their lot. In all this, while one might deplore the unwillingness of physicians to get their hands bloodied and consider the regulations inspired by a Lange or a Caius as an unfair intrusion by physicians with the ear of a powerful sovereign, one cannot mistake the burning sincerity of their crusade. Their zeal for humanist anatomy, for proper standards, for safe drugs, was one that was shared by many levels of the medical profession. It was an ideal that could particularly appeal to a surgeon, especially one with a university education and some language skills, as something that would mark him off effectively from the group beneath him. 'The smell of the barber's shop', to use Lange's phrase, was equally offensive to an opulent surgeon and to a theoretical physician, and, particularly at the higher levels of the speciality, surgeons were on remarkably good personal terms with physicians. Clowes' praise of his contemporaries, like Bullein's, makes little distinction between doctor and surgeon.[86]

This tradition can be found throughout Europe, from Portugal to Poland, as a reading of Gurlt will show. Yet its strength varied from area to area; Lange's surgery was less influential than that of Tagault. But it appears in some unfamiliar places, and its sheer flexibility was one of its greatest strengths. In 1597, Peter Lowe, a Scotsman, trained in France as a graduate surgeon, returned to England where he published his *Discourse of the Whole Art of Chyrurgerie*. A friend of George Baker, he too was concerned to preserve the authority of surgery by stressing the distinguished past and by removing 'cosoners, quacksalvers, charlitans, witches, charmers and divers other sorts of abusers'. In an appendix he published the first ever English translation of the Hippocratic *Prognostics*, whose aim and intended audience are clear from one frequent circumlocution. Each time that the Greek has   , 'doctor', Lowe adds 'or surgeon', and the object of Hippocrates' advice, who is infrequently mentioned in the text itself, except as 'he', is constantly called the 'mediciner Chirurgian'. This translation thus shows, at the end of the sixteenth century, a surgeon deliberately laying claim on behalf of his art to a share of the classical tradition. It was an argument powerful enough to convince James VI, of Scotland, who in 1599, at Lowe's request, gave permission for the creation of a Faculty of Physicians and Surgeons in Glasgow, in order to put an end to the 'ignorant, unskillit and unlernit personis, quha under the collour of chirurgeanis, abuisis the people to their plesure, passing away but tryel or punishment, and thairby destroyis infinite number of oure subjectis'.[87] Though the language is Scots, the sentiments could be found throughout the learned medical world, from Bohemia even to Mexico.[88] Although even sympathizers might now doubt the wisdom of a perpetual prejudice in favour of antiquity,[89] the humanist tradition in surgery as well as in medicine was by no means lifeless, and its ideals, if not its doctrines, could still inspire and instruct.

5

Pharmacy in the republic of Venice in the sixteenth century

RICHARD PALMER

In the sixteenth century the study of *materia medica* offered exciting prospects for the renewal of therapeutics. The renaissance ideal of improvement through the revival and emulation of antiquity had a profound impact on this field, and particularly on medical botany. In addition, there was scope for optimism in the arrival of novel drugs from the New World, and in the investigations of chemical therapies pursued by Paracelsus and his followers. The dynamic for change came largely from learned physicians. In Italy it was they who published the influential books, formulated the civic pharmacopoeias, and supervised the production of the principal drugs. Often physicians condemned the ignorance of pharmacists, or exposed their cunning frauds in works such as Giovanni Antonio Lodetto's *Dialogo de gl' Inganni d' alcuni Malvaggi Speciali* (Brescia, 1572). Yet it was pharmacists who purchased, composed and dispensed medicines, and it is hard to believe that any substantial change in therapeutics could have occurred without their active cooperation. In assessing the practical impact of renaissance pharmacology, the physician–pharmacist relationship is therefore of great importance. This chapter, which concentrates on botanical research and chemical therapies, aims to explore the question of how far intellectual currents among physicians influenced pharmacists and their drugs in the republic of Venice.

In the dedication which he wrote for the 1548 edition of his commentary on Dioscorides, the physician Pietro Andrea Mattioli outlined his views on the state of *materia medica*. Mattioli had been convinced by reading Dioscorides that medical botany had fallen into decay since classical times. Many important plants known to the ancients could no longer be identified. At the same time, mistaken identifications had led to the use in pharmacy of the wrong plants, and even of poisonous ones. Ignorance too, had opened the door to malpractice – the falsification of drugs imported from the Indies and the Middle East, and fraudulent pharmaceutical practice within Italy.[1] The revival of interest in classical botany, led by the

100

recovery in the fifteenth century of the works of Dioscorides and Theophrastus[2] prepared the way for a renewal in pharmacy. The prospect
offered was that of recovering the astonishing curative properties of
ancient drugs, as well as amazing aphrodisiacs, which, as an awed Mattioli
learned from Theophrastus, would allow one to make love seventy times
over.[3]

By the time Mattioli published the second edition of his *Dioscoride* in
1548, he could look back with satisfaction to the philological achievements
of early commentators on Dioscorides such as the Venetian Ermolao
Barbaro, to the tradition of botanical study at Ferrara begun by Leoniceno
and continued by Manardi and Brasavola, to the work of Frenchmen such
as Ruel (on whose Latin translation of Dioscorides he relied) and Germans
such as Fuchs and Brunfels. The first chairs of *materia medica* had been set
up in the Italian universities. Luca Ghini, teaching at Bologna from 1534
and at Pisa from 1544, was educating a whole generation of botanists and
natural historians which was to include Anguillara, Falloppia, Maranta,
Cesalpino and Aldrovandi, and introducing new aids to study such as the
herbal of dried plants.[4] Two universities, Padua and Pisa, had recently
established botanical gardens, while botanical field work, both to collect
plants for the new gardens and for research, was increasingly commonplace.

In all this the Venetian republic played a prominent part. If the revival
of *materia medica* depended on recovering the plants described by Dioscorides – for the most part plants of the eastern Mediterranean – then
Venice had unique opportunities and responsibilities. It ruled islands such
as Crete and Cyprus, which were considered to have been the herb gardens
of antiquity, and it had unrivalled trading relations with Constantinople,
Syria and Egypt. Small wonder that Mattioli called on the Venetian Senate
to procure from all parts of the world where its galleys sailed the true
herbs, liquors and minerals so urgently desired.[5] A start was made with the
foundation at Padua in 1533 of the first chair of *materia medica*, held first by
Francesco Bonafede,[6] and later in the century by Gabriele Falloppia,
Bernardino Trevisan and Prospero Alpino. This chair was subsequently
described, in 1589, as a lectureship on Dioscorides, whose *Materia Medica*
was evidently the set text.[7] In 1545, responding to pleas from students and
teachers alike, the Venetian Senate founded the Paduan botanical garden as
a collecting point for plants and minerals from Crete, Cyprus and wher-
ever medicinal simples were to be found.[8] The garden became an important centre of study, despite students who, familiar with body-snatching
for anatomy, were given at first to uprooting the plants and carrying them
off.[9] Under Melchiorre Guilandino, who was in charge from 1561, the
garden was given a formal role in teaching. Afternoons in May, year after
year, were given over to teaching and demonstrating there. Giacomo
Antonio Cortusio, Guilandino's successor, who carried on the tradition,

claimed in 1602 to have an audience on these occasions of anything from 400 to 700, 'with such applause, love, and reverence as would be hard to express.'[10] Many of the plants were collected on field trips. The work of Luigi Anguillara, the garden's first custodian, took him throughout northern Italy and overseas.[11] Guilandino, in the years before he succeeded Anguillara, had travelled extensively in Egypt and the Middle East, and had only been prevented from going on to the East Indies by falling into the hands of corsairs.[12]

Yet research into *materia medica* was by no means confined to university circles. Interest was general amongst physicians by the mid-sixteenth century, and particularly well placed for research were those serving as doctors to Venetian colonies in the eastern Mediterranean, in the Venetian fleet, or in consulates such as those in Damascus or Cairo. Nicolò Sanmichele of Como, who practised medicine in Venice, and who was described by Anguillara as a 'most perfect botanist' (*semplicista*), and a 'great investigator of Levantine plants', introduced new plants into Italy on his return from Greece and Crete, probably following his service in the Venetian fleet in 1539. He also extended his knowledge of the Levant with the aid of another Comasco physician practising in Venice, Michiel de' Muti, who sent him botanical specimens from Aleppo in Syria where he was physician to the Venetian consulate in the 1550s.[13] Prospero Alpino, a pupil of Guilandino, used his years as doctor to Giorgio Emo, the Venetian consul in Cairo (from 1581 to 1584), for research towards his books on the plants and medicine of Egypt, which, in turn, opened the way for him to succeed Cortusio as custodian of the Paduan garden.[14] Even barbers and surgeons could be drawn into botanical research. Mathias de Lobel was delighted to receive roots of *colchicum syriacum alexandrinum* from one Domenico, a surgeon in the Venetian fleet, who added it to decoctions of guaiac for the treatment of syphilis,[15] while Prospero Borgarucci was no less grateful for seeds of *nasturtio* brought to him in 1564 by a Venetian barber-surgeon, Battista Ceschoni, from Constantinople.[16]

In Venice one doctor, Maffeo Maffei, established his own botanical garden, which was visited by Mattioli.[17] Others were owned by Venetian patricians. Particularly famous among botanists were the gardens of Pietro Antonio Michiel in Venice[18] and Lorenzo Priuli in Padua,[19] while Conrad Gesner also had lavish praise for the garden on Murano of Girolamo Cornaro, a former governor of Cyprus, who had brought rare things from Crete, Egypt and elsewhere.[20] Gardens such as these, together with the presence of merchants and traders in *materia medica* from East and West, made Venice a forum where the latest botanical news could be discussed and new specimens examined. The Venetian presses, whose productions included the Valgrisi editions of Mattioli's commentary, added a further stimulus. Venice was, according to Pandolfo Collenucio, the defender of Pliny against Leoniceno, 'that great centre for the diffusion of information as well as commodities',[21] so busy a centre of communication that one wonders how men like Valgrisi found the time to print in between forwarding plants from Calzolari in Verona to Aldrovandi in Bologna,[22] or passing on consignments of Mattioli's favourite cheese *en route* from Siena to Trent.[23] Certainly few cities can have been so much visited by leading botanists and natural historians. Pierre Belon was amongst them, supplying plants for Michiel's garden at S. Trovaso.[24] Antonio Musa Brasavola showed his first-hand knowledge of Venetian pharmacies on page after page of his *Examen Omnium Simplicium* (Rome, 1536), whilst Valerius Cordus used his stay in Venice in 1544 to build up a store of important medicinal simples unavailable in Germany.[25] Conrad Gesner also spent a month in Venice in 1544, studying and drawing fish,[26] and Rondelet may have followed similar interests.[27] Ulisse Aldrovandi was in Venice in 1554, 1558 and 1571,[28] and Mathias de Lobel in the 1560s.[29] Mattioli was another visitor, both early in his career and towards the end of his life.[30] Foreign students in Italy, like Joachim Camerarius,[31] inevitably included Venice in their itineraries, while for their part teachers at Padua like Anguillara, Guilandino, Falloppia and Cortusio, were in constant touch with the capital.

Writers on *materia medica* from the days of the early medical humanists claimed that their interest was not merely academic, but concerned with the improvement of therapeutics.[32] Mattioli, as we have seen, was particularly emphatic that his aim was the reform of pharmacy. The Venetian Senate took this very seriously. In founding the garden at Padua, it followed the advice of Paduan doctors that the garden would increase knowledge of simples and so do away with errors and frauds in pharmacy which were causing the deaths of patients.[33] What impact, then, did the upsurge of interest in botany in the sixteenth century have on the practice of pharmacy? How far were pharmacists involved, and how far did their training allow them to participate in the activities of physicians and scholars of natural history?

Pharmacy in Venice was a highly developed trade, controlled traditionally by the magistracy of the *Giustizia Vecchia*, though with the rival involvement from the 1520s to 1548 of the *Provveditori alla Sanità*.[34] In 1565 owners of pharmacies formed themselves into a *Collegio degli Speziali*.[35] At its early meetings some seventy one distinct pharmacies were represented. By 1617, though the population of Venice had fallen from about 172 000 to about 142 000, the number of pharmacies had risen to over a hundred. New regulations had to be brought in that no one might open a pharmacy within a hundred paces of another.[36] The trade, it seems, was flourishing. The pharmacist was trained by apprenticeship. According to the statutes of the College, no one was to open a pharmacy (*bottega medicinale*) unless he had been an apprentice (*garzone*) for five years, and had served a further three in dispensing and composing medicines (*per giovane ad esercitare il*

dispensare et componere).[37] In practice, apprenticeship could begin at any age
from about twelve to eighteen, and lasted four to five years. In a typical
instance in Venice in 1582, Santin, the twelve-year-old son of Pietro di
Murari, was apprenticed for five years to Domenico Aselli at the sign of
the two columns at S. Canciano. Aselli was to provide clean lodging,
maintain Santin in health and sickness, and teach him his craft. In return,
Santin's father was to pay, in the first year only, three Venetian *staia* of
flour, and six Paduan *mastelli* of good wine.[38] At the end of the apprenticeship an examination was conducted by the officers of the *Collegio degli
Speziali*, and a licence to practise issued by the *Giustizia Vecchia*.[39] An
apprentice might broaden this training by reading. Prospero Borgarucci,
in his *La Fabrica degli Speziali* (Venice, 1567), urged pharmacists to learn
Latin from boyhood and to read Dioscorides, Galen, Serapion, Mesuë,
Avicenna and others. At the same time he recognized that many pharmacists were not sufficiently skilled in Latin, and to these he recommended
recent authors and translations.[40] Amongst others he had his own book in
mind, for the *Fabrica* was a practical manual for pharmacists, built up in
part from his visits to Venetian pharmacies, and containing nine hundred
pages of advice on how to recognize, gather and preserve simples, how to
stock a pharmacy, and how to manufacture the twelve types of medicines
in use. The *Fabrica* was published in Venice by Valgrisi, who also
published Mattioli's commentary, similarly issued first in Italian for
pharmacists ignorant of Latin.[41] In addition a pharmacist could broaden his
education by travel and visits to well-known pharmacies. Giorgio
Melichio, born in Augsburg, was tempted to Italy by the reputation of its
pharmacies. He travelled to Rome, various Lombard towns, and to
Dalmatia and Greece, serving voluntarily in famous pharmacies such as
that of Girolamo dalla Luna in Padua. Finally Melichio settled in Venice,
where his pharmacy at the sign of the ostrich (*Struzzo*) became one of the
most celebrated of the later sixteenth century. There, too, he published his
book, unlike Borgarucci's a book written by a pharmacist for pharmacists
– *Avertimenti nelle Compositioni de'Medicamenti per Uso della Spetiaria* (Venice, 1575). A number of the better-known pharmacies in Venice appear to
have taken in young men concerned to broaden their education. Giovanni
Battista Fulcheri, as we know from his thirty four letters to Ulisse
Aldrovandi, spent the years 1565–6 in Venice, gaining experience at the
Coral kept by Galeazzo Corniani.[42] While there he enjoyed the friendship
of Jacques Raynaudet, who came to Venice in 1566 after visiting Gesner in
Zurich. Both men left Venice in 1566 to gain reputations as owners of
botanical gardens as well as pharmacies, Fulcheri in Lucca, Raynaudet in
Marseille.[43] Another correspondent of Aldrovandi, Domenico Caravallo,
stayed at the same pharmacy, the *Coral*, from at least 1571 to 1572, when
he returned to Piedmont to a career in pharmacy.[44] Marco Orselini, from
Massa Carrara, was in Venice from 1554 to 1559, at first at the pharmacy

at the sign of the *Medico*, kept by another branch of the Corniani family, and later at the *Campana* kept by Giusto di Mei (or, di Megi), an associate and friend of Nicolo Massa. Writing to Aldrovandi in 1559, Orselini also asked for help in finding a place for a year or two in a Bolognese pharmacy, indicating the sort of way in which a pharmacist could broaden his experience during his years as a *giovane*, between apprenticeship and owning his own shop.[45]

Particularly formative for the pharmacist were his relations with local physicians. Drug prices in Venice, as in other towns in the Republic such as Padua and Bergamo, were fixed each year, in Venice by the *Collegio degli Speziali*.[46] The pharmacist's success therefore depended not on his prices, but on his reputation for quality, and on his contacts with local physicians. The physician–pharmacist relationship was crucial for both partners. Scipione Mercurio, who was encouraged to start a medical practice in Venice in the late sixteenth century, was told that a physician needed to know only two things to make a great career in the capital – how to make women fertile, and how to get on well with the pharmacists.[47] The pharmacy was, in effect, the centre of medical practice in the community. Doctors, and even surgeons, met in the pharmacy and probably saw patients there as well as making home visits. Prospero Borgarucci expected the doctor to order drugs personally on the patient's behalf. He urged the pharmacist to listen attentively to the doctor's instructions, to record carefully in his prescription book details of weight, dosage, method and times when medicines were to be taken, and then to read the whole back to the doctor as an extra precaution. If a pharmacist lacked an ingredient, this was the opportunity to discuss it with the doctor, who might name a substitute.[48] Physicians frequently attached themselves to particular pharmacies. Bartolomeo Agolante was described in 1543 as practising at the *Coral*,[49] and so too was Giovanni Andrea Bentivoglio of Bologna in 1545.[50] Prospero da Foligno based himself at the *Medico*,[51] while Nicolò Massa regularly ordered drugs for his patients from the *Campana*, run by Giusto di Megi, who was named as executor in Massa's will made in 1562.[52] Girolamo Donzellini, the humanist physician later drowned by the Venetian Inquisition for his views and extraordinary carelessness with his prohibited books, made at once for the *Sarasin* in the Merceria on his arrival in Venice in about 1547. Donzellini, it may be noted, took a keen interest in botany and was part of the Mattioli circle, while the Fenari brothers, Marco and Ippolito, who ran the *Sarasin*, were amongst the most botanically-minded Venetian pharmacists. From this time, as Ippolito was to relate, Donzellini was offered the use of the pharmacy (*noi comenzassemo proferirli la bottegha*).[53] According to longstanding Venetian law, no physician might have a financial interest in a pharmacy, and in one case, in 1541, Girolamo Rizzo was specifically forbidden to order medicines at the pharmacy of his brother Domenico on Murano.[54] Yet, as the statutes of the

Collegio degli Speziali make clear, abuses continued, with pharmacists giving doctors large presents to keep them attached to their own shops.[55] It was also standard for doctors of the pharmacy to receive medicines for their own households free of charge. Drugs supplied to Silvestro di Silvestri in 1572 from the *Cerva* were not even entered in the prescription books.[56] This was a well-established practice, also referred to in the will drawn up in 1540 by Valerio Superchio, one of the most prominent Venetian physicians of the first half of the century. Superchio noted that he had been with the *Anzolo* from its outset, never paying for medicines for his household, though giving medical treatment in return. He left ten ducats to the numerous children of the pharmacy.[57] These were the children of Cechino Martinelli of Ravenna (d. 1535), who had served prominently as *Soprastante delle Spitiarie* on behalf of both the *Giustizia Vecchia* and the *Provveditori alla Sanità*.[58] The Martinelli sons are particularly interesting since they demonstrate in themselves the close connections between pharmacists and physicians, including, as they did, two physicians, Pietro and Andrea, and two pharmacists, Zuan Alberto, who continued at the *Anzolo*, and Cechino, who became well known for his botanical research in the Middle and Far East in the 1560s.[59] Through their close day-to-day contacts, physicians and pharmacists could provide a mutual stimulus. Giorgio Melichio paid special tribute to the doctors of his shop (*miei medici*) in his *Avertimenti*, not surprisingly, since they included Andrea Marini, an editor and commentator on Mesuë (Venice, 1562), and Giovanni Paolo Mongio, who edited the works of Avicenna jointly with Giovanni Costa, and who also encouraged Costa towards his edition of the Junta Mesuë.[60] Another of Melichio's physicians was Decio Bellebuono, who was possibly a follower of Paracelsus. Greatly praised by his friend Leonardo Fioravanti,[61] Bellebuono owned a distillery for medicinal waters at the Frari, as the Holy Office discovered, though he ran the business in his brother's name to circumvent the law against the involvement of physicians in pharmacy.[62] Clearly he had much in common with Melichio, who was also praised by Fioravanti as a great distiller.[63] A shop such as Melichio's could thus be a centre of discussion and even of innovation. Paolo di Romani, Melchio's pupil and successor at the *Struzzo*, was, for instance, the inventor of a method of reducing syrups to solid form while preserving the aroma and virtues of the herbs from which they were made. The result was said to be less nauseous to the patient.[64]

Whilst, therefore, the pharmacist lacked the intellectual background of the physician, he could still be directly involved in the development of *materia medica*. This is clear, for instance, from the twenty four unpublished letters of Marco Fenari at the *Sarasin* to Ulisse Aldrovandi, from 1569 to 1573. Fenari had been in contact with Luca Ghini, who had sent him botanical specimens from Bologna and Tuscany. From Aldrovandi, too, he requested various seeds and bulbs, presumably for his own garden in

Venice. In return he supplied Aldrovandi with seeds, bulbs, and plants from Cairo, Crete and elsewhere.[65] His brother Ippolito Fenari, the first Prior of the *Collegio degli Speziali*, likewise took a leading role in planning a public botanical garden in Venice in 1566. In August of that year fourteen Venetian pharmacists, including, as well as Fenari, Galeazzo Corniani of the *Coral*, Melichio of the *Struzzo* and Zuan Alberto Martinelli of the *Anzolo*, pledged a total of forty six ducats a year for the rent and maintenance of a garden to be established on Murano or the Giudecca which was to contain plants from all parts of the world for the benefit of medical education.[66] Though there is no evidence that this pledge was put into effect, it is clear evidence of the pharmacists' commitment to botanical research. Pharmacists themselves could take a direct role in searching out the true Dioscoridean plants and in reintroducing them into pharmacy. Antonio Musa Brasavola was amongst those who became convinced that the rhubarb in use in the pharmacies did not correspond to Dioscorides' description. Nevertheless in Venice he discovered true Dioscoridean rhubarb (*rhaponticum*), brought all the way from the banks of the Volga by the pharmacist at the *Campana* [probably Giusto di Megi] who, according to Brasavola, spared no expense on his drugs.[67] Naturally such an example was soon imitated. Mattioli, too, noted in the 1540s that true rhubarb (*rhapontico*) was beginning to be imported from the Bosphorus – he himself had bought it several times in Venice at the *Medico*.[68] Mattioli's works, like those of most writers on *materia medica*, make frequent reference to the reappearance of classical simples in Venice. 'It is not long', he wrote, for instance, in the 1548 edition of Dioscorides, 'since true Cretan dictamnus began to be imported into Venice'.[69] Physicians who wrote on *materia medica* therefore relied heavily on the pharmacists, with Prospero Borgarucci particularly indebted to Melichio, 'an exceptional botanist' (*semplicista*), and to Zuan Alberto Martinelli 'a famous pharmacist and worthy botanist'.[70] Martinelli benefited particularly from the research of his brother Cechino, who, during the 1560s (approximately 1564–7) travelled via Crete, Cyprus and Syria to the Indies.[71] From there he sent home rare plants, including important ingredients for theriac, to Mattioli, and, above all, to his brother in Venice. This made the *Anzolo* a centre of interest. While de Lobel was there he was shown, amongst other things, *satyrion erythronium* sent from Aleppo, an aphrodisiac so potent that its mere touch filled Cortusio with desire, to the entertainment of de Lobel who thought that Martinelli had got the wrong plant.[72]

Most famous of all the republic's pharmacies was the *Campana d'oro* in Verona, kept by Franceso Calzolari.[73] Few pharmacists were so respected and admired by leading natural historians, many of whom joined him on botanical expeditions to nearby Monte Baldo. Calzolari's *Viaggio di Monte Baldo* (Venice, 1566) claimed to supplement two other publications from the Valgrisi press – Mattioli on how to identify simples, and Borgarucci on how to use them to compose medicines – with a third work on habitat and how to find plants in nature. Calzolari also built up a much-admired natural history museum, with animal, vegetable and mineral exhibits.[74] Mattioli, an intimate friend, was one of its visitors. He spent over a week with Calzolari in 1573. Aldrovandi paid a visit in 1571, leaving behind on his departure a distraught Calzolari, melancholic to the point of madness because he had forgotten to display his sample of true *cinnamomo*.[75] Mattioli trusted to Calzolari to manufacture drugs of his own invention, such as his oil of scorpions, and had the highest praise for Calzolari's theriac and mithridatum, which he said were the best that could be had.[76]

Theriac and mithridatum were indeed the prestigious drugs on which a pharmacist's reputation could be gained or lost. The ambition – not to say the race – to produce a perfect theriac stimulated pharmacists throughout Italy. Botanical interest came together here with hopes of financial rewards in what was, for Venice especially, an important export market.[77] In antiquity, according to Maranta, theriac was never known to have failed, its virtues being attested by clinical trials on criminals condemned to death.[78] Essentially theriac was an antidote to poisons, but it was also considered to be a remedy for an infinite variety of diseases, and a prophylactic for preserving health. Orazio Guarguanti, who claimed in 1596 that the best theriac was made in Venice at the *Struzzo* and the *Campana*, gave a list of its uses more than fifteen pages long, covering everything from dropsy, epilepsy, melancholy, plague and paralysis to worms and ulcers.[79] Maranta, too, thought it was good for all illnesses.[80] Yet although it was made in large quantities in the sixteenth century,[81] several doctors expressed doubts about its efficacy, at least in comparison with the theriac of the classical age. In the 1548 edition of his *Dioscoride* Mattioli wrote that if good theriac could be found, then there would be no need to look further for antidotes to poisons. But, he implied, so many of the ingredients used in classical times were now unavailable that modern theriac was scarcely worth having.[82] The same thought stimulated him, by 1559, to devise new antidotes of his own composition.[83] Maranta blamed the ignorance of doctors and pharmacists in post-classical times for the failure of theriac to produce the effects it once did.[84] Guarguanti noted with dismay that many doctors, even in Venice, had given up prescribing it,[85] while Prospero Alpino asked what doctor in his day would trust solely to theriac or mithridatum to cure the bites of vipers or scorpions or remedy the effects of poison.[86] Yet despite these misgivings, the overall tone was optimistic. Theriacs, it was believed, were getting better and better as botanical research progressed. As more and more classical plants and simples were rediscovered, it became possible to use fewer substitutes (*succedanei*) for missing ingredients. Already, in the 1540s, Mattioli was reporting the rediscovery of plants which were amongst the 81 ingredients of theriac.[87] Cretan dictamnus, and rhubarb, already mentioned, were amongst them. Yet in 1548 the list of missing items was still a long one, including *cinnamomo, balsamo, petroselino macedonico, mirrha, folio, meo, chalciti, amomo, aspalatho* and *calamo aromatico*.[88] The effect was probably to dampen enthusiasm for the drug, and indeed, in 1548 when Galeazzo Corniani of the *Coral* told the Venetian College of Physicians and the *Giustizia Vecchia* of his intention to make theriac, it was said that it had not been made for many years.[89] Particular progress was made between the 1550s and the 1570s. Mattioli claimed in 1565 to have rediscovered the mineral *chalciti*.[90] Calzolari, in his theriac made in May 1566, included four newly rediscovered ingredients, *acacia, costo, amomo* and *aspalatho*. He made a point of having his ingredients approved not only by the College of Physicians of Verona,[91] but also by Gesner and later by Mattioli. His ingredients then went on public display to the sound of trumpets and drums, and a permanent exhibition was included in his museum.[92] The provenance of Calzolari's new ingredients remains unexplored, though it is possible that the *acacia* came from Cechino Martinelli, since in 1568, presumably immediately following his return from the East, Martinelli gained the approval of the Venetian College of Physicians for 48 jars of a thick juice which he claimed was *acacia*.[93] Ferrante Imperato of Naples, who was, like Calzolari, a pharmacist, botanist and museum owner, was also soon using true *costo* in his theriac. He noted that it was now available from Venice, and that he had received a sample from Guilandino.[94] Imperato was also soon growing another missing ingredient, *petroselino macedonico*. According to Maranta the seeds had come from Venice from the pharmacist Marco Enario[95] – evidently a mistake for Marco Fenari of the *Sarasin* who also sent *petroselino* seeds to Aldrovandi in 1569.[96] Prospero Borgarucci credited Cechino Martinelli with the recovery of true *calamo* – his brother Zuan Alberto used it in his theriac in 1565, and so, too, did Giorgio Melichio.[97] In this way botanical research was making a definite impact on pharmacy. Borgarucci noted in 1567 that it had once been necessary to use twenty or more substitute ingredients in theriac, but now only five or six were needed.[98] Ferrante Imperato, who was prepared to spend years collecting his ingredients, used ten substitutes in his theriac made in 1557. His second theriac, made in 1561, contained only eight, and, a decade or so later, his third theriac contained only six.[99] But even this did not match the achievement of Calzolari, who could boast certificates from the College of Physicians of Verona that whereas his first theriac made in 1561 included six substitutes, his second, made in 1566, contained only three.[100] The scepticism about theriac which Mattioli had expressed in 1548 gave place, in 1568, to a paean of praise for Calzolari, whose theriac was now hailed as equal to that made by Galen for the emperors.[101] The search continued for the remaining lost ingredients, above all for that wonder drug of antiquity, balsam. Though there was room for controversy here, the College of Physicians of Verona felt able to approve a sample of opobalsam acquired by Giovanni Pona of the *Pomo d'oro* for his theriac in 1595,[102] perhaps under the influence of Prospero Alpino's *De Balsamo Dialogus* (Venice, 1591), which argued that the balsam currently to be had from Egypt was the true balsam of antiquity.

I have concentrated at length on theriac because it provides evidence of the impact on pharmacy of the search for classical drugs, which I take to be the central preoccupation of sixteenth century Italian writings on *materia medica*.[103] This was a quiet revolution in simples, scarcely to be detected in the civic pharmacopoeias which were increasingly compiled in the second half of the sixteenth century.[104] Classical plants and minerals were coming once more into use. At the same time, changes in plant identifications brought the replacement of some pharmaceutical substances with others, even though continuity of names made this far from obvious. So, too, as the Mattioli programme had foreseen, harmful substances mistakenly in use were being replaced. Cortusio, for instance, was amongst the first to realize that the plant used in pharmacy for the Arabic *doronicum* was actually a poisonous one, which he identified as Dioscorides' *aconitum pardalianches*. Cortusio discovered that doses of *doronicum* administered to wolves, dogs and pigs proved fatal in all cases.[105] Calzolari, Borgarucci and Mattioli, to whom Cortusio reported this discovery in 1565, all carried out their own tests, producing a steady toll of chickens, wolves, dogs and pigs as the news spread. Mattioli concluded that pharmacists' *doronicum* should rather be called *daemonicum*, for he believed it could kill men as well as animals.[106] Castore Durante followed him in urging pharmacists to banish *doronicum* and substitute *galanga* or *zedoaria* and, while serving as *Protomedico*, he succeeded in removing *doronicum* from the pharmacies of the Papal States.[107] Gesner, for his part, was sceptical that *doronicum* was fatal to humans. He tried two drachms on himself and survived, though he was ill for two days. Yet even he accepted that pharmacists' *doronicum* was not the true Arabic *doronicum* and he too instructed them to use *galanga* or *zedoaria* in its place.[108] Botany in this way was having a practical effect in the pharmacy, with Arabic simples being drawn into the discussion alongside classical ones.[109]

But if Italy was at the forefront in the development of botany, the same cannot be said of another influence on pharmacy, namely chemistry. It is tempting to think of Italian medicine in the sixteenth century as so wedded to humanism and the Galenic tradition as hardly to have been touched by events north of the Alps, and only recently has any attempt been made to trace the existence of a Paracelsan movement in Italy.[110] There were certainly factors which discouraged Italians from adhering to the Paracelsan cause. Amongst these was the continuing strength of medical humanism, and, in pharmacy, sustained enthusiasm for botanical research, represented in the early seventeenth century by the work of Prospero Alpino. Botanical studies were sufficiently complex and demanding to fully occupy a student of *materia medica* – hence, according to one critic, the reason why Ruel, Fuchs and Mattioli were so notoriously inept in medical practice.[111] We cannot rule out the possibility that Paracelsus exerted a personal influence in Italy, since he studied and travelled there, and is said to have been employed by Venice as a military surgeon in 1522.[112] Nevertheless his writings were not readily available in Italy. Many were written in German, and most were only published from the 1560s onwards, in the Tridentine era which placed barriers in the way of the free circulation of printed books.[113] The Paduan anatomist and surgeon Nicolò Bucella, for instance, had his baggage confiscated by the Venetian Holy Office in 1574 while *en route* to become doctor to Stephen Bathory, afterwards King of Poland. It was later released minus works by Paracelsus, which were judged heretical (*detractis tamen quibusdam libris Teophrasti Paracelsi tamquam haereticalia continentibus*).[114] Claudio Textor had a similar brush with the Holy Office in Venice in 1587, over prohibited books which included works by Ramon Lull and Guglielmo Gratarolo, and Paracelsus' *De Summis Naturae Mysteriis*.[115] Alchemy, too, a potent influence on the Paracelsan movement, was formally banned in Venetian territory, together with all alchemical equipment. The Council of Ten had passed a law to this effect in 1488, and, though it may not have been much enforced, it remained on the statute book a century later.[116] Perhaps in consequence, we know little about alchemical practitioners in the republic. Who, one wonders, were the *chymistae* to whom Falloppia frequently referred in his lectures *De Metallis atque Fossilibus* in 1557, but whom he never mentioned by name?[117] Finally mention must be made of the Italian Colleges of Physicians whose control of professional life favoured orthodox practice. Collegiality – in the fullest sense which included the physicians' practice of consulting together in particular medical cases – was very important in sixteenth-century Italy. Joint consultations could account for a substantial part of a doctor's income. This would be jeopardized if a physician openly favoured Paracelsan views,[118] for, as Orazio Augenio pointed out, it would be absurd for a Paracelsan and an orthodox physician to consult together since they differed both in principles and practice.[119]

Yet despite all the efforts of the Colleges of Physicians, unorthodox practitioners continued to flourish. Mainly they were on the fringes of society, but sometimes they took on a more central role, attacking orthodox medicine in a flow of racy, and, it would seem, saleable vernacular publications. Prominent in Venice in the first half of the sixteenth century was Angelo Forte, a native of Corfu, who was the author of a dozen short books on alchemy, astrology, magic and medicine published in Venice between 1525 and his death in 1556.[120] Forte practised as a physician, though, when challenged, his degree certificate proved to be conveniently mislaid, somewhere in Corfu or in Syria. He had links with the Titian circle, which produced two of the best-known renaissance diatribes against doctors, from the pens of Aretino and Nicolò Franco. His own works did nothing to reassure the Venetian College of Physicians, all of whose members were, he claimed, his enemies. The author of two books concerned with the early history of medicine, Forte presented a picture of Hippocrates groping after truth but working from false premises, followed by Galen, Avicenna and others who only compounded errors and stultified free investigation. As a result, medicine was lost in confusion – thick forests of infinite lies, wooded with books. Forte believed that wisdom was to be sought through a personal investigation of nature, and in travel and dialogue with local people in various countries. Rejecting Galenic physiology and pathology – especially the concept of natural heat, ideas concerning the generation of the humours, and the possibility of putrefaction within the veins – he developed novel theories of his own. In therapeutics he condemned vigorous venesection and purging, and excessive dieting, arguing that orthodox doctors weakened and even killed their patients in this way. Instead he sought to strengthen the governing virtue of the body in order to allow it to overcome disease, though he recommended mild evacuations if he thought them necessary. He also relied on the virtue of the doctor, which, he believed, reflected the secret and all-ruling powers of the heavens. Little is known about Forte's pharmaceutical armoury. He invented drugs (*magistralia*) of his own, stating that they should be composed of subtle substances, quintessences, which bore a relationship to the secret powers of the heavens, and which for that reason could strengthen the virtues governing the human body. But their nature remained secret, despite the pleas of one disciple, Simon Arborsellus, doctor of arts and medicine and rector of the university of Padua from 1541 to 1542, whose studies under Vesalius, Montanus and others had merely convinced him of the inability of orthodox medicine to cure disease.[121] We know however, from later evidence concerning Simon da Udine, the pupil who inherited Forte's secrets, that the remedies included pills, oils and powders, some of which seem to have had analgesic and soporific properties. Though Forte's investigations of Nature began in about 1520, when he could just conceivably have had contact with Paracelsus, the similarities between them are more probably to be explained by common influences. Currents of heterodox medicine nevertheless prepared the way, and were drawn into, movements directly influenced by Paracelsus. A chance reference in the records of the *Provveditori alla Sanità* shows that Forte's remedies (*sigilli . . . magistral de m. Anzolo de Fortis*) were available in Venice from Sabbà di Franceschi, pharmacist at the *Orso* at Santa Maria Formosa. Franceschi, as we shall see, was a close collaborator of Leonardo Fioravanti, whose admiration of Paracelsus was openly acknowledged.[122]

Fioravanti's stay in Venice, where he published all eight of his books, spanned the years from 1558 to the 1570s,[123] and therefore coincided with the period which Thorndike termed the Paracelsan revival.[124] Like Forte, Fioravanti urged his readers not to break their heads reading Hippocrates, Galen and the others, for there were as many opinions as authors.[125] The secrets of nature were to be learned by travel and from country people (*villani*) familiar with the virtues of simples.[126] He encouraged his followers to forget the old method, and to cure not slowly by *regimen*, but speedily by new medicines designed to purge and restore the body. These they were to make with their own hands.[127] Fioravanti had maintained an alchemist while in Palermo in 1548, in order to learn distilling,[128] and most of his remedies were distillations of animal, vegetable and mineral substances. Amongst them were his *quinta essentia*, made from successive distillations of wine, his *elixir vite* and *balsamo artificial*, both derived from herbs infused in alcohol and then distilled, his *olio filosoforum*, *magno licore*, *olio di vitriolo* and *olio di solfo*, and his caustic made from crystalline arsenic, sal ammoniac, sublimed mercury and strong vinegar.[129] Fioravanti's attack on weak syrups which only prolonged illnesses, and on complex drugs with contradictory ingredients, won him the hostility of Venetian pharmacists as well as physicians.[130] He was attacked by what he liked to call a conspiracy of doctors while in Rome in 1557,[131] and thrown into prison at the instance of the doctors in Milan in 1573, accused of causing the deaths of his patients.[132] In Venice in 1568 the College of Physicians tried to get him banned from practice on the grounds that he did not have a degree, though, surprisingly, Fioravanti was able to confound them by graduating at Bologna.[133] His drugs are unlikely to have found a place in many pharmacies, but he had two centres of distribution in Venice, the *Fenice* at San Luca, and the *Orso* at Santa Maria Formosa.[134] The latter was still run in the 1560s by Sabbà di Franceschi, who was also Fioravanti's partner in the years 1560–2 in a scheme to make healthy and repopulate the Istrian town of Pola.[135] By 1571 the *Orso* was run by Jacomo di Torellis, who was said to prepare antimony with such expertise that it worked wonders in various illnesses, and it was also the place of work of Angelo Rizzo, a surgeon skilled in dentistry and intestinal surgery, who was also experienced in distilling secret remedies.[136] Despite Fioravanti's praise for Paracelsus as rare and divine in the alchemical art, and as the inventor of the preparation of antimony,[137] it would be wrong to describe him without qualification as a Paracelsan. Much of his thought was derived not from Paracelsus, but from a common tradition coming from Ramon Lull, Arnoldus of Villanova and John of Rupescissa, all of whom he praised.[138] He seems furthermore to have appreciated Paracelsus' general outlook and approaches to therapeutics rather than his philosophical system. Fioravanti nevertheless helped to popularize the Paracelsan cause in Italy. His influence was widespread. In discussing his influence on English medicine, A. G. Debus noted that Fioravanti praised hardly anyone but himself.[139]

In reality Fioravanti praised so many people that it is difficult to establish the exact circle of his friends and supporters. Amongst them were Alberto Cimerlino, rector of the arts university at Padua 1567–9, 'so expert in the doctrine of Paracelsus and in the art of distilling', whose conflict with the Colleges of Physicians of Padua and Verona I have documented elsewhere,[140] the Paduan Professor Albertino Bottoni, 'so expert in the things of Ramon Lull, Arnoldus, and Paracelsus, as also in our own work', who was said to instruct his students in distilling,[141] and others such as Secondo Botalli of Asti, brother of the more famous Leonardo, Prospero Bellebuono, brother of Decio, and Giulio Contarini of Turin, all of whose success Fioravanti attributed to his own teachings.[142] In addition he praised in general detail terms Giorgio Melichio, Decio Bellebuono, Prospero Borgarucci and many others.

The impression of growing Paracelsan influence given by Fioravanti's books is further reinforced by the works of Tommaso Zefiriele Bovio of Verona (1521–1609), a lawyer turned medical practitioner who wrote three works against orthodox physicians whose titles speak for themselves, *Flagello de Medici Rationali* (Venice, 1583), *Melampigo overo Confusione de Medici Sofisti che s'intitolano Rationali* (Verona, 1585) and *Fulmine contro de'Medici putatitii Rationali* (Verona, 1592). Bovio claimed to have read thirty seven volumes by Paracelsus ('a giant amongst great men') though he found the vocabulary so unusual and the ideas so obscure that he could not make sufficient use of them to call himself a Paracelsan. He nevertheless used Paracelsan remedies and borrowed eclectically from his work,[143] adopting, for instance, the notion of the three elements, sulphur, mercury and salt.[144] Bovio attacked orthodox doctors, who, he claimed, killed their patients with strict diets and weak medicines.[145] He preferred strong vomits and purges, especially his *Hercole*, made through various distillations from nitric and sulphuric acids, salt, gold, mercury and other ingredients.[146] How far Bovio's remedies were available through the pharmacies of Verona and Venice (where Bovio also practised for a time), is unclear. He claimed, at least, to have the approval of Calzolari in Verona, and in Venice that of the Fenari brothers, and of Francesco Teofanio at the *Dio Padre*, and said that all these had made drugs to his instructions.[147]

But it would be wrong to consider the impact of chemistry on pharmacy solely in terms of unorthodox practitioners of more or less Paracelsan sympathies, despite all their success in attracting followers. Also important were less ostentatious influences felt within the mainstream of orthodox medicine. Mineral drugs had a place alongside vegetable and animal ones from antiquity.[148] The fifth book of Dioscorides' *Materia Medica*, describing minerals used in internal as well as external medicines, was well known in the sixteenth century, and commented on, for instance, in Falloppia's lectures at Padua. A physician or pharmacist could often accept remedies usually thought of as Paracelsan by associating them with Dioscoridean mineral drugs. Melichio, for example, praised the Germans for developing preparations of antimony, while recommending Dioscorides' description of *stibium* as a guide in choosing good antimony.[149] The tradition of medicine borrowing from alchemy, which owed so much to Ramon Lull, Arnoldus of Villanova and John of Rupescissa was also well established by the sixteenth century.

Particularly influential on pharmacy was enthusiasm for techniques of distilling, providing much common ground between orthodox and heterodox practitioners.[150] Mattioli noted that distillation was unknown in antiquity and that its invention was a discovery of the alchemists.[151] Most sixteenth-century writers shared this view, but showed a readiness to study with, and learn from, contemporary alchemists.[152] Gesner praised the contribution of Geber and other Arabic writers,[153] and enthusiasm for Mesuë in the later sixteenth century seems to have owed something to the fact that, unlike classical authors, Mesuë demonstrated a knowledge of distilling.[154] In his *Liber de Arte Distillandi* (Strasburg, 1512), Hieronymus Brunschwig had argued the advantages of separating the medicinally active part of a herb or animal substance from the dross in which it was trapped or diluted, and shown how distilling could produce an extraordinary range of medicinal waters and oils. Conrad Gesner took up the same themes in the *Thesaurus Evonymi Philiatri*, published in 1552. This had enormous influence in Italy, with two Venetian publishers issuing Italian and Latin versions in 1556. Andrea Marini, physician at the *Struzzo*, in his commentary on Mesuë published in 1562, recommended the *Thesaurus* as essential reading for the elegant pharmacist,[155] and followed Brunschwig and Gesner in publishing illustrations of distilling apparatus. The *Thesaurus* was also read enthusiastically by Borgarucci, who noted in 1567 that 'Such is the growth of this fine and delightful art of distilling that it is no wonder that the quintessence (as the Alchemists call it) should be extracted not only from various simples, but also from many composites'.[156]

The 1550s and 1560s in the Venetian republic certainly witnessed a remarkable upsurge of interest in distillation and improved distilling techniques, furthered no doubt by the presence in Venice of physicians such as Matthias Guttich of Bamberg, an alchemist praised by Falloppia for his skill in investigating the substance of medicines by sublimation.[157] Mattioli brought out his *Del Modo di Distillare le Acque da tutte le Piante* in 1565, with fine illustrations of distilling apparatus, especially of the favourite *balneum Mariae*, and he also used distillation to produce his own new drugs such as his oil of scorpions.[158] At Padua Cortusio was famous for his knowledge of distilling. He taught Borgarucci[159] and others, and was praised by orthodox and Paracelsan practitioners alike. Cortusio argued that the bare knowledge of simples was only a beginning. His work, night and day, went on to investigate the virtues placed in them by

God, proceeding in this 'not empirically, but (as wrote Theophrastus Paracelsus) spagyrically and judiciously'.[160] Typically, one of Cortusio's first innovations on taking charge of the Paduan botanical garden was to build a series of rooms to contain not only a museum, but also distilleries.[161] Amongst pharmacists well known as distillers were Giorgio Melichio and Francesco Calzolari, who used the same apparatus to produce not only vegetable oils (oils of nutmeg, aniseed, guaiac wood and others), but mineral ones such as oil of v triol.[162] Given, however, the almost industrial scale of some of the apparatus illustrated by Mattioli, it would seem unlikely that every pharmacist kept his own distillery. Conditions favoured the growth of specialists. Bellebuono, as we have seen, owned a specialist distillery in Venice at the Frari. Fioravanti appears to refer to another, at S. Gregorio, run by Giovandomenico de Fabii.[163] From the 1580s the records of the Venetian *Provveditori alla Sanità* become full of petitions from distillers and mountebanks to sell medicinal oils and waters,[164] and by the 1640s Venetian distillers emerged as a separate subsidiary trade, which the *Collegio degli Speziali* tried to discipline and tax.[165]

Much sixteenth-century Italian distilling was concerned with vegetable and animal substances, and was readily accepted within orthodox medicine. Orazio Augenio, for instance, who saw no common ground between Galenic and Paracelsan physicians, nevertheless wrote to the Senate of Piedmont to defend the right of Giulio Contarini as a physician to practise distilling and manufacture his own medicines.[166] But with a Paduan noble like Cortusio, physicians such as Mattioli, and pharmacists like Calzolari, acquiring equipment which continued to be thought of as alchemical and setting themselves the task of investigating new drugs through distilling, it was inevitable that their interests should lead them on to a fuller range of medicinal chemistry. This was particularly apparent in the republic from the last decade of the sixteenth century onwards, for instance, in the *Discorso della Vecchia et Nuova Medicina* (Venice, 1592) of Giovanni Bratti of Capodistria, and in the *Clavis Medica Rationalis, Spagyrica et Chyrurgica* of Zaccaria Dal Pozzo (Venice, 1612). Dal Pozzo, who graduated in Venice in 1593 and practised there for a time, demonstrated familiarity with a range of Paracelsan writers, including Quercetanus, Rulandus and Libavius, and praised his friends in Venice, Girolamo Brochino, pharmacist at the *Grifio*, whom he described as an expert chemist, and Alberto Stecchini, pharmacist at the *Struzzo* who had made up for him the laudanum of Quercetanus as well as a range of chemical antidotes, extracts, elixirs and cordials.[167] Quercetanus was especially influential in Italy through the Venetian editions of his *Pharmacopoea* published in Latin in 1608 and in Italian translation in 1609, and his attempt to show that Galenic and spagyric medicines were complementary seems to have been particularly appreciated. Galeazzo Cairo, whose experience of the inefficiency of medicine in Venice during the plague of 1576 led him to propose an academy for plague studies, recommended that chemical remedies should be a prime object of study, since they alone might be swift enough in their action to resist the plague poison.[168] Valerio Martini, deputed for the sick in the parish of Sant'Eufemia during the plague of 1630, had come to a similar conclusion, recommending in his *Trattato della Curatione della Peste* (Venice, 1630) various oils, spirits and quintessences drawn from the works of Croll, Quercetanus, Wecker, Libavius and others. By 1642 the official price list for drugs sold in Venetian pharmacies included a section, two and a half pages long, consisting of an *Index medicamentorum hermeticorum spagiricorum sive arte stillatoria paratorum*.[169] Chemistry had gained an accepted place in Venetian pharmacies, while at the same time the large number of distillers in Venice outside the pharmacies was explained in 1640 in terms of the popularity of chemical medicines, 'since today spagyric medicine is in use'.[170]

The influence of chemistry in the republic seems thus to have been felt at first, especially from the 1550s, in the application of distilling to produce an increased range of mainly traditional medicines. This opened the way, from the 1590s, for a fuller appreciation of Paracelsan remedies, which were increasingly used in the first half of the seventeenth century. The process can be followed in detail within the life of one Venetian pharmacy, the *Struzzo*. Giorgio Melichio, who ran the pharmacy from at least the 1560s until his death in 1585, seems to have been fairly traditional, for all his reputation as a distiller and his contact with the Bellebuono brothers, friends of Fioravanti. His *Avertimenti*, published in 1575, contained only a few chemical drugs, such as the preparations of antimony. His pupil and successor Paoli di Romani died too soon to reveal much about his views, though the point of his solid syrups patented in the 1590s – that they were pleasanter for the patient – reflected at least one aim of pharmaceutical chemistry. Romani's son-in-law and successor Alberto Stecchini, on the other hand, who ran the pharmacy from at least 1605, was, as we have seen, manifestly involved in producing Paracelsan chemical drugs. He also produced a new edition of the *Avertimenti* (Venice, 1627), with a commentary of his own, which announced that he was also producing a complementary collection of spagyric remedies. This seems to have been unfinished at his death in 1631, and it was taken up by his successor at the *Struzzo*, Antonio de Sgobbis. The result, Sgobbis' *Nuovo et Universale Theatro Farmaceutico* (Venice, 1667), containing nearly a thousand folio pages, described twin pillars of pharmacy – the ancient pharmacopoeia, Greek and Arabic, on the one hand, and, on the other, spagyric medicine as revealed by Croll, Hartmann, Libavius, Paracelsus, Quercetanus, Sennert and others. Sgobbis criticized those who relied on Galenic or spagyric medicines alone, and urged his readers to consult Mesuë if they wrongly believed that spagyric preparations were a new invention. By the mid-seventeenth century chemical drugs had thus acquired an honoured place in Venetian pharmacy, not replacing, but supplementing, traditional remedies.

6

Explorations in renaissance writings on the practice of medicine

ANDREW WEAR

Summary

In this chapter I discuss the general characteristics of a genre of renaissance medical writings which dealt with the practice of medicine (the *practica*). To begin with I trace how the *practica* changed over time and consider how humanistic values with their emphasis on classical purity of language and of source material altered the *practica* as did the needs of educationalists. At the same time I point out the continuation of a medieval tradition alongside the new renaissance products. I shall set out a case example drawn from the *practica*, that of vertigo. Most historians when discussing the nature of a particular type of medical literature concentrate on the general structure of the books in question and on their author's intentions as seen in prefaces and introductions and rarely look at the subject matter in any detail. I also begin with this approach but then, by looking at the topic of vertigo in detail, I show how the general conclusions regarding changes in the *practica* can be illustrated by a specific example. At the same time, the material on vertigo can be briefly analysed to discover how internal pathological processes taking place within the body were described by writers on practical medicine, and I hope to bring out the extent to which such causal accounts of illness based themselves on localized events taking place within the body rather than on a generalized imbalance of the humours. Finally, I touch upon some of the problems associated with fitting new explanations of disease into the methodical framework of Galenic medicine; and I point out how, although the application of method in medicine was suited to teaching Galenic medicine, it posed difficulties when innovation was envisaged. The chapter is exploratory and more concerned with sketching out and reporting findings in a largely unresearched area than producing an argument around a single issue.

Introduction to the renaissance practica

If a student or practitioner wanted to have information on the practical side of medicine – (diagnosis and treatment) he could use the writings of Hippocrates, Galen, Avicenna and other writers. However, in addition to these disparate sources, there was also available to him the frequently published (and presumably frequently used) *practica*. Yet with one notable exception[1] hardly anything has been written on the sixteenth century *practica*.

The *practica* were books used as primers for medical students and handbooks or 'vade mecums' for the practising physician. They followed the format of the medieval *practica* and taught 'particular' diseases in a head to toe order *a capite ad calcem* and they also dealt with the 'universal' diseases of fevers; in addition there might be separate sections on plague, arthritis, dislocations etc. The *practica* were related to university teaching in that the professors of the practice of medicine followed the same format in their lectures.[2]

The medieval *practica* continued to be available in the sixteenth century at the same time as renaissance writers were attempting to 'humanize' and reform them. They had dealt with the affections of the body in a reasonably brief manner, giving the causes (though not always) and the signs which would identify the disease and then detailing its treatment. The new renaissance *practica*, on the other hand, became increasingly verbose and concerned to define, divide and discuss their subject matter. It is not surprising therefore, that medieval *practica* continued to be printed in the renaissance (and also that a partial reaction set in later in the century deploring the concern with words and rhetoric). The *Praxis Medicinalis* of Arnald of Villanova (1240?–1311) was printed in 1585 and included his *Compendium Medicinae Practicae* which was also published separately in 1586[3] and in German in 1619. The *Practica* of Johannes Savonarola (1382–1462) was reprinted in 1559 and that of Marcus Gatinaria (d. 1496) in 1560.

The *De Medendis Humani Corporis Malis Enchiridion* or 'Vade Mecum' of Petrus Bayrus the personal physician to Charles III Duke of Savoy gives us a sense of how a renaissance editor might view his medieval material for it was edited and brought to publication in 1561 by the Swiss humanist physician Theodor Zwinger. It was frequently reissued in the following fifty years. Zwinger viewed Bayrus as a medieval writer though he had died in 1558, and he wrote, in typical humanist vein, that his language and mode of argument was not in keeping with the times. Yet, Zwinger found something of value in his author and wrote in his dedicatory letter:

He is barbarian I admit, but speaking in this barbarous manner he will be better understood than if he were forced to stammer in Latin, especially by those who can read without distaste Savonarola, Montagna, Gatinaria and the other writers of the

same ilk. I am sending you this Medicina of Bayrus put together in twenty-four
books, never before printed, with the odious repetitions of distinctions and
tractates excised.[4]

For Zwinger the positive virtues of Bayrus lay in his attempt to join the
dogmatic and empirical approaches together (a desideratum of any
humanist and Galenist), though he did not know 'if the attempt was
greater than its success'.[5] He also praised his method which consisted in
setting forth 'shortly and succinctly as necessity seemed to demand the
nature and essence of all diseases, the causes, signs, differences, prognostics'.[6] Method here was not the complex hydra of Montanus drawn from
Galen's *Ars Parva* and the *Methodus Medendi* but was, in effect, the medieval
way of writing a *practica*. Such a view of method was always possible in the
renaissance since the word could be equated with brevity and a 'methodus'
was often a synonym for a compendium. However, as we shall see Bayrus
in practice was often so brief that Zwinger's hopeful advertisement that the
nature, causes, signs of disease would be considered was misleading.

Another medieval *practica*, the *Rosa Anglica* of John of Gaddesden
(*c.* 1280–1361) was first printed in 1492 and 1502 and reissued in 1595 by
Phillip Schopfius. The *Rosa Anglica* was the exception to the rule of *a capite
ad calcem* and Schopfius remedied this by putting the contents of the book
into the traditional order. Schopfius felt that there was a market for the
book and he wrote that a new printing was necessary as copies of the
original printing were no longer available and people could not understand
its abbreviated print.[7] His comments on the text itself show how he
produced a compromise between humanistic values and the intrinsic
usefulness of the original text. He wrote that he corrected the Latin 'lest
men of more polished literary tastes should be detracted from reading it'.
However, he emphasized that 'we have left unchanged some technical
words and formulae although they are rather rough, lest we should lose
truth in our zeal for elegance of language or lest we should interpret the
author's intention less correctly'.[8] The ultimate justification of the *Rosa
Anglica* for Schopfius was based on the claim that the medieval writers
were better than the modern ones:

Now to come to the age immediately preceding our own I believe that there is
no-one so unjust or bold as to prefer the writings of the moderns of our time to the
memorials of those most excellent physicians I mean Valescus, Arnaldus de
Villanovus and John the Englishman seeing that these men in treating diseases
methodically, in prescribing remedies and setting out and solving questions
applied such care, labour and diligence as no other applied or will apply.[9]

This inversion of the normal renaissance view of things might be
explained by the date of the publication – 1595. The first flourish of the
renaissance was coming to an end, even for science and medicine which
had been late starters. Elegance of language was becoming less important

(see also the attack on humanistic rhetoric by the later editors of Avicenna's *Canon* which is discussed by Nancy Siraisi) whilst that of content, of attention to the 'things themselves' was increasing. Schopfius wrote:

There are many who are unable to read the writings of the medical barbarians who lived in an earlier age because these writings are very far from the purity and elegance of the Latin tongue and because they produce disgust and nausea to students of that tongue. This is true but it is not everyone who feels this way but the majority, and especially of those that are best in judgment, think that one should place more of one's energy in the discovery and examination of things rather than in mere elegance, splendour and charm of language.[10]

In the renaissance an attempt was made to transform the manuscript *practica* which had evolved during the middle ages within the Arabo–Latin tradition into a humanistic production. By looking at one or two writers it is possible to find out how this change was envisaged. In 1539 the German humanist physician Leonhard Fuchs produced a *practica* whose title expressed its purpose *De Medendis Singularum Humani Corporis Partium. A summo capite ad imos usque pedes Passionibus ac Febribus.* In the dedicatory letter Fuchs set out his aims. He not only wanted to revert to a pure and uncorrupted medical terminology (that is, classical), but he also wished to produce a method or *ratio* for treatment which would reflect Galen's views, especially as they related to the indications for cure.[11] Jerome Bylebyl has written at length on this topic: how some renaissance writers tried to replace medieval indications of the cause of an illness with those of Galen and how others sought to introduce Galen's idea of indications arising from the individual patient as an input into treatment. (As Bylebyl has covered the ground so well I will leave the subject of the indications rising from the patients to one side.)

Fuch's love of all things classical and his dislike of the Arabs and of the 'barbarians' (the medieval writers) further emerged when he wrote that his book was written for those who were frightened away by the great length and difficulty of the works of Galen and of the Greeks, and who consequently forsook Galen's reputation for the Arabs and for 'the most inept mob of barbarian doctors'.[12] Here Fuchs must have recognized that neither Hippocrates nor Galen – with the questionable exception of *De Locis Affectis* – had produced a compendium which could provide a doctor with a handbook for easily recognizing and treating an illness. The medieval *practica* did fulfil precisely such a need, but for a humanist doctor such *practica* were, because of their origin, corrupt. Fortunately, classical alternatives were at hand and the works of Aëtius and Paul of Aegina provided the materials from which a compendium based upon classical sources could be produced. Both Aëtius (fl. *c.* 500) and Paul (625–90) had extracted and summarized previous Greek writers, and both in a sense had produced a *practica*. The third book of Paul's *Libri Septem*,[13] in fact, had the same head to toe order as the *practica*, whilst the second dealt with 'universal fevers' which were also to be included in the *practica*. Moreover, Paul had the further advantage of being very close to Galen, Conrad Gesner reports that Manardi called him Galen's ape ('Galeni simiam'). Guenther von Andernacht, who was to become a translator of Galen and a prominent humanist and anatomist in Paris, had seen Paul's merit and translated him into Latin in 1532.[14] His reasons for doing so were to help the *practici* whom he recognized as a specific group:

Among others I first tackled turning the whole of Paul of Aegina into Latin, an excellent writer of medicine and one who was missing for a thousand years, for this cause and reason: that next to those full doctrines of Galen our schools should have some compendious author from whom they could reliably learn that way of healing which they call practical. Since Paul indisputably excels all recent writers from Galen in compendiousness, order, skill, perspicacity and doctrine. Add to this the fact that he treats of many things with erudition which are either left untouched by others, or even unknown to them.[15]

Fuchs wrote that his own *practica* or method of healing was 'conflated from the works of Aëtius and Paul who follow Galen for the most part', and that it had been composed so that men who had forsaken trustworthy judgement and rashly followed anyone could return to virtuous goodness and hence reform.[16] Fuchs' new *practica*, by going back to the Greeks, would revert to a new *prisca medicina* even if not using the original and 'prolix' words of Galen. Here the humanistic ideal of reverting to the classical world for one's knowledge and the pragmatic necessity for brevity went hand in hand.

Fuchs gave two foundations for his method of treatment:

. . . the method of the treatment of the ancients is composed especially from two things, from precepts of course, which show whence the indications for treatment are to be sought, and in medicines which repel illnesses.[17]

With regard to indications Fuchs stated that he followed the ancient Greek writers, who had set them down 'most correctly', rather than the Arabs and barbarians.[18] In contrast to indications, knowledge of medicines could not be recalled to its pristine state:

For there are many medicines both simple and compound which they used in overcoming diseases which escape the knowledge of all who live to-day and therefore cannot be recalled to use. So we are, as it were, compelled by necessity to make use in their place our own habitual remedies, especially those of which the forms and faculties are known to us.[19]

Moreover, Fuchs wrote, in order to be understood by the apothecaries he had sometimes to use words which were not in Latin but which were familiar to them.[20] The humanistic programme of retrieving ancient knowledge could not always be carried out, and the restoration of linguistic purity sometimes had to bow to the needs of business. The medical humanist could be very aware of the claims of the here and now. An example of this was Fuchs' use of well-tried local remedies in his *practica* rather than ones drawn from exotic far away places. He wrote:

I have been on my guard against exotic and expensive medicaments and those which are difficult to prepare only because there is a danger of many of these being adulterated, since they are insufficiently known either by those that sell them or by those who buy them. And the merchants in extracting them (such is their insatiable avarice) are principally concerned to sell inferior ones, and while they do this those which are good being kept too long or eaten by mould and maggots become worse. Now the apothecaries, almost all of them being no less eager for profit than the merchants and paying out money, buy only the worst ones. And although even amongst this kind there are good men to be found nevertheless, because, for the most part they are unlearned and ignorant of better things, they purchase only the familiar materials which are for the most part adulterated for making up their medicines. Wherefore, I am not able to give my approval to the practice of foolish and unlearned physicians who in practising use no medicines except those which they compose from the four parts of the world.[21]

Although I do not consider treatment in detail in this paper a cursory reading of the *practica* shows that there might be broad agreement on what was necessary in treatment but its detailed implemention could vary very much. So that if purgatives were prescribed the ingredients making up the purgative varied from author to author. The element in the *practica*, therefore, which escaped the hold of the ancients lay in the prescriptions given in the sections of the *practica* on treatment ('curatio').

After Fuchs many renaissance *practica* became more methodical and philosophical, partly in response to educational needs and practices. Fuchs himself in his *Institutionum Medicinae* (1555) produced a book which began with the theory of medicine and ended with its practice. The contents included the definition of medicine, the division of medicine, the elements, qualities, humours, the parts of the body, its actions, a description of the non-naturals, the causes and definition of illness, brief accounts of fevers and a short exposition *a capite ad calcem* of the affections of the body and then a discussion of signs and diagnostic matters such as uroscopy and the taking of the pulse. The format of the book reminds one a little of Avicenna's *Canon* which contains both the theoretical and practical parts of medicine. However, Fuchs in his *Institutiones* concentrated more on theory and on explaining the theoretical underpinning of concepts such as symptoms used in the practice of medicine, which the traditional *practica* took for granted and had seen no need to explain at length. On the other hand, the central element of the practice of medicine, that concerned with the nature, recognition and treatment of diseases was reduced by Fuchs to a mere enumeration of the names of illnesses and of their definitions.

Writers like Montanus, Altomari, Capivaccio and Massaria wrote at much greater length and with more concern for theory when producing their *practica* than had their medieval predecessors, and were more concerned with educating medical students than providing handbooks for practitioners. (Montanus did not write a *practica* but lectured on the *practica* of Rhasis.) Bates and Bylebyl[22] have also pointed out that such men attempted to transform the *practica* into treatises of methodical therapeutics following the example of Galen's *Methodus Medendi*. Apart from the wish to restore Galenic teachings and to educate students, one motive for this may have been to bolster the claims of university-trained doctors over the providers of medical expertise in the renaissance, namely: priests, wise-women, magicians, herbalists, travelling empirics and so forth. In an age when licensing and regulation of doctors was lax, a claim to have a proper 'method' of healing which only the properly educated could practise could be a means of excluding outside competition. The renaissance physician could use as a model Galen's attack on the empirical sect and his praise of the dogmatic[23] physician who knew the causes of diseases as well as its signs. When Montanus lectured on Rhasis' ninth book *ad Almansorem*, which listed diseases *a capite ad calcem* and formed one of the models of the medieval *practica*, he castigated Rhasis for writing empirically and contrasted this with his own approach which was 'dogmatice et methodum' and a few lines later 'dogmatice et ex methodo'.[24] The reform of the practice of medicine was not to be undertaken only by method but also by the allied but much wider concept of dogmatism or rationalism (the latter being concerned to cure by discovering the causes of disease, the former curing by rational indications derived from the patient). That knowledge of the causes of disease and knowledge of disease from the patient himself came to be linked together as representing expert knowledge and opposed to the ignorance of the empiric can be seen in one of Johann Lange's letters where he attacked the ignorance of empirics and uroscopists. He wrote that the method of healing consisted in the knowledge of the causes of diseases, whilst:

> . . . the ignorant and inexperienced crowd of philosophers, seduced by old women's superstition and by the impostures and false appearance of knowledge of the Jews and pseudodoctors whose effrontery knows no bounds, thinks falsely not that the causes and the natures of illnesses can be discerned by pathognomic symptoms or by dyscrasia of the affected part or organ . . . but that the natures of the illnesses can be discerned by a mere inspection of urine.[25]

Lange went on to say that the uroscopist also ignored the way of life of the ill patient. Uroscopy, where the practitioner could be sent the urine without seeing and examining the patient, set at nought the lengthy education of the university physician and the Galenic mores of knowing the causes of a disease and taking into account the patient's specific nature.

As such it was an obvious target for opposition by the rational physicians of the renaissance.

Sentiments such as Lange's, attacking the competition and defending the virtues of the Galenic doctor, can also be found in the introductions to some of the renaissance *practica*. The Frankfurt physician Johann Hartmann Beyer, in his dedicatory letter to the *Practica Medica* (1594) of his former teacher at Padua Girolamo Capivaccio, quoted Galen to the effect that the physician defeats disease by being instructed by reason and that 'the best doctor is a philosopher'. At the same time Galen was cited as commending experience by means of which the precepts of the theoretical part of medicine were confirmed.[26] Beyer considered *ratio* and *experientia* and wrote that though he liked both he would have to give the palm to reason.[27] Then, from this rather abstract discussion of reason and experience he moved to the empirics and the quacks, and he clearly saw his support of reason as a defence against them. For, he wrote 'what is more cheap than empirical physicians' and every place was full of well tried (medicinal) recipes:

You can see that mad, deaf, toothless witches, priests, barbers, porters, Jews, murderers and criminals who are deserving the cross and further people who are bereft of reason, are all rich with remedies so that the waters could more easily fail the Rhine than empirical remedies fail this class of people.[28]

How far this fear of empiricism was real and how far it was an ancient literary device should become clearer from other chapters in this book. However, it is possible that the opposition to empirics made for a conservatism in which reason (that is, Galenic doctrine) was defended to the exclusion of new knowledge gained by experience.

Beyer contrasted Capivaccio with the empirics and praised him as being most studious about method and order and 'he leans everywhere on the solid foundations of philosophy'.[29] As we shall see later on Capivaccio certainly applied a philosophical approach to his *practica*, so much so that it is doubtful if it was much use as a *vade-mecum*; brevity, which is one sense of 'methodus', being sacrificed for the prolixity of philosophical distinctions.

Peter van Foreest (1522–97) the town physician of Delft wrote at the end of this period a series of medical observations arranged in the head to toe order of the *practica* (medical observations, *consilia*, *consultationes* were the practice of medicine brought to the level of the individual case and formed a counterpart to the general approach of the *practica*). Foreest, the 'Hippocrates of Holland' was a practical physician par excellence and in the prefaces to his books of medical observations we get the views of someone looking back, rather dispassionately, at a panorama of medical views. He made it clear that his intention was to make doctors rather than orators[30] and that he preferred knowledge of treatment to eloquence, the thing itself rather than the decoration of words.[31] He was not therefore a humanist who would exclude the Arabs and the medieval writers. He admitted that he did 'not fear to bring forward now the Greeks, now the Latins, now the Arabs or even the Barbarians and on occasion to follow these same people'.[31] Although Foreest wrote a violent diatribe against uroscopists and empirics[33] he was willing to acknowledge that within 'proper' medicine there had been criticisms and disagreements. He listed some of the comments made against particular philosophers and physicians, when he came to Galen he wrote that he had been attacked for excessive prolixity and for the fact that he had written in 'a certain order which is not suitable for practise'. He continued:

Furthermore, quite a number of people embrace Avicenna and neglect Galen. On the other hand, others reject Avicenna because of the barbarous medical terms. They receive Galen with both arms. Or rather the ears of some people are so fastidious that they admit no other doctor unless one who has written in pure language, Greek or Latin, and that briefly. But they turn away from all practici (*practicos*) as though they were barbarians and loath them. So, that they do not deign even to read the Arabs however much they might have produced remedies for us. All the same the Arabs and the barbarians have each their reputation, they have been more fertile in remedies than the Greeks themselves and there are certain people who just as they blame the prolixity of Galen so they blame the brevity in Paulus of Aegina and not a few consider him an ape of Galen.[34]

From this passage it is clear that the humanists had not been able to have it all their own way. There still remained an undercurrent within medicine which, paying less attention to ornament and more to the things themselves, valued the Arabs and the traditional *practici*. The attraction of the new, reforming, movement within medicine and the articulateness of humanist physicians has meant that more attention has been paid to them than to the old-fashioned practitioner and his needs. Nevertheless, Foreest made it clear that such people did exist, and that he himself was not so besotted by classical eloquence that he would reject what could be of use.

Francis Bacon felt that the middle ages and the renaissance could be characterized as having too much empty argumentation to the detriment of the study of 'substance'[35] and too much elegance of style so that 'men began to hunt more after words than matter . . . Then grew learning of the schoolmen to be utterly despised as barbarian'.[36] We have also found these generalizations in the medical writers cited above. However, like all generalizations they were too exclusive. The Arabic and medieval writers were valued by some physicians despite the attempt by renaissance writers to reform the teaching of the practice of medicine by 'humanizing' its language and by producing a philosophically based (that is, concerned with causes) and methodically ordered form of *practica*.

Continuity is equally strong in the structure of the *practica*. Firstly, the traditional order of classical origin, *a capite ad calcem*, is found not only in

Galen[37] and Paul of Aegina but also in Rhasis, Albucassis and Avicenna amongst the Arabs and in Constantine the African, Gariopontus and Petrocellus in the Salernitan period and in writers such as Gilbertus Anglicus, Arnald of Villanova, through to Sylvius, Fuchs and then to Capivaccio and Massaria at the end of the sixteenth century. It was not until Theophile Bonet in 1682 wrote his *Mercurius Compilatitius* that an alphabetical listing of diseases was produced as a substitute to the head to toe order. The latter had distinct advantages. It ordered the body into regions such as the head, the upper chest, belly, sexual organs and so forth. Within these sections one could list the illnesses or affections that could befall those areas of the body. (Affection or illness is a better word to use than disease, as some affections could be symptoms of an underlying disease.) Secondly, the list of affections remained reasonably constant over time and kept recurring in nearly all writers up to the end of the sixteenth century. So, for instance, headache, migraine, vertigo, phrenitis, epilepsy and melancholy would almost certainly be found in any medieval or renaissance account of affections of the head. The existence of a new disease such as syphilis might be admitted in the renaissance but in general the list of possible disorders remained remarkably constant from Greek times to the renaissance.[38] As I explain below, in my study of vertigo, the question of whether an affection was a disease (*morbus*) or not could arise, but apart from such issues which were meat and drink to the men applying method to medicine in the renaissance, there was no attempt to discover new illnesses unless they were thrust into the consciousness of physicians.

Vertigo and the description of illness

There was nothing novel about vertigo for the medieval and renaissance writers. It was a condition known from Greek times and was one of the affections regularly discussed in the *practica*. In other words, it was ordinary and well established, and although lacking the interest of a new disease like syphilis for contemporaries and historians, it can be used as a representative example of what was contained in a *practica*.

A difficulty faced by anyone undertaking a case study of this sort is how much space to devote to questions of provenance and how much to an analysis of the material in its own right. Such was the derivative nature of medieval and renaissance medicine that if a particular slice of medical knowledge is studied it will inevitably involve a consideration of its provenance. This is a proper way of proceeding since both medieval and renaissance writers were concerned to draw their knowledge from past authorities, and the latter often took great care in detailing the sources that they used, so that by tracing the provenance of a piece of medical knowledge the historian is engaged in the same sort of activity as the writers that he or she studies. Yet, such an approach can have its dangers.

For instance, we may find that the description of say, migraine goes back in all its essentials to an account by Galen and consequently we may ignore its content or meaning leaving that to people who write on Galen – although such an account would not have lost meaning for the middle ages and renaissance merely because it was derivative. It is notorious that analysis of the content of ideas is undertaken by philosophers and historians at their point of origin, and only some innovatory ripple within the calm sea of tradition – for instance, developments in anatomy – stimulates an investigation of content. In my discussion of vertigo I will consider provenance but I will run counter to the normal trend and also look briefly at content. I want to bring out three things. First to demonstrate the change-over from medieval to renaissance *practica* and the developments that occur within the latter. My specific example will mirror the general points made in my introduction to the *practica*. Secondly, by briefly analysing Arnald of Villanova's explanation of vertigo I give an exposition of humoural medicine which contradicts some commonly held assumptions. Lastly, I hope to give the reader some taste of what was in the *practica* and this means that I have included more material than is strictly necessary.

The Arabic and medieval writers

Rhasis' ninth book *Ad Almansorem* was frequently used in the middle ages and commented upon in the renaissance. The *Articella*, which formed a basis for medieval medical teaching was often printed together with it. Rhasis' account of vertigo did not discuss the provenance of the information given – though some was ultimately derived from Galen – and it had little if any discussion of causes, but instead it was concerned with identifying the affection in its various forms and giving instructions as to treatment. The chapter on vertigo began:

When someone sees what is before him move in a circle and his eyes are darkened and he wants to fall down and his face and eyes grow red at the same time and the veins also which are behind the ears swell prominently you must perform venesection, and cupping glasses must be placed on his neck and shin-bones. But if the aforementioned veins do not appear and the face is ruddy the blood is to be lessened by drawing it from the basilic vein and the cupping glasses must be applied to the shins.[39]

As Montanus and Massaria[40] realized Rhasis proceeded empirically; there was no discussion of the causes that produced the symptoms. What we are given are the visible signs to be found in the patient and instructions on how anyone with those signs is to be treated. However, other Arabic and medieval writers did discuss the causes of vertigo and should not be stuck with the label of empiricists.

Avicenna wrote at length, in a vein of natural philosophical enquiry, on how external impressions could impress themselves within the subject's brain so that when one saw a rotating wheel its impression would remain within a susceptible individual (such as a sick person) even when it was no longer being sensed. Another explanation concerned vertigo produced by someone going round in a circle; in this case Avicenna thought that the vapours in the brain were given a sort of momentum so that they continued moving in the brain even after the motion had stopped. These explanations drawn from reasoning in natural philosophy were not taken up by later writers. Avicenna also wrote, in more of a medical manner, of vertigo which occurred from causes within the body. Vapours, either from bile or phlegm originating in the stomach or in the womb, could rise up and affect the animal spirits within the brain. Avicenna differentiated vertigo from epilepsy by its greater duration and lack of spasm, but he wrote that when vertigo came from phlegm it was close to epilepsy (epilepsy being thought to be produced by phlegm). He went on to write about the signs which preceded vertigo such as pains in the head, tinnitus and heaviness of the head, he also gave the differentiating signs which would distinguish whether the humour involved was phlegm or bile. Finally, Avicenna detailed the treatment for vertigo.[41]

Avicenna's account of vertigo was very unlike that of Rhasis and certainly combined reason and experience in a manner that the renaissance should have approved of. Avicenna's ability to look at the phenomena from more than one point of view is not untypical of medieval authors, though their renaissance successors tended to oversimplify the tradition by seeing all medieval medical writing as an undifferentiated whole.

Constantine the African gave an account of vertigo which combined a discussion of its causes with an account of the signs of the condition in its different forms.[42] The shadowy Salernitan writer, Gariopontus, on the other hand, seemed to favour the approach of Rhasis. His discussion of 'scotomia' (darkening of the eyes, black-out) or vertigo began in an empirical fashion with no discussion of causes: 'Those people who suffer from scotoma have these signs . . .'[43] However, in the next chapter he again discussed vertigo, but this time did write something on its causes. He wrote that scotomia arose in bibulous men and in those who frequently cleansed (*purgant*) their heads in the sun. According to Gariopontus when the head was heated its veins opened up and haemorrhoids in it would be inflated. In a more general sense, he saw vertigo as resulting from bile coming from the top part of the stomach to the head and in that case the stomach had to be cured.[44] Elsewhere in the book the empirical approach based on signs and treatment, and the dogmatic founded on causes, signs and treatment alternated.

Other medieval writers discussed the cause of vertigo as well as its signs and treatment. Arnald of Villanova tried to grapple with the causes of vertigo, and his attempt is worth analysing. First of all Arnald used his imagination to describe the inner happenings of the body. The distinction between a sign and an internal cause in all the writers that I discuss is that a sign was visible whilst a cause was invisible. Therefore, in the case of the latter one had to produce a description of something that could not be observed but which, nevertheless, was believed to be taking place in the body and producing visible signs. However, the story was not totally imaginary. It was given shape by reference to well known, if invisible entities, such as the animal spirits, vapours in the body, and hidden but known structures such as the optic nerve, and by the use of concrete analogies drawn from the visible world to explain the hidden world inside the body. For Arnald, vertigo was a revolution of the spirit in front of the eyes (in the anterior ventricles of the brain?) or an enveloping of the brain whereby the spirit of vision was impeded. First the definition, then came the cause. This was from some material existing in the brain itself or coming from the stomach. Smoke was formed from material in the stomach and coming up to the optic nerve it closed it up. This blockage in the optic nerve produced a change in the essence of the animal spirits and the interactions of smoky vapour and the animal spirits produced a circular motion in the optic nerve just as when two winds of equal force create a whirlwind.[45] This was essentially a story, a narrative of generally unverifiable events and it was given verisimilitude by the references to generally-agreed-upon structures within the body; the imaginative part had been to produce a narrative of happenings within the body that would account rationally for the visible manifestations of the condition; hence the trick was to show how the animal spirits themselves could be put into a motion analogous to the spinning motion that people feel while they have vertigo.

This analysis, I would argue, holds for most accounts of illness in the medieval and renaissance period. A point that emerges, and which I will develop later is that even if the ultimate cause of an affection was humoural there was, nevertheless, a very specific and localized element to causal explanations of illness (one effect of this would be to allow identifiable conditions to be defined, not only from signs, but from causes). One can also note that many writers referred to external causes of vertigo. These were specific rather than general and also, by the very fact that they had an external origin, they run counter to the internal causality that is usually thought to have been required by humoural medicine.

Some accounts may have been more persuasive or rational than others (though how contemporaries could judge the matter is usually impossible to tell). In the *Rosa Anglica* of John of Gaddesden the explanation of vertigo is less convincing (to me) because there was no clear connection between what was said to be going on inside the body and the outward signs of vertigo. John wrote that in vertigo the cause was a more subtle material than in scotoma (he was one of the few to separate the two). This material was trapped with flatulence inside a humid viscous matter that had no exit, and so went round and round just as children are used to do when they spin themselves round like wheels.[46] John's analogy between the motion of children who, of course, produce vertigo by their action, and the motion of the subtle material is blurred because we are not given enough details as to what happens to the subtle material in the body: where is it situated? how did it arise? what is its nature? how is it set in circular motion? and so on. From the analogy of children spinning themselves dizzy John came to his conclusion:

So vertiginous man, when he sees a wheel revolving or water rushing in a torrent or in a revolution as occurs in whirlpools in water or moving clouds swiftly driven by the wind, thinks that he is being swung round with them and therefore he grasps onto things near at hand because he absolutely must sit down or fall down. Hence in scotoma and vertigo there is a corruption of the vision and an injury to the procreation of images . . . as if the optic nerves have been shaken and consequently injury is produced in the common sense and as a consequence judgement is corrupted in the imaginative (faculty).[47]

Neither the 'So' at the beginning of the passage nor the 'Hence' towards the end is justified, for the two conclusions have little connection with the antecedent material. In a sense John of Gaddesden was not, at least in this case, a convincing or rational story-teller and perhaps this partly explains why some medieval writers thought poorly of him.[48]

In the renaissance there was a similar method of giving an explanation of what was going on inside the body. However, the story becomes more uniform and this is because the three sources of Galen, Aëtius and Paul of Aegina, although not always agreeing with each other, provided the materials from which a causal account of the affections of the body could be produced. The Arabic and medieval writers, of course, also ultimately drew upon Greek writers[49] but the derivation was not so clear cut and, as the differences in their accounts of vertigo show, there was no agreed explanation of the condition, though the description of the outward signs of the condition was reasonably uniform.

The Greek sources for renaissance writers

At this point it is necessary to give a brief exposition of the opinion of Greek writers on vertigo as this will help to put the renaissance writers into context.

In *De Locis Affectis* Galen wrote[50] that scotoma and vertigo occurs on trifling occasions. This was often repeated, as was his next comment that people subject to vertigo fall down after one rotation whilst it takes many spins to make other people fall down.[51] Galen wrote that vertiginous persons also get dizzy watching someone else spinning round, or when they see a wheel turning or something else in a circular motion or when they look at whirlpools. The vertigo occurs more readily if they have been exposed to the sun or if their heads have been overheated for some other reason.[52] Galen went on to argue that in normal people the effect of dizziness or spinning round many times is produced by an irregular, turbulent and disordered motion of the humours and the spirit.[53] Therefore, logically, the same should occur in the disease condition. The affection, Galen argued, could be primary and situated in the head or it occurred by sympathy with the opening in the stomach[54] (a view found later in Avicenna and some medieval writers), and he cited Archigenes to this effect. Galen also repeated Archigenes' differential signs: vertigo which was a primary affection of the brain produced tinnitus, pain and heaviness in the head, whilst vertigo originating at the stomach was preceded by *cardiogmon* (pain in the heart area) and by nausea.[55]

The two compilers, Aëtius and Paul of Aegina, differed in one or two instances from each other. Aëtius, who drew his material from Archigenes and Posidonius, argued that hot and acrid vapours carried to the brain disturbed the animal spirit,[56] whilst Paul stated that:

The affection of vertigo arises when a cold glutinous humour occupies the brain whence men even fall down straight away on the slightest occasion as when they see certain things outside them going round such as wheels, whirlpools or when they spin themseves round.[57]

Aëtius described similar precipitating causes:

If the ill persists they are affected with vertigo from a slight cause so that they sometimes fall down, especially when they spin round in a circle, for what befalls others as a result of many revolutions befalls them from one revolution. But also if they see someone else spin round they are affected with vertigo, or if they see a wheel or something of that kind going round they suffer the same thing.[58]

The similarity in the descriptions by Galen, Aëtius and Paul of what external causes brought on the condition is striking. In the Latin editions of Galen and Aëtius the same adjectives were used to describe what happened to the humours and the spirit when they were excited by an outside cause – 'inaequalem et turbulentem et inordinatum'[59] – and the renaissance writers often repeated them.

The renaissance

In the renaissance as in the middle ages there was no uniformity in discussions of the affections of the body. Some writers, especially in the second half of the sixteenth century, might write at length on causes whilst others could be very brief. The intention of the writers also differed and some concentrated more on treatment and giving prescriptions than on detailing the causes of the conditions, which others, more concerned with education than practicalities, emphasized.

Sylvius, the Paris humanist and Galenist, in his *practica*, rather surprisingly only alluded to the causes of vertigo and was more concerned with treatment. He divided the causes of vertigo into external and internal, the former consisting of spinning round and of getting drunk, the treatment being to stop the activity in question, and additionally in the case of drunkenness the applications of clysters.[60] An internal cause could be produced by the immoderate and disordered movement of spirits and for that Sylvius advised staying in a dark room and gave a detailed prescription consisting of cold ingredients for quietening and settling the turbulent motions of the spirits.[61] Sylvius' real interest lay in treatment and he went on to advise that the patient should be given external applications to repel the material flowing into the head; he also prescribed remedies for vertigo caused by the different humours.[62] In effect, what Sylvius did was to assume that his reader already knew the causes of vertigo and would understand his allusions to them. In other words, he was not concerned with educating his reader in the theoretical part of medical practice.

In the *practica* of Bayrus, as edited by Zwinger, the explanation of the cause of vertigo was minimal. The chapter was organized on the lines of: 'if vertigo arises from bloody matter there should be cut first the vena basilica' and so on through each of the four humours with a final section devoted to the treatment of vertigo arising from 'foetid vapours'.[63] What was important was the treatment; how to recognize which humour was involved was left to the reader who might need to have recourse to some other *practica* to find this out. Yet, despite Zwinger's complaint, this is no barbarian *practica*; for the author was aware of Galenic teaching since he quoted the one piece of advice concerning treatment to be found in the chapter on vertigo in *De Locis Affectis*.[64]

Rather than taking the renaissance *practica* to be an undifferentiated whole we should see them as having a range of interests and approaches. Bayrus (via Zwinger) had the clear intention of producing a *practica* in which treatment ('curatio'), the essence of practical medicine, was more important than 'causa', even though the lack of the latter might condemn an author with the label of empiricism. (Zwinger's doubt as to whether Bayrus succeeded in his attempt to unite dogmatism and empiricism was more than well founded, as Bayrus had hardly anything on the causes of disease.)

Leonhard Fuchs, on the other hand, being a good Galenist and a student of method in medicine and a humanist to boot, produced in his *practica* a totally different account of vertigo from that of Bayrus. His chapter was structured in the following manner. There was a discussion of the name σκότωμια which he held to be Greek for the Latin 'vertigo', and he pointed out that the 'barbarians' had corrupted the word to 'scotomia'.[65] This was a typical opening to a renaissance-humanistic *practica*, reflecting the concern to produce a correct and pure terminology. The chapter then dealt with causes, signs, regimen, treatment, venesection, purgation, local remedies and cautery. It would be tedious to go into much detail, but Fuchs followed Galen's account in *De Locis Affectis* and also used Aëtius and Paul. Fuchs mentioned how a trivial occasion could bring the condition on, and how one spin rather than many would make a person prone to vertigo fall down.[66] Also present was the idea that vertigo is either a primary affection of the brain or came by sympathy from the mouth of the stomach with the excretions in the stomach producing vaporous exhalations which drove the animal spirits round.[67] Fuchs used the same adjectives – 'turbulentus, inequalis, inordinatus'[68] – as had Galen and Aëtius to describe the motion of the spirit and the humours. The account was not totally derivative for some creative work was involved in producing agreement where one's sources clashed with each other. The contradiction between Paul and Aëtius on what were the humours which caused vertigo was resolved by Fuchs when he described the humour as 'thick and slow' from which a vaporous spirit was released by the heat of the ill person.[69] In this way the cold glutinous and the hot acrid humours of Paul and Aëtius respectively were reconciled. There was, however, no explicit discussion of the issue and Fuchs' *practica* like many others did not involve lengthy argument, with the juxtaposition of conflicting authorities and the solution of contradictions so beloved of medieval and renaissance writers. Although, as we shall see, the *practica* did not always retain their claim to brevity, there yet runs throughout the genre the style of assertion rather than of dialectical argument.

The regimen that Fuchs advised was explicitly rational, for there was a connection between the cause of the condition and its avoidance and treatment. Food should lack 'flatus' and everything steamed should be avoided (so that vapours causing vertigo could not be generated – though Fuchs did not spell this out) and things going round in a circle should also be avoided.[70] As for venesection, Fuchs repeated the advice of Aëtius and recommended that only a small amount of blood be let since people with vertigo fell on the slightest occasion.[71]

Fuchs had produced a brief and rational account of illness. From the time of Montanus onwards there was an effort to apply the idea of method to therapeutics. As I mentioned before, Jerome Bylebyl[72] has discussed how the indications arising from the individual patient came to be included in the discussion of what should be the correct treatment. In what follows I will concentrate on the question of the cause of the affection and its signs rather than on indications from the patient. I do this in order to illustrate the general point that the philosophical/logical approach applied to therapeutics was also co-existent with discussions of method. Leoniceno and Manardi had explored the instruments of method – definition, division, demonstration and resolution and the three orders of resolution, composition and definition, but they did not apply it to the practice of medicine. Montanus, however, also produced interesting ideas on the question of method and order in medicine, and he did go on to apply method to the practice of medicine.

The contrast between Fuchs and Montanus is quite striking. This is partly because when Montanus wrote on vertigo it was in a lecture course commentating on Rhasis' ninth book and not in a *practica*. He, therefore, explicitly pointed out the contradictions between Aëtius and Paul, gave the opinion of modern writers – that all the humours could cause vertigo – and from various passages in Galen concluded that Galen's opinion was that it was caused by a cold humour.[73] Montanus' solution to the conflict of opinion was that vertigo fixed in the head was caused by a cold humour, his reason being the Galenic one that because of a lack of heat the excrements could not be properly concocted and consequently vapours would be produced which agitated the animal spirits. On the other hand, vertigo which was not fixed in the head could be caused by any humour, as in cases of drunkenness, or of too much blood or bile in the stomach.[74] This discussion and conciliance of previous views shows how the past served as a repository of knowledge out of which one could arrive at one of the objects of method in medicine, that of definition. Montanus wrote:

From this the correct definition of vertigo is obvious: vertigo is a disordered motion of the spirits in the anterior ventricles of the brain which motion arises because of the thick and confused vapours in them.[75]

What is significant here is that Montanus, the great teacher of clinical medicine at Padua, drew his knowledge of the causes of vertigo not from his experience but from the ancient authorities. This perhaps was inevitable, because to have knowledge of causes was to be rational, and reason as we have seen was sometimes contrasted and opposed to experience (and by extension to the empirics). The reliance on authority meant also that whatever might have been the potential flexibility of the humoural system for a writer producing an explanation of illness, in well recognized affections at least, physicians like Montanus did not have a great deal of freedom, for in practice they did not go beyond previous authorities.

The application of method to practical medicine involved both logic *and* experience – despite my comments above. In the case of logic, Montanus pointed out that vertigo was a symptom or accident and not a disease. It resulted from the action of the humours, and as the animal spirits were injured so the many actions which depends upon them were also injured.[76] This concern to have a proper classification was a characteristic outcome of the renaissance concern with method. At the same time the method of division brought the physician close to experience (that is, in his examination of the patient). Montanus produced a 'syndrome of signs' to be found in the patient from which the physician could deduce which particular humour was causing vertigo. The signs common to all types of vertigo were the feeling of everything going round, blacking out, hearing ringing in the ears and a corruption of the motive faculty so that the sufferer thinks he is falling.[77] But the signs which allow one to distinguish between the different causes producing vertigo were according to Montanus of three kinds: those arising from the injured function, those seen in the excrements and those found in the common accidents (or qualities).[78] The signs from the injured function originated from the animal faculties and could be divided into sensitive and motive signs, and the sensitive was further divided into interior and exterior.[79] Montanus continued in this vein and argued that if blood was the cause of vertigo the natural functions of the patient will make him imagine cheerful things, he will be inclined to sleep, he will feel heavy in the head and have happy dreams as did those of a sanguine temperament 'and in this way you will know from the internal operations of the brain what it is that has dominion'.[80] Montanus went on through the different division of signs:

So far as the vital functions are concerned you have the pulse which is felt to be great, vehement, resisting the touch, soft to the touch, full rapid, infrequent so that it would demonstrate to those that were blind the predominance of the blood . . . As far as the excrements are concerned they must clearly indicate the predominance of the blood, the urine is thick, red, which is the perpetual property of blood, the stools are concocted and the excrements which descend from the head are somewhat moist and if there are tears in the eyes they will be hot but not stinging and trickling down. And besides this, coming down to the mouth, the mouth will be somewhat sweet, and if it is the blood that predominates he will have ringing in the ears and heaviness in the head.[81]

Montanus then enumerated the signs taken from accidents which consisted of the first qualities, namely the habit and disposition of the patient, and of the secondary and tangible qualities such as the gentle heat felt on the patient's head.[82] Montanus concluded 'From all these things you will have so clear a syndrome of signs that you cannot be in error. You will say absolutely the same about bile . . .'[83]

One can see how the methodical approach of Montanus, by using the method of division, allowed him to fulfil Galen's requirement of applying universals to particulars. Moreover, it also helped the student (for Montanus had him in mind) and the physician to infer systematically rather than in a haphazard way what particular form of illness affected the patient. It also gave further verisimilitude to the explanation of the cause of the affection; for by means of the syndrome of signs one moved from the visible to the hidden, and inferred what was going on inside the body. Of course, the inference is not a real one, for what is happening is that the syndrome of signs reflects the causal account and without the latter's pre-existence would make no sense. In reality, the signs are not a research tool, independent of theory whereby new causes are discovered. For, as we saw, the causes are to be first established by an examination of ancient opinions and were not discovered *de novo* from signs in the patient. The signs merely indicated which amongst a set number of predetermined causes is the operative one. Montanus' general discussion of signs confirms this interpretation.[84]

Whether the signs were drawn at all from contemporary clinical experience is difficult to say. Some of them were clearly traditional such as the feeling of heaviness in the head, others such as ringing in the ears could be read in Galen and found in clinical practice. From Montanus' *Consilia* it is pretty clear that the signs were not only run through in a set order, but that their interpretation was uniform. In the case of the Venetian senator Bernardo Naugerio, Montanus went through the three types of signs and he was guided by authority not only in his choice of what signs to look for (for example, the colour of the face) but also in his interpretation of them (as in the case of the senator's urine).[85] This should not be too surprising, for not only was the modern idea of progress alien to the renaissance physician but we are here faced with the practice of medicine, a practice, moreover, to be undertaken methodically. Now, even the modern practice of medicine tends to be conservative in approach and revolves around well-tried methods and this was certainly the case in the renaissance where the distinction between teaching and discovery was unclear, and discovery often consisted in uncovering and teaching the proper views of the ancients.[86] Classification, as seen in Montanus' methodical approach to a problem, where he defined it and divided it up, was also essentially conservative, as the categories used were normally well established ones.

To end my case study of vertigo I will look briefly at the *practica* of Capivaccio and Massaria. Montanus exemplified a thoughtful application of philosophy and method to practical medicine; Capivaccio and Massaria who followed in Montanus' footsteps as professors at Padua show how the methodical approach could be taken to extremes, and how the *practica* were being changed from handbooks for practitioners to teaching texts for students.

Capivaccio's account of what happened inside the body is less graphic in detail and more ponderously abstract, being almost baroque in style:

> . . . the animal spirit which resides in the ventricles of the brain is affected with a morbid motion so that when this morbific motion tends towards the circular the brain is affected in repect of the heat of the imaginative faculty, so that the substance of the brain is affected by an affection which does not produce darkness as in melancholy, which is not fiery as in mania, but is circular. Hence the imagination is corrupted so that the patient imagines that objects are going round . . .[87]

Perhaps Molière had this sort of writing in mind when he considered the medicine of his time. Capivaccio went on to give the definition of vertigo and then took each term of the definition and differentiated it:

Vertigo therefore is a corruption of a principal function of the anterior brain along with injury of the vision and of the motion of the whole body dependent upon a circular affection of the brain. The function is said to be corrupt as differentiated from being destroyed and removed. The function is said to be principal as differentiated from non principal. It is said to be a function of the brain as differentiated from any other of the viscera . . .[88]

There is a certain sense of Aristotelianism about this which is confirmed by Capivaccio defining the 'form' of the vertigo.[89] This application of logic to medicine was the sort of thing that Ramus might have objected to; certainly it lacked the sense of enquiry and concern with substance that one finds in Montanus' application of method to medicine (in fact one might argue that the injection of Aristotelianism into medicine in the second half of the sixteenth century tended to produce a frame of mind which was at home with forms, specific qualities and occult qualities and would make something which appears abstract to us seem concrete – perhaps this is how we should see Capivaccio's 'morbific motion' and 'circular affection'.)

Massaria also applied logic in his discussion of what vertigo was. Whereas Montanus asserted that vertigo was a symptom, Massaria wanted to prove it (in fact his 'proof' was also close to an assertion):

Now since vertigo is a thing contrary to nature and the things contrary to nature are threefold, namely disease, cause of disease and symptom the question is under which heading it is to be placed. First of all it is not a disease because it is not a dyscrasia and not a lesion in the continuity of the body nor an abnormality in the composition of the body. Secondly, neither is it the cause of a disease since there is no disease produced by it and so it remains, as it should be, a symptom. Now since symptoms are of three kinds, injuries of the functions, change in the excrements, change in the qualities, it is obvious that the excrement is not changed nor the quality, therefore it will be an injury to the action. But once again since functions are threefold, the natural, the vital and the animal and since in the present case neither the vital nor the natural function are injured it does follow of necessity that it is an animal function which is injured. But since functions of this kind are threefold . . .[90]

This type of argument explains why the renaissance writers found it convenient to use tables to encapsulate the information they wanted to communicate (that is, moving from the general to the specific by the use of inclusive brackets as in a family tree but horizontally left to right across the page). However, clear as such *practica* might have been to the reader they tended to put great emphasis on theory and its sytematic presentation and less on treatment. Capivaccio had little on treatment in relation to the space that he devoted to discussion of the affection itself. It is a moot question if practising physicians found such *practica* useful, as they were designed more for teaching students (Massari's *practica* was produced from his lecture notes) to acquire a philosophical and methodically ordered knowledge of medicine (note how the ordering of the information in the passage above into three becomes a mnemonic device for students). Furthermore, the question could be raised: what happened to new ideas or findings which could not be fitted into the categories that the application of method to medicine had produced? The *practica* at the end of the sixteenth century, therefore, seemed not only to have restored Galen's teaching but to have codified it in such a way that the original purpose of the *practica* was being lost sight of, and at the same time a potentially inflexible system was being raised inimicable to innovation. Before discussing the last point I turn first to the question of how the causes of illness were described.

The description of disease

So far, with the exception of my discussion of Arnald of Villanova, I have discussed the approach rather than the content of the writers of *practica*. A look at content may prove worthwhile, for it will show that whatever might be the ideal explanation of illness, in practice it contained a specific and localized element which is at variance with the commonly accepted view that medicine until the nineteenth century was holistic and concerned with general disorders within the body.

Certainly the latter might at first sight seem to be the case. In the passage above from Massaria a disease was defined as either a dyscrasia (humoural imbalance) or, a lesion in the body or an abnormality in its composition (this was a standard definition).[91] Most internal illnesses appear to be produced from a general cause since they would fall under the heading of dyscrasia or ill temperament (the varieties of ill temperament were eight plus a ninth, the neutral state). The treatment of dyscrasia could involve other general considerations such as the habits and disposition of a patient. Furthermore, although symptoms were specific they were clearly differentiated by renaissance writers from diseases for, as Manardi wrote in his letter on the principles of medicine, we recognize diseases from symptoms.[92] At first sight, therefore, the specificity of symptoms should not be seen as extending to diseases. Yet in a sense it does, for there was a continuity from the symptoms to the diseases. As Manardi put it symptoms were more readily apparent and it was this that allowed us to infer what disease was involved,[93] but it is clear that for this to happen the symptom must be connected with the disease. The bridge between the two was the story of the hidden events in the body that were producing the symptoms. These events could ultimately be caused by a qualitative or humoural dyscrasia such as too much heat or blood in the body. This pattern, from symptom to hidden event to dyscrasia can be seen in the 'curatio' of the renaissance *practica* in which many of the remedies were not only concerned to treat the dyscrasia but also to treat the symptoms and to rectify the internal course of events (for example, Fuchs' advice to avoid the sort of food which could produce vapours that might affect the brain, and Lange's prescriptions).[94] In fact, a great deal of treatment was concerned with altering what was occurring in the body, and this is a sign that importance was attached to local pathological events and not only to the underlying humoural balance. Moreover, the dyscrasia itself could be localized rather than general, Montanus stated:

The vapours can ascend from any humour existing in the stomach or the spleen or the liver or the bladder and the whole body as well . . . But that this symptom (falling) arises from a quality, this you have from Galen book 3 chapter 7 of *De Locis Affectis* where he gives two cases, one of a child of thirteen years of age from whose shin a certain quality begun to rise which he did not know how to name which arose from part to part as far as the brain and at length he fell down. In the other case, a youth, from whose large toe a cold quality ascended to the brain . . . and which produced and caused epileptic fits.[95]

Here the origin of the dyscrasia itself was a local one though its ultimate cause might be of a general nature; and although Montanus did not go into detail, its journey to the head was localized for it 'arose from part to part'.[96]

It is understandable, given the nature of the *practica*, that renaissance writers should have held not only a general concept of illness but also a specific view in which localized events within the body produced symptoms. The *practica* were concerned with *particular* affections. These were given specific names such as 'lienteria', 'dysentery', renal stone, phthisis, dropsy and others, and they were often explained in semi-mechanical, concrete terms. As we have seen in the case of vertigo, these explanations tended to be uniform, especially after the retrieval of Greek medical texts. Jerome Bylebyl has pointed out that writers like Montanus tried to make treatment less standardized (that is, they were against the view of one treatment for one condition). However, the dogmatic tradition within medicine (which held, against the empiricists, that hidden causes produced disease) ensured that there was always a tendency to emphasize the causes of the illness rather than the indications originating in the patient and thus to conceive of illness in universal rather than individualistic terms (Montanus' phrase 'dogmatically and methodically' thus expressed a hidden tension as well as agreement).

New diseases and new explanations

Vertigo was a well-known affection, but how did the renaissance deal with a new illness? Here I will turn away from the *practica per se* and I will briefly look at Montanus' influential explanation of syphilis. I then consider how new explanations could be seen to fall outside of the ambit of methodical medicine and this will illustrate the difficulty that Galenic medicine as codified by the methodical *practica* faced in accepting innovation. My comments are very limited and exploratory.

A new disease like syphilis could be easily assimilated into the *practica* tradition. Montanus employed the same techniques to explain the newly arrived disease as he and others had used to describe well-known conditions. Story-telling, a localized and detailed account of what took place in the body to produce syphilis, was the key to Montanus' explanation.

Montanus first stated the dogmatic proposition that in order to teach the treatment of syphilis its nature and essence had to be discovered,[97] he continued 'I say that it is a bad hot and dry dyscrasia impressed in the liver by means of contagion.'[98] From this assertion or definition Montanus went on to unfold his story. The disease begun with intercourse with an infected person from whom emanates a certain poison 'in which exists that evil and poisonous quality'.[99] This attaches itself into the foreskin or to the mouth since these parts are loose (permeable) and more suitable for receiving the poisonous quality. We now proceed on a journey to the liver. Montanus wrote that gradually the quality creeps to the small veins then to the larger ones until it arrives at the liver. Once there it takes over and changes the liver's natural temperament. Because the liver is so changed it burns all the humours which are in it, which are transmitted to all parts of the body for nourishment. However the parts of the body do not accept these humours, the body then becomes full of sharp excrements which produce ulcers, blisters, joint pains and infinite other symptoms.[100] Montanus went on to give other graphic details of the action of this bad quality upon the body.

Montanus was telling a story with a beginning (intercourse, and the permeability of the foreskin), a middle (the liver) and an end product (the symptoms). Verisimilitude is given to the journey of the bad quality by referring to the bodily structures passed along the way, the permeable skin, the small and large veins, and the liver. The enormity of the disease is stressed by the damage it does to one of the primary organs of the body. In Galenic theory the liver was the source of nutriment to the body, changing chyle to blood, with the different parts of the body attracting blood as food for themselves as needed. The arrival of the 'mala qualitas' at the liver, and its destruction of the liver's natural temperament made the consequences fully understandable to Montanus' readers, given their knowledge of the liver's function.[101] In other words, not only did Montanus use anatomical points of reference but also ones drawn from theory. In fact, his whole account is within the ambit of Galenic qualitative theory.

However, the qualities involved could be either manifest (that is, those we can feel such as hot, cold, dry and wet) or occult. Occult, hidden qualities were often associated with the concept of *tota substantia*[102] that is discussed in Linda Deer Richardson's chapter. Both concepts were used to explain the inexplicable. The action of poisons, drugs, the magnet, the electric discharge of the torpedo fish were unexplainable in terms of manifest qualities so recourse was had to hidden qualities or to the action of the total substance (that is, the action of a poison might appear far greater than might be expected from its manifest quality, hence either a hidden quality was at work or the poison acted by its whole substance). Here was an addition to traditional theory (albeit having its origins in Galen). However, Montanus did not accept occult qualities as an explanation of disease. Those who teach nothing, he told his audience when lecturing on plague, flee to two things: to occult qualities and to unknown and obscure names.[103] Montanus did, rather grudgingly, consider the possibility of occult qualities in pestilential fevers stating that Galen 'your teacher and mine' advised that occult qualities should not be neglected if the manifest qualities could not be discovered.[104] As, however, Montanus believed that he had found out a manifest quality for plague the discussion was academic. Similarly, for syphilis Montanus gave a manifest 'hot and dry' quality as the cause, rather than an occult one. Yet, he stated that remedies for syphilis could operate either by manifest or by occult qualities. He excused this inconsistency over occult qualities by recourse to Galen.[105]

Why was someone like Montanus so hesitant to use occult qualities and *tota substantia* as explanatory concepts? After all a 'mala qualitas' transmitted by contagion has a similarity to the action of the magnet. Apart from the obvious point that in using occult qualities one was employing the unexplainable to explain the inexplicable, which is what Montanus implied in his castigation of those who teach nothing, there were more concrete objections.

Montanus raised a problem related to the practice of medicine. He stated that those who taught that pestilent fevers were caused by an occult quality derived knowledge of the different types of fevers from unknown differences in the qualities. Furthermore, if the differences in the qualities were unknown how could one discover the proper treatment?[106] As we have seen, in the methodical practice of medicine the different qualities could produce different forms of an illness, and unless the particular quality was known (and by definition an occult quality was unknown) no rational treatment could be given.

Apart from Montanus' very practical objection there was a more general problem. For some physicians occult qualities and the concept of *tota substantia* did not fit into the general scheme of methodical medicine. Moreover, for the rational physician the two concepts were tainted, for they seemed only to be known by experience. (Cesalpino, in his chapter on poison in the *Artis Medicae*, in fact tried to show that such a charge was unfounded.)

Argentarius, one of the *bêtes-noir* of the Galenic establishment, was by no means hostile to the idea of *tota substantia* but he was also very much in favour of the methodical approach of Montanus (he joined Montanus with Vesalius as a man who had to suffer much opposition at first before his views prevailed).[107] When, therefore in *De Morbis* Argentarius discussed how many different kinds of diseases were to be put into the category of *tota substantia* he was perplexed. He stated that although the different types of diseases arising from the four qualities were eight (that is, the eight types of dyscrasia) the diseases produced by the pestilential air and by poison were diverse and as yet unknown. A definite number of diseases could not be assigned to *tota substantia*.[108] Argentarius continued and developed a line of thought from Galen:

> To this is certainly relevant the fact that Galen is accustomed everywhere to write that the remedies which are beneficial through the *tota substantia* are discovered through experience alone, but are not established by any reasoning. But of things for which there is no reason there can be no definite species.[109]

Occult qualities and *tota substantia* did not fit into the rational, classificatory scheme of methodical medicine and this in a sense reflects the latter's conservatism. Of course, as with any scheme accommodations could be made. Thomas Erastus in a letter to Capivaccio wrote that he agreed with him that when we consider the genus or the differences of diseases, that a disease of *tota substantia* could not immediately fall into the realm of methodical doctrine. But Erastus went on to say that this was not because of any inherent difficulty in fitting an anomaly into a classificatory system as his correspondent thought, but because a disease of *tota substantia* did not exist anywhere and never had.[110]

Erastus then embarked on an interesting line of thought. Some people, he wrote, believed that diseases of *tota substantia* are known by experience and did not fit into methodical teaching. He denied this, and argued that everything found by experience had been placed within the method of medicine.[111] This claim contradicted the dichotomy and tension between experience and reason in renaissance medicine that I have been pointing to in this paper. Galen, of course, had written at length on the need to unite experience and reason, and renaissance authors were aware of his teaching (though the fear of empiricism could make a writer prefer reason). It was natural, therefore, for Erastus to feel that methodical medicine, as one might call the systematic practice of Galenic medicine, should always be able to include any findings from experience. However, as with all systems, methodical medicine was not open-ended but structured around the mainstream of Galen's theories. Therefore, a bad mixture of the qualities rather than an occult quality *had* to be the beginning of the disease process. Anything that did not fit into the standard eight combinations of the qualities did not fit methodical doctrine.

Erastus' solution in his letter was to integrate and assimilate the new ideas of disease causation embodied by *tota substantia* and seeds of disease into the old system. His example was the older disease of plague. He wrote that a method for treating the plague could be produced even though it was believed to be a disease of *tota substantia*. He argued that a 'morbus seminarius' (he seems to equate it epistemologically with *tota substantia*) did not act directly by pouring itself across from an infected person to someone else and then extinguishing his spirit and innate heat. Instead, the seeds of disease first affected the temperament or balance of the humours.[112] Erastus' solution thus brought one back to familiar territory for once the temperament was involved, therapy proceeded normally and rationally with the physician trying to discover the variety of ill temperament and initiating treatment accordingly.

Erastus' union of experience and method was a one-way process, with the latter altering the former into its own image. Perhaps the problem was that *tota substantia*, occult qualities and seeds of disease were not purely matters of experience but had a theoretical element alien to standard Galenic medicine. They could either transform Galenic medicine, they might themselves be transformed back into orthodoxy or the two could exist side by side.

By the end of the sixteenth century university teachers had bound the *practica* together with method. The benefits of this for them were that the practice of medicine could be systematically taught, and also differentiated from empiricism; at the same time, the localized element in explanations of illness which had been present from early on gave them detailed and specific material to classify and methodically digest. If there had been only a generalized notion of a humoural dyscrasia to account for illness it would have been difficult to produce the detailed differentiae of diseases and their treatments which gave such confidence to renaissance physicians. (Method was frequently associated with the avoidance of error.) Another benefit of localism was that a new illness could be placed within Galenic medicine. This was not so much because of the vagueness and flexibility of the humoural system, but because the techniques of telling quite a complex story could be applied to a new disease. The corollary of this was that, despite new ideas within establishment medicine such as occult qualities, the practice of methodical medicine might for some writers act as a barrier to change.

Conclusion

The keystone of Galenic practical medicine in the renaissance remained the list of fevers and affections contained in the renaissance *practica*. I have traced some of the changes that occurred in the *practica*. These were concerned with the restoration of Galenic medicine, and with the development of a methodical approach to the practice of medicine which was designed to codity Galenic knowledge and to show how, in a logical manner, it could be put into practice. The brief excursion into new illnesses and new explanations illustrated how the need to have a rational methodical medicine might exert a strong conservative force dampening innovation. As I have shown, the writers on the practice of medicine could be creative and were far more specific and detailed in their explanations of illness than is sometimes thought, but ultimately they were constrained by the overall qualitative theories of Galen. Innovation did exist but its only systematic development lay amongst Paracelsus and his followers.

I thank Marie and Rupert Hall and Vivian Nutton for their helpful comments when I was preparing the chapter, the participants of the Cambridge Conference for their very constructive discussion, and especially Iain Lonie for giving a great deal of help in a short time.

7

Jacques Dubois as a practitioner

GERHARD BAADER

Paris is usually regarded as the centre of the renaissance of Galenism of the sixteenth century. One of the most famous masters of this period is Jacques Dubois (Jacobus Sylvius). Born of humble origin near Amiens in 1478 he was educated in Paris. He first studied arts at the Collège de Tournai, where his brother François was professor and principal; he afterwards studied medicine, but without taking a degree. He graduated MB in Montpellier in 1529 and MD in 1530. Returning to Paris he was incorporated MB in 1531. He taught medicine at the Collège de Tréguier and took examinations for the licentiate. From 1536 he lectured, until his death in 1555, in the faculty itself.[1]

Dubois is well known as a teacher of anatomy.[2] He performed his own dissections and was also the arch-Galenist of Paris, trusting entirely in Galen's medical knowledge. He maintained the superiority of Galenic anatomy and replied to criticism of it by insisting that the human body had degenerated since Galen's times. This appears principally in his posthumous *In Hippocratis et Galeni Physiologiae partem Anatomicam Isagoge* of 1555. His invective against his former pupil Vesalius, whose *Fabrica* (of 1543) he could not accept, is famous.

Most of his writings are part of his academic teaching. This is true not only of his anatomical work but also of his introductory treatises: his *Ordo et Ordinis Ratio in legendis Hippocratis et Galeni libris*[3] of 1539, and his prolific commentaries on Hippocrates and Galen, for instance on Hippocrates' *Elementa*,[4] on Galen's own commentary on the Hippocratic *De Natura Hominis*,[5] and on Galen's *De Ossibus*.[6] At first sight Dubois' therapeutical and pharmaceutical treatises also seem to be part of his teaching. We must see if this is really the case.

In his pharmacological texts Dubois often states emphatically that Galen is the only reliable author on the topic. No doctor ignorant of Galen has any idea of medical practice, wrote Dubois in book two of his *Methodus Medicamenta Componendi et ab aliis Composita Expendendi ac Judicandi* (1541). Anything praiseworthy in this book, continued Dubois, should be attributed to Galen, and anything imperfect to Dubois, the author.[7] The *simplicia*, simple drugs, were of the utmost importance for the new practical medicine to a physician of the renaissance like Dubois; and he dealt with them in the first book of his *Methodus*, which he intended as a practical guide for doctors rather than for apothecaries.[8] The presence of Arabic elements in the *simplicia* did not dismay Dubois, for he held that in relation both to the simples and the complex drugs into which they were compounded, the Arabs had been followers of Galen and had added their knowledge of practical medicine to his.[9] But it was in respect of compound medicines that the modern Arabists, said Dubois, differ from the trained and qualified Galenists, for Galenic remedies were short and composed mainly of simples. Dubois held that in contrast the Arabists, unworthy of the name of physician, added more and more new simples to produce elaborate and expensive receipts that brought greater profit to the apothecary. In thus showing a lack of consideration for the patient, these modern Arabists, said Dubois, depart even from the advice of their leader Avicenna, who had recommended the prescription of cheaper and simpler medicines. Even worse in Dubois' eyes was the false claim of the Arabists to be followers of Galen; for in fact, he said, they adulterate Galenic medicines and insert pseudo-Galenic receipts into the pharmacopoeias. Another reason to know Arabic simples was the discovery of Arabic compounds.

In fact, although Dubois tried to return to Galen, he was no more able than any physician of the time to ignore Arabic *materia medica* and compound medicines in his own practice. Many Arabic compounds, like electuaries and syrups, are to be found in the fourth book of his *Methodus*. Often Mesuë is his authority, and so it is not surprising that Dubois in 1542 added to the *Methodus* a commentary on the so-called *Mesuë* itself.[10] An added justification for the study of Mesuë, as Dubois remarked in his preface to the commentary,[11] was that Mesuë himself was a follower of Galen, and that in consequence his writings reflect the true Galenic doctrine of drugs or develop the doctrine in a Galenic way (unlike the Arabists and moderns). For these reasons then, although Galen was the unassailable authority for Dubois, he could not do without the Arabic tradition in his medical practice.

This can be shown not only in the pharmacological treatises of Dubois, but also in his books on therapy and on causes and symptoms. Here again at first sight he follows Galen alone. Dubois' first book on causes is more or less a commentary on a semiotic treatise of Galen. In the preface of this *Methodus sex librorum Galeni de Differentiis et Causis Morborum et Symptomatum* of 1539 Dubois attacks contemporary physicians who no longer, he said, have any knowledge of medicine, but buy their degrees. Dubois states that in Montpellier every mountebank of this sort is ignominiously expelled from the city.[12] For every well-trained physician, on the other hand, there can be only one real authority, Galen; for he is the only real doctor. But because Galen's semeiology (which has its origin in Hippocrates) is dispersed into many books, Dubois tries to summarize it into one, in order to make it available also to persons trained in medicine at a lower level. Thus his treatise is directed to the average practitioner as well as to the student of medicine.

In his commentary on fevers, on the other hand, Dubois writes for the layman as well as for the practitioner. As he states in the book's preface, it should be useful not only to the physician as a guide to the correct treatment of fever, but to the layman as well, as a guide to its prevention. But if after all the layman should fall ill with fever, the book would put in him a position to assess the doctor's therapy.[13] Apart from such new ideas Dubois shows himself a strict Galenist in this commentary on fevers. He draws its doctrine from Hippocrates and Galen and from nobody else, because all other authors, whether Greek or Arabic, drew their knowledge from these authors alone and often merely corrupted it. In conforming with such ideas Dubois also commented upon Galen's *De Differentiis Febrium*.[14]

From all this it might seem reasonable to conclude that in discussing causes, symptoms and therapy, Dubois was as strict a Galenist as he was in anatomy. This conclusion would seem to be confirmed by his first printed treatise, written in 1530 while he was at Montpellier.[15] Champier and Montuus, then both still Arabists, had advised giving wine to patients suffering from fever. Dubois on the other hand disagreed with this treatment and tried to use the texts of Hippocrates and Galen to solve the question. To decide whether to give wine as diet to a patient, Dubois wanted to know his strength, his age, his condition as well as the violence of the illness. That is pure Hippocratism.

But on some matters Dubois found that the doctrine of Hippocrates and Galen was not sufficient. In the first place it was not sufficient for the treatment of plague[16] and *sudor anglicus*,[17] to each of which maladies Dubois devoted a small separate treatise. On plague, he follows medieval tradition. Thus he quotes Gentile da Foligno's first *consilium* against plague, which had been followed by the medical faculty of Paris in the 'Medical Opinion' upon plague which it gave in 1348; and on this 'Opinion' too Dubois is largely dependent. Although he tries to integrate into his treatise such classical authors as Thucydides in his description of the plague of Athens, and although he refers, for the use of opiates, to Dioscorides, Galen, and Pliny, these authorities are not sufficient for him. For the use of opiates against the plague he also refers to the practice at Montpellier, and finally, from his own experience, he gives his own recipes for opiates, electuaries and pills for the prevention of plague. He also knows of remedies which had been used with success in Paris against the plague. But often – as he says – it is only God who can help.

The question to be asked here is whether this dependence of Dubois on medieval (that is, Arabic) medicine in therapy is an exception occurring only in connection with diseases unknown in antiquity and in the middle ages, or whether Dubois normally used Arabist authorities besides Galen for medical practice, as he did for pharmacology. One treatise can help us to solve this question. In 1545 his *Morborum Internorum prope omnium Curatio brevi methodo Comprehensa ex Galeno praecipue et Marco Gatinaria*[18] was published; in its preface Dubois points out that after he had published his *Methodus sex librorum Galeni de Differentiis et Causis Morborum et Symptomatum* in 1539 for general therapy a compendium of special therapy was still needed. It is strange that Dubois thought that he could not take Galen as his guide in this topic as he had done in general therapy, although Galen's *Methodus Medendi* was already well known at this time. One has the impression that – like many other compendia on therapy of the middle ages and the renaissance – Galen's treatises on special therapy were too prolix for Dubois to be helpful either for study or for practice. Therefore he chose an author of the fifteenth century as his guide for the treatment of internal diseases, Marco Gatinaria, who had written a manual on therapy *De Curis Aegritudinum Particularium noni Almansoris Practica uberrima.*[19] Gatinaria, an Arabist professor of medicine in Pavia, had written this treatise on special therapy in 1462 and, as the title indicates, it is simply a commentary on the ninth book of Rhasis' *Liber ad Almansorem*. Gatinaria's book went through eight editions up to 1575. Although Gatinaria's manual shows – as Dubois remarked – many errors typical of his time, Dubois seems to have chosen it for its brevity.

He simply made its language conform to humanistic taste, and superficially added some passages taken from Galen. Gatinaria did not only use Arabic sources; he was a good practitioner and often quoted contemporary *practici*, and from time to time facts won by his own experience as well. The fact that his main Arabic source, Rhasis, had also been a famous practitioner of his time, may be one of the reasons that Dubois had chosen Gatinaria as his source in special therapy. We know from Vesalius in his preface to his paraphrase of the ninth book of Rhasis' *Liber ad Almansorem* that he had learnt from his teacher Dubois that Rhasis was to be considered as taking the first place among the Arabs. This ninth book of Rhasis' *Liber ad Almansorem*[20] is simply a manual of diseases in an order frequent from antiquity, *a capite ad calcem*, starting with headache and mental diseases and ending with the diseases of the legs like sciatica. In general, Gatinaria follows Rhasis only in diseases of the eyes, of the ears, of the nose, of the teeth and of the mouth, sometimes reducing the original by omitting paragraphs or whole chapters. Sometimes Gatinaria introduces his own differentiation into diseases treated by Rhasis. He differentiates headache, for example, according to its origin from different humours, into bloody, choleric or phlegmatic, into a headache of general origin or headache caused by staying too long in the sun. In dropsy he uses the ancient division into ascites, hyposarca and tympanites. Here as well as in other points Dubois follows Gatinaria. Gatinaria himself not only follows as his main source, the text upon which he is commenting, but also quotes the *Continens* of Rhasis, the *Canon* of Avicenna, parts of the *Articella*, the *Antidotary* of Nicolaus, and works of Mesuë, William of Saliceto, Taddeo Alderotti, Matteo da Grado and other contemporaries, as well as those *practici* whom he summarizes. In general Gatinaria's treatise has the character of commentaries produced in the north Italian universities of the fifteenth century; the chapters show exact dispositions in single *intentiones* and where necessary also theoretical passages are inserted. The commentary itself is limited to therapy. The knowledge of the diseases as found in Rhasis is assumed as known without being mentioned in detail. Dubois' own work may be illustrated by a few examples taken from his descriptions of different species of headache and of mental diseases.

First, in most of the chapters Dubois starts with a definition of the diseases in a form not found either in Rhasis or in Avicenna. Dubois defines for example inflammation of the brain, phrenitis, as 'erysipelas of the membranes enclosing the brain, a very acute disease with very violent symptoms',[21] a definition derived from the Hippocratic aphorism 4, 10 (from the *Articella*); apoplexy as 'a strong disease that has its origin out of too much respiration';[22] catalepsis is defined in agreement with Galen as an excessively cold and dry concoction within the brain; by the physicians it is called freezing in general. It is a disease that is different from κατοχή or 'sleeping awake', for catalepsis is cold and dry and shows an inefficient respiration of the soul without the involvement of substance; 'sleeping awake' is produced from a surplus of yellow bile combined with more phlegm in the brain. It is therefore warm and dry and involves substance qualitatively and quantitatively.[23]

Secondly, Dubois often changes Arabic or Latin words into Greek and vice versa: *soda* into *cephalalgia*, *subeth* into *caros* ('heavy sleep'), *congelatio* into *catalepsis*, *spasmus* into *convulsio*, *debilitas visus* into *visio imbecilla*, *cataracta* into *suffusio* and *guidem* into *venae iugulares*.

Thirdly, most of the Arabic references in Gatinaria are omitted by Dubois, except for Gatinaria's references to Rhasis, Avicenna, and Mesuë.

Fourthly, although Dubois says that he has made many additions from Galen, there are only a few to be found. Occasionally he gives a direct quotation from *De Methodo Medendi*, as for instance when he quotes a passage in which Galen says that if somebody has a headache, he should not have a crowd of visitors, because the air of the room where the patient lies would be warmed by their perspiration.[24]

Fifthly, in general one can say that Dubois shortens the text of Gatinaria, simplifies the style and makes it more understandable. These are the usual modifications made by humanists in paraphrasing Arabist texts.[25]

Sixthly, as far as the content is concerned, it is made more suitable for practice. In the treatment of phrenitis for instance Avicenna recommends abundant use of phlebotomy.[26] Gatinaria, quoting him, had already expressed caution about this therapy[27] and Dubois himself gives direct contra-indications: the patient should not be bled if the stomach is still filled with food.[28] In the case of apoplexy, thought to be caused by an abundance of blood, Gatinaria recommends phlebotomy of the *vena cephalica, vena saphena* and *vena basilica* as initial therapy.[29] Dubois omits the phlebotomy of the *vena saphena*, but recommends massage of all parts of the body, bandaging of the afflicted parts, warm baths, the use of cupping-glasses together with scarification of different parts of the body. Also where Gatinaria gives a choice of recipes,[30] Dubois gives one recipe alone.[31] Quotations from Avicenna that can be found in Gatinaria[32] are omitted by Dubois if they have nothing to do with medical practice. On the other hand he often makes a recipe more precise, as when he recommends for example that one should change a hot compress before it gets cold. In summarizing the aspects of Dubois' work which I have tried to point out, one could say firstly that Dubois allows a place to Arabistic authors in therapy as he does in pharmacology. Secondly, his purpose was to purify and paraphrase the text to make it more readable for his own time. Thirdly, in doing this his motive was to publish a text which was needed for medical practice at the time and lastly, the text also reflects the medical practice of Dubois himself, as was the case with his pharmacological writings.

These pharmacological and therapeutical treatises of Dubois give us an impression of the medical practice of one who is mostly known as an anatomist. It is of interest to have a look finally at his dietetic treatises. There are four of these. The content of one is sufficiently indicated by its title: *Schema rerum omnium ex quibus Alimenta Hominum depromuntur, de quibus tribus libris de Alimentis Galeni disputavit.*[33] This treatise must have been one of the texts which Dubois used to teach medicine. The other three are interesting testimonies of everyday life and of social conditions in France in the sixteenth century. These are the *De Victus Ratione facili ac salubri Pauperum Scholasticorum libellus* of 1542, the *De Parco ac Duro Victu libellus*, probably of the same year, and the *Adversus Famem et Victuum Penuriam Consilium* of a few years later. The first treatise, that of 1542, is addressed to poverty-stricken scholars,[34] a class to which Dubois himself had belonged. For his origin was humble, which may have been reflected in the avarice which was one of his traits. He refused to teach until he had received his salary in advance, and even on the day of his funeral a scandal was caused by the publication of certain verses which lampooned his greed.[35] On the other hand we can see from this short dietetic treatise his sympathy with penurious scholars. These scholars very often suffered – as Dubois remarks in the preface – from serious diseases, because they followed a faulty diet and especially use medicaments at the wrong time. It was therefore Dubois' idea to write for them a convenient dietetic work so that they might better resist the causes of disease; for it is more desirable to avoid a disease than to cure it. But if after all they should be taken ill, they should not hesitate to ask the physicians which medicaments they should take to prevent the disease becoming chronic. To make the work useful to anyone who cared to follow its prescriptions, Dubois followed the daily round, from getting up to going to bed and included advice about reading precautions against chill, and advice about eating and drinking. Although Dubois' prescriptions in one way or another depend upon humoral pathology, this work is in the tradition of the *regimina sanitatis* of antiquity and still more of the middle ages. Quotations of authorities, like Mesuë or Galen, are rare. For the most part the work consists of practical hints on how to organize the course of the day: one should not get up, if the stomach is still full of undigested food from the day before; one should only put on warm clothes. Massage and frictions are useful as well as bodily exercise. If one is reading one should have a sufficient light from the left; the letters should not be too small. One should read especially Quintilian, Budé, Erasmus and Vives. The lectures of the master should be copied and repeated at home. One should always take care to keep sufficiently warm; one should wear warm clothes and shoes, the study and the library should be heated, so that it is warm enough, while the bedroom should be heated only moderately by an hypocaust. However, Dubois gives most of his attention to the right diet in a stricter sense, to food and drink; every meal should be cooked well and cut into little pieces that it may be digested well. Only inexpensive dishes should be cooked. Meat should be eaten only rarely, for it is too expensive; also one may drink beer instead of light wine, if one cannot afford wine. Bread and broth are recommended. Fish, vegetables, mostly in brine, eggs, no mushrooms, no pastry – these are Dubois' proposals for a right diet. It is very doubtful whether everything that Dubois recommends in this book would be available to a poor scholar. For – as Dubois himself says in a poem at the end of the treatise – if you want to get that desired welfare of your body, then you must have sufficient means.

In another dietetic treatise *De Parco ac Duro Victu Libellus Elegans*, probably written in the same year,[36] Dubois deals with the situation of the poor in general. He cannot give any hope of a real change in their situation to those who – as he says in his preface – suffer a hidden poverty at home out of shame or who get their subsistence out of robbery. He tries only to give them advice on how to conduct their life and preserve their health as far as it belongs to diet, to eat the right food and to have shelter against cold, so that they can endure their poverty more easily. Whether this book was likely to fulfil Dubois' hope that the poor could use it to avoid diseases, or, if taken ill, they could learn from it remedies against disease in order to survive longer in good health, is even more doubtful than in the case of his treatise for the poor scholars. What we learn from Dubois' remarks is the real situation of the French working class of this period. The most common food for the poor was bread, made of barley rather than of wheat. Most of the meals of the poor were made of bread, such as gruels made out of bread and water, of bread and milk, or at the best bread and broth or bread and beer. Sheep's blood or pig's blood boiled down with onion and fat might provide a thick soup. No meat, but only the intestines are recommended. A common meal for farmers and workmen was made from gristle, small bones, tendons and sinews minced together and cooked. In preference to water, the poor drank, instead of wine, beer, hydromel and other mixtures. But all this had a good aspect according to Dubois: the poor avoid the faulty and unhealthy nourishment of the rich by using these foods and drinks. Also, as opposed to the rich, one need not recommend bodily exercise to the poor; they are used to hard work. What they must avoid is sudden chilling, if they sweat after having finished their work, for instance by cold drinks. Dubois also gives some precautions against chill similar to those he gave to the poor scholars. How the poor could achieve all this, Dubois cannot say. More to the point is his last recommendation: that against all buffets God is the only refuge.

The poverty described here by Dubois was a problem general to this period. France, which had been a wealthy country in the fifteenth century fell under the reign of Francis I, into an increasingly deplorable economic state. Financial disaster, especially after the unsuccessful wars against Charles V and Henry VIII, which ended in 1544 and 1546 led to a situation which Dubois described in his last dietetic treatise, his *Consilium perutile adversus Famem et Victuum Penuriam.*[37] Everything grew still worse – as Dubois writes in his preface. Diseases, shortage of money and resources, the lost wars and the scarcity of foodstuffs, especially of grain, induced Dubois to attempt to advise the poor on how to improve their chances of survival. His aim is to lighten their burden so that they can regain their health, which is imperilled by all these external circumstances. Dubois knows that he cannot alter the conditions themselves. Only God who has sent these evils can help us and we must have faith that nobody without guilt is punished by God with the scourge of calamity. But Dubois cannot give the poor real hope. That is even less possible for him than in his previous dietetic treatises. So he seeks refuge in the ideas of humoral pathology. He tries to show that hunger and thirst do not have their origin in the bad situation of France, but in a disturbed equilibrium of the humours. Only in this way can he do anything about the situation or make recommendations which might alter it. For the only reason for hoping that hunger and thirst may be brought to an end is the assumption that the quantity and quality of the substance of things can regain their balance. Hence everything must be done to restore equilibrium to the elements – solid, humid, and gaseous – and to their attributes – dry and wet, warm and cold, thick and thin. Therefore Dubois recommends for instance stopping up the pores of the body and removing excessive heat by dietetic methods in general, avoiding sweet foods such as sugar and seeking refrigeration. One must try, if possible, to live only on gaseous, not on humid and solid food. The examples which Dubois gives verge on the incredible.

His assertion that there were in Germany people of a melancholic quality who could live without any food and drink or who lived only on perfumes, shows how desperately low food production in France must have been at that time. The only thing that Dubois can advise is to take nothing else than drinks, for which he gives detailed dietetic prescriptions. He mentions water with different aromatic admixtures, the mixtures themselves, buttermilk, blood, bran-water, and if possible wine. Because weakness and fatigue of the stomach follow this sort of nourishment, one must sleep and avoid every form of bodily exercise. This humoral-pathological approach of Dubois merely shows that he did not know of any way by which the situation of misery and distress in France at that time could be improved. In his first two treatises for poor scholars and for the poor in general, Dubois could still give the impression that if the outward situation was not too bad, dietetic measures could have some success. Now the outward situation must have become so bad, that it was only possible for him to retire to a theoretical position which no longer had anything to do either with reality or with medical practice.

To summarize, Dubois, generally known as an arch-Galenist, an anatomist and as an academic, can be seen as a practitioner of the same kind as his contemporaries in his pharmacology and therapy. For the renaissance of Galenism in sixteenth-century Paris, of which Dubois was a notable representative, could not suffice for him when he turned to the actual practice of medicine. As a practitioner Dubois was able to frame a pharmacology and therapeutics of his own, consisting of elements of medieval Arabist medicine as well as of those of the new Galenic medicine. The limits and possibilities of the renaissance of Galenism in the sixteenth century in Paris become still clearer when we look at his dietetic treatises. While it had been possible for Dubois by making a synthesis of medieval and renaissance medicine to arrive at a system of pharmacology and therapy suitable for medical practice, he did not improve dietetics in a similar way. His recommendations, which stand in the tradition of the medieval *regimina*, reflect only the universally bad situation of the poor in France in the sixteenth century and it is doubtful whether any real alteration of that situation was possible. It was therefore inevitable that as the economic situation grew still worse from 1545 onward he had recourse to a merely theoretical humoral pathology remote from any practical application.

8

The 'Paris Hippocratics': teaching and research in Paris in the second half of the sixteenth century

IAIN M. LONIE

The rest led the uneventful life of academics, lectured, annotated, read much and (with a few exceptions) wrote little. They still lead a shadowy life in their prefaces and are duly recorded in the pious tributes of local historians and bibliographers

Richard J. Durling, *A chronological census of renaissance editions and translations of Galen.*

Just as the University of Paris was the largest in Europe in the sixteenth century so too was its Faculty of Medicine. It was also prestigious, and, through the large number of foreign students who attended it, influential outside France. Yet the men who taught medicine at Paris during the century and who determined the direction, preoccupations, and tone of medical teaching there have on the whole a very small place in history books and biographical dictionaries. This fact causes no problems for those whose interest in the history of medicine at this time is primarily in anatomy and who see Paris as the stronghold of a reactionary Galenism: it is appropriate that reactionaries should be sterile, obscure, and small. These Paris Galenists are suitable predecessors of the men who refused to accept Harvey's demonstration, or who were satirized by Molière for their unintelligent pedantry. But whatever we may think of Paris medicine in the seventeenth century, in the sixteenth at least its teachers were men of great eminence not merely in their own and their pupils' estimation, but in that of outsiders as well.[1] And this admiration extended into the next two centuries. Giorgio Baglivi, pupil and assistant of Malpighi and himself a devoted experimental investigator of the new anatomy, a man who was in regular correspondence with the most progressive spirits of his age, praised the Parisians of the previous century for their progressive attitude.

155

For although, as he says with befitting patriotism, it was the Italians who were the first to 'shake off the yoke of Arabic medicine', they were

followed by the French, and, above all others from the noble Academy of the Parisians, Duret, Baillou, Houllier, Jacot etc. (who) . . . turned all their energies to the restoration of the pristine wisdom of the Greeks in medicine . . . By planting out this doctrine in almost all the universities of Europe they stimulated other scholars of the time to enlarging it and confirming it.[2]

Not petty and obscure reactionaries, then, but mighty spirits who determined the tendencies of an age. And Baglivi confirms his expressed admiration for these men by frequent quotation from their works.[3] Baglivi's judgement was echoed by the historian Sprengel, who set these same men in an impressive historical contest in which they, with kindred spirits in Italy and Germany, joined forces to defeat medieval barbarism and darkness. It was, wrote Sprengel of such men, the spirit of Hippocrates which inspired them to accomplish 'the restoration of good taste and judgement'[4] in medicine. The two results of this revolution in taste were actual changes in therapy and a new interest in observation which was prompted by the reading of Hippocrates' *Epidemics*.[5] The enthusiasm of Baglivi and Sprengel echoes, while placing in a new interpretative context, the enthusiasm of sixteenth-century contemporaries who regarded the teaching of these men as something rare, precious, and new.

The men whom Baglivi names, Houllier, Duret, and Baillou, and with whom I shall be concerned in this chapter, published practically nothing in their lifetimes, and their fame did not depend upon the publication of their work which came later and was a consequence of that fame. In other words they were felt to be great men by their admirers because of their teaching or the research work which they communicated in teaching. But when we look at their posthumously published writings, the testimony and reflection of this teaching, we find it, unless we are profoundly and perhaps perversely addicted to such material, very dry and unpalatable stuff. That is, if we are looking in it for the great ideas of medical history. For it is hard, matter of fact, bread and butter commentary on the most routine and technical matters of pathology and therapy. It is practical medicine (which sixteenth-century writers defined as diagnosis, prognosis, and therapy), an area which we find particularly inaccessible because of its detail and because of a lack of ready-made questions which might give us entry to it. This was not so for earlier historians: Baglivi and later, Sprengel, still read the work of the Parisians for practical purposes, and the practical issues which that work raised were quite clear-cut and very much alive for them. Thus Sprengel, as an historian, was able to give a masterly account (upon which everyone has depended since) of the early sixteenth-century Brissot controversy about bloodletting, partly because as a doctor he practised a medicine in which bloodletting was regularly used and could be justified.[6]

That kind of access is not available to us, and would not necessarily be an advantage, although it was the main reason why historians from Le Clerc to Sprengel wrote histories of medicine. But without some kind of access to practical medicine and its teaching we are in danger of ending with a history of medicine which includes everything except the craft of medicine itself. In the case of teaching it is worth trying to see what it was that such men as the Parisians taught, what their aims were and why they thought they had achieved them; and what it was about their work that inspired enthusiasm for it among their pupils. I confess that I do not yet properly see how this can be done, for all those welcome but rare moments when one's historical imagination has let one in by a back door to a clamorous sixteenth-century lecture hall; and this paper is intended only to convey a few impressions which I have gained by reading the published works of these men. I have not investigated any manuscript sources, if they exist; nor have I gone, except in a general way, into questions of institutional history. It is of course important to be aware that throughout the sixteenth century, as in earlier and later centuries, the Paris faculty waged unremitting war upon outsiders of all kinds – non-academic practitioners, mountebanks and charlatans. The writers whom I examine and the students who edited their work frequently draw attention to these matters, and they represent their own scholarly and university-based medicine as the only protection against pernicious error.[7] Thus the heavy investment of their work in linguistic and scholarly skills might be partly explained as a response to institutional and social pressures. I shall not however be concerned with this important aspect in this chapter, but instead I shall try to characterize the work itself and to suggest some reasons for its popularity and success.

The men named by Baglivi and Sprengel were successive in time and in training: Louis Duret was the most eminent among a number of pupils of Jacques Houllier, all of whom carried on his work, while Guillaume de Baillou was a pupil of Duret. I confess that my initial interest in these men was prompted by their special relation to Hippocrates, but as it turns out this relation does not make them untypical of Paris medicine. Instead, it was due to the tone which they set that for a time in Paris medicine and *doctrina Hippocratica* were synonymous. They gave a special meaning to that 'medicine of Galen and Hippocrates' which was a shibboleth to most faculties of medicine, and it was a Parisian, Maurice de La Corde, who was the first as far as I know to use in print the word 'Hippocratism' to express an ideal standard to which medicine should aspire.

Jacques Houllier, the first of these men, was born around 1510, as I infer from statements that he 'flourished' in 1550 and that his death in 1562 was regarded as premature, and from the fact that he graduated as bachelor in 1534 and as doctor in 1536.[8] From his graduation to his death his name appears regularly in the minutes of the meetings of the faculty, of which he was dean in 1546 and 1547. He was appointed one of the two ordinary lecturers in the faculty in November 1538, and seems to have taught publicly as well as privately from then on.

Houllier received his medical education at a time in which Paris was the centre of the industry of editing and translating the classics of Greek medicine, especially Galen, although the scholars who were most active in this industry were gradually disappearing from the scene. Wilhelm Kopp had died in 1532 and had ceased teaching for some time before that; Guenther of Andernach left Paris in 1537; Jacques Dubois however was still active, and so was Jean Vasses, who died in 1550. Houllier was unlike these men in that he did not himself edit and translate Greek texts.[9] But he shared their values and their belief that a return to the Greek classics was the only way to end uncertainty and error in the practice of medicine. His pupils testify to this belief and to Houllier's brilliance in interpreting Greek medicine.[10] The teaching in which this brilliance was displayed is represented principally by three posthumous works: his practical lectures, published as *De Morbis Internis*, and his two commentaries upon the Hippocratic texts *Coan Prognoses* and *Aphorisms*.

Houllier's own work seems to have served as a focus for the work of those who possessed copies of his notes or transcripts of his lectures.[11] This is illustrated by the publishing history of his lectures on internal diseases. These were first published in 1565, along with other minor works, three years after his death, by two former pupils, Didier or Desidère Jacot and Christophe Bourgeois, under the title *De Morborum Curatione*.[12] These two men shared lodgings in Paris in the winter of 1564/65 and among other things attended the lectures of Louis Duret, the most eminent of Houllier's pupils. The project of publishing Houllier's work seems to have grown out of this association.[13] The 1565 publication consisted of Houllier's very brief and schematic treatment of each internal disease in top to toe order, of which the largest part is recipes, supplemented by more discursive scholia on each disease which Jacot represented as his own. This work was republished in 1567 by another of Houllier's pupils, Antoine Valet,[14] this time with the addition of material taken from Duret's lectures – presumably those which Jacot and Bourgeois had attended – on practical medicine. What is interesting here is Valet's statement that Duret had actually chosen Houllier as a text to lecture upon. In Valet's 1567 edition and in a new edition which he published in 1571,[15] the material taken from Duret's lectures appears only in the form of brief marginalia glossing words used by Houllier.[16] In the 1571 edition, for which he wrote a new introduction, Valet claimed that the scholia published by Jacot as his own in 1565 were in fact taken from Houllier's lectures, as Valet had discovered when he came across them in an autograph manuscript.[17] The layout of this 1571 edition consists of Houllier's brief text on each disease, giving its name, its symptoms, and a list of recipes, all without explanatory discussion, followed by Houllier's more discursive scholia, which discuss and explain symptoms and treatment; these are followed in turn by Valet's own *enarratio* or commentary upon the text. The margins are embellished with the brief notes taken from Duret's lectures.

Neither the form nor the content of Houllier's work clearly reveals to us why it should have been reprinted so often (including one version published without Houllier's name in 1565 by Caspar Wolf), nor why his lectures should have aroused so much enthusiasm. The recipes which form such a large part of his formal treatment of each disease seem to be fairly traditional. Indeed Sprengel criticized him for retaining so much from the Arabs in his prescriptions.[18] Presumably we should look in the more discursive scholia for evidence of Houllier's attractiveness as a teacher. These represent the moments when Houllier, having satisfied formal requirements, felt free to expatiate in a less formal way on each disease, giving his students the benefit of a wide knowledge of classical authorities, of his own practical experience, and of that ability to convey the essence of a matter with memorable simplicity and clarity which is the talent of a good teacher.

Houllier's pupils praised him for his knowledge of the classical sources, and it may have been this aspect of his teaching which struck them most forcibly and made them feel that they were getting something much better than was available from other expositions of practical medicine. In his scholia Houllier does quote very extensively from the ancient sources: mainly from the Hippocratic *Aphorisms*, which were of course not new in the teaching of practical medicine, but also from other Hippocratic works such as the *Epidemics* (apart from *Epidemics* 6), which were new, and from Aëtius, Paul of Aegina, and Alexander of Tralles, whose works had become available only recently. He quoted and discussed Greek words, and demonstrated their relevance to the students' understanding of the matter in question. For example in chapter 47 of Book 1 ('retention of urine')[19] he discusses in his scholium the Greek terms *strangouria*, *ischouria*, and *dysouria*, which were applied to various forms of this condition, and explains the differences between them. Houllier states that his distinctions are based upon many passages in Galen, and he accuses a recent commentator upon the *Aphorisms* (Leonhard Fuchs) of a serious confusion between *strangouria* and *dysouria*. We must never, he says solemnly, confuse the words of the ancients in this way. He goes on to discuss the differential cause of these conditions. In this example, lexical distinctions depending upon a wide knowledge of the Greek sources are directly applied to practical medicine as diagnostic concepts, to yield a practical knowledge *which was not to be obtained in any other way*. This, as we shall see, was the essence of Parisian practical medicine.

Houllier's general approach to the exposition of a disease may conveniently be illustrated from his discussion of apoplexy in book one, chapter

seven of *De Morbis Internis.*[20] His text begins with treatment, and he gives
a long list of prescriptions. After this practical beginning, he discusses the
disease in more general terms in his scholium. He begins with the
observation – which we, as perhaps did Houllier's students, perceive as a
Hippocratic touch – that it is likely to occur in a 'cold and southerly
constitution of the air'. He supports this observation by referring to a
number of individual cases in his own experience, with names or other
identifying circumstances: one of these cases is from the year 1545. He then
describes different varieties of apoplexy, and their causes. For treatment he
recommends bleeding, referring to dissensions in this matter between
Arab and other writers. The Arabs prefer to bleed from a small vein, and
one which is remote from the head, the seat of the condition. Houllier
disagrees. But he does commend the Arab practice of bleeding from the
jugulars, although he expresses caution because of the danger of haemorrhage.

What Houllier says about apoplexy may not be startlingly different
from what one might find in the lectures on practical medicine of other
teachers of the same period. We, of course, notice the reference to the
weather and the adducing of individual cases, especially if we have been
reading historians who share Sprengel's view that the influence of the
case-histories in the Hippocratic *Epidemics* was crucial to the development
of sixteenth-century medicine. But it may have been quite other aspects,
not apparent to us, which moved the enthusiasm of Houllier's audience. It
is not easy to find words to describe the differences between sitting in a
stuffy room and sitting in the same room after the windows have been
opened, but for all that the difference is real enough.

We are faced with the same interpretative difficulty over Houllier's
commentary upon the *Aphorisms.*[21] In the eyes of contemporaries Houllier's Hippocratic commentaries were his finest achievement. He commented, according to Valet, on *Aphorisms, Coan Prognoses, Prognostics,* and
Epidemics, although only the first two were ever published.[22] The commentary upon the *Aphorisms* was published by another pupil, Jean
Liébault,[23] in 1582. Liébault had obtained an autograph of Houllier's
commentary from Alexis Gaudin, a former pupil of Houllier, who was
now a royal physician. Liébault edited this manuscript, adding extensive
scholia for which, as he says in his dedication, he drew upon the lectures of
Louis Duret, also adding his own comments. Thus the commentary on the
Aphorisms has the same composite and inbred form as that of the books on
internal diseases.

Houllier's commentary is one of a recognizable group of 'modern'
commentaries upon the *Aphorisms,* of which the first to be published was
that of the Flandrian Jérémie Dryvère, who had been educated and became
Professor at Louvain (book one, 1538; the remaining books in 1551),
followed by those of A. M. Brasavola (1541) and Leonhard Fuchs (1544).[24]

At least some parts of Houllier's commentary are later than that of Fuchs, to which he refers frequently, but then Houllier might have taught the *Aphorisms* at any time in his career, and he probably did so more than once.

Dryvère, Brasavola, and Fuchs explicitly contrast their commentaries with the scholastic ones of Taddeo Alderotti, Jacopo da Forlì, and Ugo Benzi. They condemn these commentators for their 'barbarous' Latin, for their ignorance of 'good', that is to say Greek, authorities, and because they overloaded their commentaries with irrelevant 'dialectic', by which they mean the formal discussion of *quaestiones*.[25] Houllier himself did not compose a preface in which he might have drawn attention to the absence of these undesirable things from his commentary; it would however have been very clear to his contemporaries in Paris, where Jacopo's commentary was still read.[26] He in fact succeeds better than Brasavola or Fuchs in producing an uncluttered, straightforward, and practical exposition of the text. This exposition is clearly directed to the needs of the young and inexperienced student of medicine. Through his comments Houllier introduces him, avoiding all unnecessary complication, to the basic principles of purging, venesection, and diet, which he illustrates by devising simple imaginary examples. In reading Houllier's comments on particular aphorisms it is easy to forget the elaborate treatment given to these same aphorisms by the earlier scholastic commentators, especially when Houllier manages to cover the same points in much briefer compass and simpler style. This simplicity however does not preclude the discussion of Greek words, their meanings and distinctions of meaning, which here again is a prominent feature of Houllier's approach, and which he uses, as he does in *De Morbis Internis*, to establish practical distinctions in diagnosis and therapy.

Apart from his excellent teaching method, Houllier's comments convey a striking sense of the relevance of Hippocratic medicine to the future practical needs of the modern student. Houllier is able to do this precisely because he is conscious of the geographical, chronological and historical differences between the situation of the Hippocratic author and that of his audience, who will be practising in the Paris region in the mid-sixteenth century, confronting diseases which often behave differently from their counterparts in Hippocrates, and possessing modern means of therapy. Houllier is sensitive to environmental, particularly climatic, factors, and he often uses these to account for disparities between Hippocratic statements and modern experience.[27] These variables are indeed the means by which Hippocratic medical practice can be adjusted to modern practice. There is a typical example in Houllier's comment on *Aphorisms* 1, 2. After mentioning an observation of Galen and Asclepiades that at Rome and Athens, which face south, venesection is bad for pleuritic cases, while in Paros and the Hellespont, which have a northerly aspect, it is good, Houllier remarks that the physicians of Narbonne and Lyons blame the

Paris physicians for using venesection too freely: 'but in Paris men tolerate venesection easily, because Paris is exposed to winds from the North'.[28] Regional and climatic co-ordinates help, as it were, to locate sixteenth-century Paris in the map of the ancient world. I put it in this way, because there is an eager tendency discernible in Houllier's pupils to identify themselves with the ancients: to emulate them in their writing, to see themselves in ancient rôles, and to assume analogies between the Paris faculty and Hippocrates' school of Cos. Such identification with the ancient world, which simultaneously implies a consciousness of historical distance, can no doubt be paralleled in other areas of French cultural, especially literary, life. There are indeed links between these Parisian doctors and the world of literature, and they may be looked for in the poems, written in Greek as well as in Latin, which ornament the preliminary pages of the most technical medical publications.

Houllier's other surviving Hippocratic commentary, that upon *Coan Prognoses*, was edited and published by Didier Jacot in 1576, in a bulky folio volume of over 1200 pages.[29] The bulk was provided by Jacot's scholia which, as we are told elsewhere, plagiarized material from Louis Duret, who also lectured on this text. Houllier's own comments are quite terse.[30]

This Hippocratic text, *Coan Prognoses*, is of great importance for an understanding of the aims of the Parisians and an appreciation of the kind of medicine which they thought valuable. Both the text itself, and their work upon it, were at the very heart of their endeavour. This work seems to have occupied various members of the group over a period of twenty years. It was inaugurated by Houllier, and was carried on after his death; it was Houllier's pupil Louis Duret who was responsible for the final product, a new text, translation, and commentary. It was a work quite new to the syllabus: no medieval Latin translation is recorded, and the Greek text was a renaissance discovery. Galen had written no commentary upon it, and indeed spoke slightingly of the work: in elucidating it therefore the Parisians had to rely almost entirely[31] upon their own knowledge of Hippocrates and Galen and of the principles of Galenic commentary. It was a daunting task, and one for which there was no immediately obvious motive. An answer to the question why, in that case, they invested so heavily in it, leads us to the heart of Paris medicine. The answer must be sought in the nature of the text itself.

Coan Prognoses[32] is an unorganized collection of 'sentences' (*sententiae*), which describe clusters of signs and symptoms, and state what these clusters forecast (prognosis in the modern sense), or the condition which they indicate, or other symptoms which are likely to occur along with such clusters. The two latter kinds of statement are included in the Greek sense of prognosis, which like prophecy was an insight into 'things which are and are to be and things which were before'. There are over six hundred of these clusters and together they comprise almost all the symptoms and conditions known to Hippocratic medicine. A considerable number of them are found in other Hippocratic texts as well, especially *Prognostics*, *Aphorisms*, and *Prorrhetics*.

There were two ways in which a commentator might approach such clusters. He might simply accept them as statements of empirical fact, or he might attempt to find causal explanations of their concurrence. Galen's policy in commenting upon the three texts named above was to search in humoral theory for explanations why such signs should occur together, and why they should signify what they were claimed to signify. Where he was unable to find such a causal explanation, he condemned the cluster as a particular and accidental combination of signs, the result of inexperienced observation, and therefore probably not written down by Hippocrates who was interested in setting down only truly universal combinations, such as could be justified by causal reasoning. This assumption of Galen was part of his belief that Hippocrates was a 'rational' physician, and of his campaign against the empirical school who explained all such Hippocratic sentences as the result of repeated observation, for which no causal justification need or could be found.[33] This Galenic version of Hippocrates was accepted without question by the Parisians, as indeed it was by all sixteenth century medical writers with the notable exception of the Paracelsians. The Galenic procedure of connecting and explaining symptoms by reference to humoral theory was, moreover, a regular part of giving an account of a disease, whether in a textbook or in a *consilium*. Hence to comment upon *Coan Prognoses* would not have seemed to the Parisians a philological activity peripheral to the main business of teaching practical medicine: it was that business.

The reason the Parisians were so interested in this particular Hippocratic work – in editing and translating its Greek and making it accessible, through a commentary, as it had never been before – can be seen in the terms in which they describe the work. They refer to it as a 'storehouse', 'repository', 'treasury' (*thesaurus*) of medical experience and lore.[34] They accepted the tradition embodied in the title that these sentences were the collected experience of Hippocrates' pupils and associates, the 'masters' of Cos. Ancient wisdom of such provenance was likely to be invaluable, and it was important to recover it for the modern world. So the Parisians set about the task of bringing its riches to the surface, in defiance of the disparagement of the work by Galen. In undertaking this task, the Parisians may have been piqued by fancied resemblances between the corporate endeavour of the school of Cos and their own faculty. Louis Duret, in commenting upon one passage, criticizes the 'masters' (*magistri*) of Cos for not setting down a prognosis 'distinctly or appositely enough to agree with the intention of their teacher who wrote it'.[35] That some works attributed to Hippocrates had actually been written by him as notes, but arranged, edited, and published by his successors had been a commonplace of criticism since Galen. Duret here gives a contemporary twist to this belief. The *Coan Prognoses* are Hippocrates' lecture notes, published after his death by his colleagues and pupils on the faculty – as had happened to the commentaries of Houllier, Duret's own teacher. Anuce Foes, who had also been pupil to Houllier and whom Houllier had employed to hunt out variant readings in manuscripts, wrote a long separate introduction to *Coan Prognoses* in his edition of the collected works of Hippocrates. In it he associates the corporate nature of *Coan Prognoses* with the idea of a treasury of medical lore. The wealth of the treasury is explained by the fact that so many have contributed. Foes extends this idea to the corpus as a whole: it is 'a most complete encyclopaedia of the art of medicine' precisely because so many able men were adopted into the Asclepiad family and contributed to its composition. Foes' conception of the Hippocratic corpus as an *encyclopaedia* which, if properly arranged as he claimed to have done in his edition, could be transported into the sickroom and used as the basis of practice, was a novel idea. But it is easy to see how it might have grown up in the Paris environment in which Foes was trained.[36]

In his dedication to Houllier's commentary on *Coan Prognoses* (1576) Jacot states that Houllier had decided 'twenty years back' (1556) to be the first to comment on this work. This date is supported by a reference by Anuce Foes in 1560 to work which Houllier had already done upon the text,[37] and perhaps also by the publication in 1557 by the Parisian scholar-printer Guillaume Morel of the Greek text. This had hitherto been available only in the Aldine edition of 1526 or in Cornarius' Froben edition of 1538. Morel printed Cornarius' text, with corrections, in a utilitarian selection of texts without introductory matter. The edition was clearly aimed at students, and perhaps intended to meet a sudden new demand.[38]

Houllier's comments are brief and reveal little about the nature of the work he had done upon *Coan Prognoses*.[39] His work was carried on by his most eminent pupil, Louis Duret. It is not altogether clear, although probable, that Houllier lectured upon the text. But Duret certainly did, in 1570, and it was from these lectures that, according to Duret's son, Jacot pilfered material.[40]

Louis Duret (1527–86) had been awarded his doctorate in 1552, and apparently taught continuously from that time until his death.[41] His pupil and devout admirer Maurice de La Corde, writing in 1585, describes him as lecturing upon Hippocrates thirty years before, and states that he himself was his pupil for five years from 1558.[42] Duret was lecturing on Houllier's *Internal Diseases* at least before 1567, on the Hippocratic *Humours* and *Regimen in Acute Diseases* in 1565 and 1566, and, as we have seen, on *Coan Prognoses* in 1570.[43] He was appointed Professor at the Collège Royale in 1568. Duret's knowledge of Hippocrates was legendary, and he earned the nickname, given to Fernel before him, of 'The Hippocrates of France'.[44]

Like Houllier, Duret earned his eminence by teaching, not by writing. According to René Chartier, his time was so preoccupied by teaching and practice that he had no leisure to write. His students, says Chartier, published his teaching as their own, and there are many works in print today on anatomy, aetiology, prognosis and therapy, and many comments on Hippocratic texts which, if they were stripped of all that rightfully belongs to Duret, would excite ridicule by the paltriness of the remainder.[45] All that was published after his death, apart from his commentary upon *Coan Prognoses*, were his lectures on Houllier's *Internal Diseases*, and the commentaries on *Humours* and *Regimen in Acute Diseases*. The latter two works were not published until 1631.[46]

These are all practical works. It seems to have been Duret's way to use the exposition of Hippocratic texts for the teaching of practical medicine, and for establishing correct principles of practice. This was certainly his approach to the Hippocratic *Regimen in Acute Diseases*: that work, he pointed out, is not about diet, which serves merely as an example to illustrate the author's main theme. That theme is a basic principle of therapy, the principle of treating each individual appropriately. Duret comments on the text in such a way as to bring out and develop this principle.[47] Antoine Valet in 1567 hoped for practical fruits from the eventual publication of Duret's works

. . . so that the method (*ratio*) of practising medicine, now wrapped in Cimmerian darkness in the obscure books of the ancients as in the confused compilations of the moderns, may yet return to us in all its original dignity, and we may no longer wander blind, troubled, and in ignorance of what leader to follow. Then we shall leave the desolate wilderness of the Arabs . . . and with Duret as our sole guide, come at last to the trim and pleasant gardens of Hippocrates and Galen, where it shall be our pleasure to enjoy more solid fruits.[48]

The solid fruit of practice is the end of elucidation. The philologically minded Parisians always began with the word, because they believed that this was the most direct way of getting to the deed. Duret's most ambitious work, the elucidation of *Coan Prognoses*, was aimed at just such solid fruits.

Although Duret frequently emends the Greek text, and makes a new translation (the two existing ones were by Calvus, whose manuscripts did not contain the full text, and Cornarius) the purpose of his commentary is not primarily philological, and he does not discuss variant readings often. He makes very clear, both in his general remarks about *Coan Prognoses* and in his comments on individual sentences, that he values the work for its practical applications. Describing its purposes at the beginning of his first comment he says

It was Hippocrates' intention, or rather that of his disciples, who set down as many as possible of their teacher's riches and ornaments in this most ample and august theatre of medicine, first of all to explain all the manifestations which accompany fever, and after these, those of all other diseases.[49]

But the point of building up a complete picture of disease through such description and explanation is practical. In another passage he writes

Here our author considered it his duty to explain the diseases of the hypochondria, from which the causes behind these signs are derived, and to disclose the nature, symptoms, periods, paroxysms, and crises of such diseases. And indeed this passage brings wonderful returns in knowledge for procuring the indications of diagnosis, prognosis, and therapy, which are the three obligations of the physician in the exercise of healing.[50]

The way in which *Coan Prognoses* can, in Duret's belief, be used as a guide to practice is abundantly illustrated by his comments. These are necessarily long and elaborate, since Duret's method of explanation requires discussion of the meanings of Greek words and reference to many other passages. At the beginning of each of the sections into which he divides the text, Duret usually expounds the general significance and the various senses and divisions of the symptom which is discussed in that section (for example the meaning of *apoplexia* and its differences from *paraplegia* or from *paralysis*),[51] or the normal functions of the part of the body which is the subject of that section (for example the liver, in the section on hepatic symptoms). He then discusses, usually very extensively, the individual components of each sentence, explaining the causes which produce the symptoms and which make them occur together. This discussion is often illustrated with cases drawn both from the Hippocratic *Epidemics* and from Duret's own practice. Analysis of the Greek words is an essential part of the exposition.

Some of these characteristics of Duret's commentary are illustrated by his comment on book two, chapter twenty-three, 2.[52] The *sententia* to be explained reads

Those who lose control over the body after a wound recover, if fever without rigor supervenes. If fever does not supervene, they become apoplectic either on the right side or on the left.

Duret's commentary upon this is, typically, long and exhaustive, and the following is a precis of his argument with much illustrative material and repetition omitted.

In this prognosis, writes Duret, Hippocrates deals with apoplexy arising from external as opposed to internal causes. The kinds of external cause are classified by Hippocrates in a passage in *De Morbis* 4. According to that classification, *wounds* are in question in the present passage, especially wounds in the head. The word *akratees* ('without control') means those whose bodies are no longer governed by the animal faculty and animal spirit. This is because of a laxity (*atonia*) in the brain, the origin of the nerves, caused by an excess of moisture. Hippocrates recognizes this cause, for example in *Aphorisms* 3, 5, when he speaks of southerly winds (which are always wet) as 'stupefying and relaxing'. Confirmation of this interpretation is found in the symptoms of an ardent fever which, according to Hippocrates in *Epidemics* 3, 2, occurred in a pestilential constitution characterized by southerly weather: 'about the time of the exacerbations there was loss of memory with *aphesis* and loss of voice' (*Epidemics*, 3, 6), where Galen in his commentary upon *Epidemics* 3 glosses the word *aphesis* as 'a resolution and relaxation of all parts, like what happens to paralytic cases'. By 'fever' in the present passage Hippocrates means an acute fever, which is caused by bile, and bile is hot and dry. A fever arising from any other cause would only make the patient's condition worse. And the reason why he specifies that there should be no rigor, is that symptomatic rigor would be a sign of empyema in the wound, and this of course would be fatal. But when Hippocrates says that these cases *recover* if they have a fever, this creates a difficulty, for according to his book *Wounds in the Head*, the fever which arises as a consequence of a wound in the head is invariably fatal. However, there is a way of preserving the authority of the present prognosis, and this is as follows. The symptoms which Hippocrates describes in *Wounds in the Head* are all a consequence of inflammation in the brain; but that is not the case here, where the cause of the loss of control is, as we have seen, a cold distemper in the brain, along with excessive moistening of the nerves. 'Hence', Duret concludes, 'an acute fever vigorously attacks both causes of the loss of control, namely oppression of the brain and excessive moisture'. The fever, being hot and dry (bile) dries the moisture out.

In this deft exposition, Duret's main concern is to give a rational justification of the prognosis, and thus to preserve its credit or 'authority' as a truthful and valuable observation. The store of medical knowledge is to that extent increased, which satisfies the purpose of his commentary. But of course his commentary is also an interesting (though in this case fairly easy) exercise in the application of humoral theory, enjoyable for the writer and instructive for the reader. Due attention is paid to the meanings of Greek words; and the Hippocratic *Epidemics*, a difficult work recently made accessible, is referred to as a valuable source of observed fact. What Duret is teaching in the whole passage is not antiquarian philology but practical medicine, and it could hardly be better done.

In another passage Duret spells out the implications for therapy. *Sententia* 2 of book two, section on haemorrhages, reads

It is a bad sign for haemorrhage to occur on the opposite side (*anapalin*: literally 'backwards' or 'contrariwise'), as, in the case of a large spleen, on the right side. And similarly in the hypochondria.[53]

Duret's commentary begins

This prognosis puts an end to all controversy over the place of withdrawing blood for the retraction of a vigorous flux and the detraction of a flux which has come to a halt in systrophic tumours of the thorax and hypochondria. For if operations which are undertaken fittingly and under the guidance of nature afford the physician an artifice for the imitation of nature herself, it plainly follows that if haemorrhage *kat' ixin* ('on the same side' or 'in the same direction') is considered to be a good thing on that score, while the opposite is considered to be a fault, we should imitate the former and not the latter in withdrawing blood. Therefore we should cut the vein *kat' ixin*, not *anapalin* ('on the opposite side') . . .

Duret then refers to a longstanding dispute over the meaning of *kat' ixin*, which goes back to the days of the Brissot controversy over bloodletting,[54] and justifies his own translation of the word *anapalin*, on which his whole interpretation of the passage depends, by adducing two passages from the *Epidemics*. Later in his comment, Duret applies the sentence about the spleen to a practical issue which was very much alive in his own time: the question of from which site one should draw blood in the treatment of pleurisy.

Now if anyone should object that blood resides in the veins and heart only, and nowhere else, and therefore cannot be drawn from anywhere else, and that there is no vein extending from the spleen to the parts on the left side, because the liver is the origin of all the veins, then let him know that when nature is well-ordered, and especially when maturation of the splenous tumor is still incomplete, whence the blood is thinner, this blood is rapidly driven into the greater veins on the side of the affected spleen . . . Away then with the arrogance of Vesalius, who obstinately maintains that the basilic vein of the right arm should be opened in all cases of pleurisy. For there is greater force for propulsion in the distension of the part affected than there is in the situation of the veins.[55]

Duret returns to the question of bloodletting at the end of book two, where he describes the last *sententia* in the book as a 'caution against bloodletting', actually emending the text to give it the meaning he wishes, and preaching a sermon, always closely related to the text, against the indiscriminate use of venesection.[56]

Duret's commentary upon *Coan Prognoses* helps us to define the Parisian ideal as erudition in the service of practice – practice comprising, as Duret says in a passage quoted earlier, diagnosis, prognosis, and therapy. We can see too from Duret's commentary how extensive that erudition was required to be. Duret was reputed to know Galen and Hippocrates by heart, which may well have been approximately true. It was certainly necessary for him to be able to lay his hand upon the right passage in order to resolve a particular difficulty. But of course it was his critical acumen which led him to the right passage in the first place. And the word 'critical' leads us to the question of what kind of work this is, and what the criteria were for judging its success. How did the Parisians know a good piece of research in the field of practical medicine when they saw it? The answer can hardly lie in the test of successful practice, although – naturally – the

Parisians did believe that they were better practitioners, and taught better practitioners, than anyone else. The answer is rather that they judged their own and each others' work much as we judge the work of a critic of literature or the arts. We are disposed to trust the critic's judgement according to the measure of his knowledge, his personal experience or personal commitment to the subject, and his dexterity and sensitivity in bringing both these factors to bear upon a problem.

These are qualities which are manifest in the work of Guillaume de Baillou. Baillou clearly enjoyed his own intellectual virtuosity, and displayed it, for his own satisfaction, in his written work. He was also a poet who could turn out a set of hendecasyllabics quite as accomplished as those written by his poetic contemporaries;[57] and in the work of this contemporary of Montaigne[58] medical writing shows a tendency to become a form of *belles-lettres*.

Guillaume de Baillou[59] was born in 1538 and died in 1616; he is said to have been a pupil of Houllier himself, which is just possible; he was certainly taught by Duret. He graduated as bachelor in 1568 and as doctor in 1570; he was dean in 1580 and 1581, and had a successful career both at university and at court. He actively opposed a sustained attempt by the surgeons of Paris to achieve autonomy within the university, and this campaign produced the only work which Baillou published in his lifetime, a pamphlet against the surgeons.[60] The rest of his works were published posthumously by his nephew Jacques Thévart between 1635 and 1643. They consist of a work in two books of which the short title is *Epidemiorum et Ephemeridum libri duo* ('Epidemics and daybooks, two volumes'), a lexical work called *Definitiones Medicae*, three books of *Consilia*, a book on women's diseases, an essay on convulsions, a commentary on Theophrastus' *De Vertigine*, and various other medical *opuscula*.[61] Why Baillou did not publish these works himself is a mystery. They are clearly written for publication, and for some of them he composed dedications at the time of writing.

Patriotism and positivism alike have directed attention to the books on epidemics. Baillou is described in the standard biographical article as a precursor of Sydenham, in being inspired by Hippocrates to observe and record epidemic 'constitutions' and in studying the connection between atmospheric conditions and the diseases prevalent at a particular time.[62] While these statements are true in themselves, the *rapprochement* with Sydenham (who never mentions Baillou) is subtly misleading and suggests an imprecise reading of Baillou's work. We can get a more accurate impression by reading the *Epidemics* in the light of his other writings: his essays and his *Consilia*.

To begin with a fundamental matter, the 'Epidemics and day-books' of the title page is an editor's title and merely reproduces the beginning of a list of contents which Baillou gave in the proem which he composed for his work, in Greek as well as in Latin: 'Epidemics, day-books, appendices, observations, questions of note, and miscellanies'.[63] As we shall see, it is the miscellaneous and informal character of the work which is significant. Baillou himself emphasized the epidemic constitutions, but regarded their value as prognostic. He explained his intentions in an address to the reader written for the first book and dated October 1574 (at that time he apparently intended to publish the work himself). He wished, he writes, to provide an historical record which would give physicians

a knowledge of the progress of preceding and succeeding times and seasons, so that when a disease of this or that character befalls, they will not say that anything new has occurred, and be terrified by the advance and appearance of new diseases, as though by some unknown monster.[64]

Baillou makes this prognostic intention even clearer in his proem:

Since the character and dispositions of diseases . . . are easily discovered by us from observation of antecedent and present times and seasons, and since we derive according to that rule the principal factors of diagnosis, prognosis, and indeed of treatment, therefore is that physician base and unworthy of his function who has not taken these factors into account.[65]

– a passage which Baillou continues by underlining the importance of prognosis for the physician's reputation. These are commonplaces of prognosis, and it is hard to say whether Baillou was on to something else as well, which might be latent in the words 'the character and dispositions of diseases'. If he was, he did not develop it.

In structure, Baillou's book imitates the Hippocratic *Epidemics* one and three by including descriptions of the prevailing weather of a particular season and the diseases epidemic in that season, followed by individual case histories. The seasons described run from autumn 1570 to summer 1579, but Baillou also mentions events of the years 1580 and 1581. However, the descriptions of epidemics and the case histories are only a part, although a prominent part, of the content of these books, which are filled with the 'appendices' and 'questions of note' of Baillou's list of contents. The relation between these questions and the diseases prevalent in a particular season is not always obvious. Sometimes Baillou extends a question into a minor essay or *causerie* on some point of diagnosis or pathology or therapy, and here there is a distinct resemblance in matter and manner to Baillou's separately written medical essays. For example, in his account of the winter constitution of 1574 Baillou does indeed open with a description of the exanthematous diseases prevalent at that time, with remarks on the different kinds of exanthemata observed; he then describes various cases – but these include obstetric and gynaecological cases which happen to have occurred at that time; this leads him on to make some remarks about embryology, then paralysis, on certain therapeutic practices of Fernel; he comments upon rhubarb, and upon several other matters. He also examines (and disagrees with) a precept of Hippocrates on diet. Then, returning to his initial topic of exanthemata, he raises the question of when these are to be regarded merely as abscessions, and when as diseases in their own right. Throughout this whole episode he frequently quotes Hippocrates and Galen, but, just as frequently, refers to observations of his own.[66] Again, in connection with the spring constitution of 1575, Baillou enters upon a long discussion of venesection, which meanders purposefully to include a number of issues: whether venesection should precede purgation, its application where pain in the side is present but not pleurisy, the nature of sympathetic pain and various senses of sympathy, whether children should be bled (Baillou for, Galen against), and so on. The discussion, like others in the book, is left absolutely open-ended.[67]

What strikes me most forcibly about Baillou's book is its style, and style, as it often can, helps to resolve a problem of interpretation and of history. The Latin, particularly in the descriptions and case histories, but elsewhere too, is cryptic, abbreviated, with drastically curtailed sentences disconnected grammatically and full of syntactical ellipses. This is not humanist Latin: it is an affectionate pastiche of the memoranda style of the Greek *Epidemics*.[68] Baillou makes what he is about even clearer by peppering the Latin text with Greek words and phrases. Sometimes this may be because he is conscious that there is no true Latin equivalent (and like other Parisians Baillou had a finely tuned lexical sensitivity[69]), but often the Greek seems gratuitous. It is as if he was getting as near as he dared to actually writing in Hippocrates' Greek – a Greek which simultaneously perplexed sixteenth-century medical writers with its difficulty, and inspired them to admiration of its precision and rightness. To use Hippocrates' language was to identify oneself with him: Baillou's stylistic *tour de force* is an aspect of the tendency of the Parisians which I have already noted to incorporate the classical past into their own situation.[70]

Baillou's stylistic imitation also directs us to the real originality of his *Epidemics*, in which others have seen an 'anticipation' of Sydenham's endeavour. His model, the Hippocratic *Epidemics*, itself represents an early application of the technique of writing to creative speculation: the scientist's informal, private, memorandum book.[71] Baillou may have been attracted to an imitation of their form and style because he was sensitive to their possibilities as a literary tool. His *Epidemics* are a new genre in the context of sixteenth-century medical writing: something that was neither a formal textbook for the didactic organization of received opinion, nor a commentary, nor an edited collection of case-histories, but an informal medium for the entertainment of new ideas, the matching of speculation with observation, the formulation of questions in an objective context which had suggested the question and might also suggest the answer. Baillou, in other words, may have imitated Hippocratic style because he saw in it a new way of 'doing' medical science. In this new way there are three elements: (i) personal observation; (ii) free speculation; and (iii) Baillou's attempt to juggle with the different aspects of his experience and to render them coherent, comparing past with present, his own observations with his reading in Hippocrates and Galen.

But this speculation, though free, is always within the ordered garden of Galenic medical theory. He had the same encyclopaedic command of Galen as Duret; like him, he could always lay his hands on the precise passage he needed from Galen's works. The freedom of his speculation was in some ways like that of an essayist – of a Montaigne – whose mind is filled with ideas drawn from a vast reading in the classical literatures, and who uses a quotation as the starting point of a journey which permits him to revisit as many familiar sites as he wishes, to contemplate them from old vantage points and from new ones, to compare one with another, and to set them all out like items in a collection. The freedom lies in the exercise of choice among items in the writer's store, and the novelty, the originality, lies in the way the writer is able to use familiar material to achieve and express insights which are peculiar or faithful to his own vision of things. And for both writers the end may often be some kind of practical counsel. But here the resemblance ends. The value of the comparison is to suggest to us that for the medical writer the purpose of his work is not entirely reducible to the small point at which all this mental furniture is brought to bear upon a practical case. When the Parisians praised each others' work, or moved their students to enthusiastic admiration, it was not because of new discoveries and new therapies, but because of their virtuosity in explicating what was there but was not visible to every man. Baillou's work is of a kind to let us see this aspect of Parisian medicine more clearly than we can in either of the other writers.

Baillou's work is nevertheless practical. The *Epidemics* are closely related to the *Consilia* both in time of composition and in the themes which preoccupied Baillou. He must have begun taking notes for the *Epidemics*, which begins with the constitution of autumn 1570, around the time of his graduation, and the dedication to the first book was written in 1574. The *Consilia* were concurrent. Book one was completed by 1572, book two by 1574.[72] Since a *consilium* required some discussion of the case and its complexities, it could easily develop into a discursive general essay on the condition concerned. A number of Baillou's *consilia* do just this; a number, too, deal more extensively with topics which arise incidentally in the course of the *Epidemics*. There are similar cross-connections between the *Consilia* and the medical essays. Some of the latter are more elaborate and self-contained treatments of topics raised in a *consilium* in which they were attached to a particular case. For example the essay *De Convulsionibus* includes an excursus on the cause of hiccupping and an apparent discrepancy between Hippocrates and Galen. This is a question which Baillou had discussed in *Consilia* 1, 58, 'De singultu febri superveniente'.[73] Thus Baillou's *Epidemics*, *Consilia*, and essays are all of a piece, and all related to his practical work.

The essay on convulsions[74] is a fair example of Baillou's manner. Its topic is the question, which Baillou says is regular or commonplace (*solennis*), 'why are those who are injured on the right side of the head convulsed on the left side of the body?' This, he says, is a notorious crux in Hippocrates' *On Wounds in the Head*, which many before himself have attempted to solve. Baillou begins by citing a number of passages from Hippocrates, most of them occurring in the *Epidemics*, to show that the thing can in fact happen. He follows this with a lexical discussion, similar to those of his *Definitiones Medicae*: does the Latin word *convulsio* correctly convey Hippocrates' meaning in the Greek word *spasmos*? Some have denied that it does, but careful investigation of the way Hippocrates uses the word in a number of passages makes his meaning quite plain. Baillou next turns to a subsidiary difficulty, the problem also discussed in *Consilium* 1, 58. This is that Hippocrates recognized only two causes of convulsion, namely inanition and repletion, but Galen appears to add a third. Baillou refers to previous discussions of this problem by his predecessors Houllier, Jean de Gorris, and J. C. Scaliger: he adopts Scaliger's solution. After these preliminaries, Baillou comes to the main question. Since upon the evidence given by Hippocrates in his *Epidemics* the fact is so, and since we are now also clear about Hippocrates' meaning, what is the cause of this phenomenon? In the rest of the essay Baillou canvasses possible explanations. He introduces the concept of *consensus* or sympathy, and a distinction drawn by Giovanni Arcolani in his commentary on ar-Rāzī (Rhasis) '*Liber nonus*'[75] between absolute and relative (*secundum quid*) sympathy. Baillou was well read in the late medieval *practici*: the reference to Arcolani here reminds us of the similarities, as well as the differences, between Baillou's essays and medieval *quaestiones*. Baillou finds Arcolani's distinction useful, but he settles the question whether there can be such a thing as absolute sympathy (or action at a distance) in a somewhat modern way, by an historical discussion of the various views on the matter taken by Galen, by Erasistratus, and the followers of Erasistratus respectively. Of the four possible explanations which Baillou considers, three involve the movement of humours or of spirits between the two parts of the body affected, while the fourth is the concept of absolute sympathy, where there is no intervening contact. This is the one which he finally selects. Baillou reaches this decision by wide reference both to classical authorities and to modern post-mortem observations, with no obvious preference for one source of information above the other. He does regard the Hippocratic *Epidemics* as a particularly reliable source of observed fact. This is not quite the same as blind acceptance of ancient authority. Baillou does not hesitate to question critically Hippocratic as well as Galenic statement or precept. But he accepts evidence from Hippocrates' *Epidemics* because there Hippocrates is reporting his own observation, and we are bound to believe him as an observer who as well as being honest is accurate above all others.

So Baillou's answer to the problem he discusses in *De Convulsionibus* is the one which he regards as best supported by the facts, the source of his knowledge of these facts being ancient as well as modern observation. But the real craft which makes this piece of scientific work good of its kind, is Baillou's talent for processing the information, which includes an ability to determine the meaning of a passage by philological techniques, and his control of the ancient sources. Presumably Baillou thought that he had been successful: if we ask ourselves why, the answer must be that he was conscious of possessing these talents and this learning and of his ability to deploy them better than others. He was a true product of the Paris school.

9

The generation of disease: occult causes and diseases of the total substance

LINDA DEER RICHARDSON

This chapter has grown out of an earlier attempt to understand the explanation of generation put forward in the writings of sixteenth-century academic physicians, in particular those of the French medical philosopher, Jean Fernel (1497–1558).[1] Like his theory of generation, Fernel's system of pathology contains certain unorthodox features, which looked as though they would be worth investigating: in particular, the notion of occult causes in medicine, and of diseases of the total substance.[2]

Further investigation showed that there was a distinct set of diseases that Fernel classified as 'of the total substance'. These were superficially very different, ranging from skin diseases, such as scabies, through phthisis to plague, venereal disease and the bite of poisonous insects and mad dogs. This classification in itself raised certain questions. What were these diseases of the total substance? How did diseases come to be included in this group? How was their action defined? What did it mean, to Fernel or his contemporaries, to say that a disease had an occult cause? What was the use of such a concept to medical theory or treatment? How did an explanation of disease based on occult causes relate to the more conventional explanation of disease, based on an imbalance of the temperaments or some physical cause, such as an obstruction? What were the origins of such a theory, and how common was it? Did other writers use the concept, and did they relate it to the same group of diseases as Fernel had?

This chapter is a first attempt at answering some of these questions. It raises a further question, too, concerning Fernel's position in the world of renaissance medicine.

Jean Fernel's reputation as a commanding authority in the medical world of his day is not in doubt. His distinction as a lecturer and practising physician made him one of the most famous medical men of his generation, and his two treatises of theoretical medicine were classics in their day and continued his influence into the following century.[3] His popularity was reflected in the numerous theses, particularly at Paris but also at foreign

175

universities, which took him as their inspiration; the large number of later medical textbooks which followed the format of the *Medicina*; and commentaries by devoted followers, including Guillaume Plancy, Jean Riolan the Elder and Jacques Aubert.

Despite this, his position on a number of major theoretical issues seems to have been a minority view. For example, Fernel's belief that the innate heat and *spiritus*, which acted, in his physiology, as instrument of the soul in the body's actions, was celestial in origin was rejected by his disciple, Jean Riolan, as well as by the more generally critical Joannes Argenterius.[4] In his treatise *De Innato Calido et Naturali Spiritu* (1626) the Italian writer Joannes Bronzerius insists that the innate heat is elemental in its nature, and, he says, he has the majority on his side;

In which opinion I find all others zealous for truth, only excepting Fernel and a few lovers of novelties.[5]

Indeed, as D. P. Walker points out, the Neo-Platonic theory of the astral body, with which Fernel seems to identify his celestial *spiritus*, 'was . . . not generally considered safe or respectable.'[6]

The same seems to have been the case with the example dealt with in this chapter: Fernel's contention that certain diseases operate, not through the action of Galenic qualities, but by their total substance – and that these powers too are celestial in origin.

We thus have a paradoxical image: on the one hand, the 'French Hippocrates', creator of perhaps the most successful synthesis of classical medicine of his generation; on the other, a promoter of suspect ideas which his contemporaries condemned as a straying from the path of Galenic orthodoxy.

Where Fernel does stray from the orthodox view, and I think that the fact he does so is unquestionable, I should like to suggest that this is at least partially a rational response to deficiencies in the explanatory force, and applicability to medical practice, of the Galenic system as taught in the universities. Plancy indeed tells us that, after taking his M.A., Fernel left Paris to study privately, and remained out of the university environment for five years.[7] In the case of the diseases which Fernel identified with the action of the 'total substance' and with 'occult' rather than temperamental causes, this deficiency was particularly marked, as we shall see.

The main body of this chapter is in three sections. It contains a brief description of the classical theory of temperament; compares this with Fernel's own theory; and finally looks at the development of the concept in the work of two of Fernel's disciples and commentators, and in a group of monographs dealing with diseases of the total substance. In particular, this final section looks at its relevance to the theory of poison action and the transmission of contagious disease.

The theory of temperament as a theory of disease action

One of the cornerstones of academic medicine, central to therapy as well as theory, was the classical doctrine of temperament, or the 'rules' governing the mixture of the elemental qualities of hot, cold, moist and dry, synthesized by Galen from the Hippocratic writings and Aristotle. The Galenic works *De Elementis, De Temperamentis* and *De Facultatum Naturalium Substantia*, in which the theory is set out, were edited and commented upon by renaissance doctor-philosophers, including two whose works were published near the time of Fernel's own *Medicina*. Jacobus Sylvius (Jacques Dubois) published short commentaries in editions of Galen in 1549 and 1550, while commentaries by J. B. Montanus were published posthumously, probably from his lecture notes, in 1554.[8]

In *De Elementis*, Galen had explained the relationship among the three sets of 'elements' which constitute the human body: the elements of nature, earth, air, fire and water; the elements of man, blood, phlegm, black and yellow bile; and the body's simple or similar parts, such as blood, flesh or bone.

Joannes Baptista Montanus's commentaries make clear the medical importance of this relationship. Temperament, as Montanus reports in his commentary on the Galenic fragment *De Facultatum Naturalium Substantia*,[9] deals with the balance of contrary qualities in the whole organism. It uses the 'qualitative' terms of Aristotelian physics, hot, cold, moist and dry, not in terms of absolute levels of heat or cold, but primarily as a system of comparisons. These comparisons are made with reference to what Galen calls the *symmetron*, the point of balance or medium between extremes of temperament in an individual, a genus, or a species.

The ideal temperament, or *eucraton*, is, mathematically, one in which the proportion of the activity of each element is exactly equal with respect to all the others. Functionally – and this is the sense which is important to the theory of disease – it is measured by the perfection of action of the species or individual. Disease is, by analogy, the result of a breakdown in this temperamental balance.

In addition, temperament is a means of explaining the differentiation from one another of the similar parts: blood, flesh, ligament and the rest. They too can be compared along two intersecting scales, one from hot to cold and one from moist to dry. The midpoint on both scales is the skin, and in particular the skin of the fingertips; it follows that the touch of human fingertips is the instrument best suited for distinguishing temperament – an important point, greatly convenient in providing a theory for medical diagnosis.

Temperament, then, is the doctor's 'way in', via touch, to the ills which afflict his patients. It is a pragmatic approach, and Galen makes clear his own reluctance to speculate on the causes which lie behind the phenomena we can see and touch in a number of his works,[10] notably in a passage from his short treatise on the substance of the natural faculty. The doctor, says Galen, is faced with a variety of conflicting answers to the question of the substance of the soul and its faculties, none of which he can reasonably accept as more than uncertain probabilities. But medically speaking, the answer to this question is irrelevant: whatever the soul's substance, and however it is introduced into the body, the latter serves it according to its own nature, which is the result of the temperament of the elements composing it. It is not necessary, therefore, to understand the essence of the soul in order to cure disease, to preserve health – or even to lead a moral life. Temperament gives the doctor all the clues he needs.[11]

Montanus's commentaries also deal with the signs of temperament, that is to say, with their actions. When the degree of heat in a living body is altered, as in fever, its functions are impaired. Just as the normal activities of the body arise from the proper blending of heat and cold, or *eucrasia*, Montanus can observe with Galen that 'the primary impairments of these activities necessarily arise from its [that is, *eucrasia*'s] derangement'.[12]

This definition links temperament with another Galenic explanatory device, faculty. Galen located faculty, as he had temperament, in the simple or similar parts of the body. As Montanus points out, there is another link too. We recognize temperaments by their actions: the same is true of faculties. Both, indeed, are drawn from the same physical evidence: the structure and function of the body in health or disease.

Jacobus Sylvius agreed: as he wrote in a marginal scholium to the 1550 edition of *De Temperamentis*, 'the essence of faculty is in temperament'.[13] Like Montanus's, Sylvius's commentary reflects the aspects of Galenic temperament theory which were of most interest to sixteenth-century medical teaching. It also reflects the overelaboration, by generations of commentators, of the nine Galenic varieties of temperament (*eucrasia*, plus imbalances of hot, cold, moist and dry temperament and of the four complementary pairs). Sylvius provides the unwary student with twelve pages of tables listing 'latitudes' of temperament. He ends up with 40 different grades of hot, and 700 categories in all, subdivided to the point of near-uselessness. Where Galen had provided a simple means of classification, Sylvius offers an infinite variety of temperamental types, each identified with the structure and function of a particular animal or plant.

Fernel, too, deals with the theory of the elements and temperaments, both in books two and three of his *Physiologia*, and in the theoretical work, *De Abditis Rerum Causis (On the Hidden Causes of Things)*. In both works, however, he makes it clear that there is for him a large and important area of physiological explanation and disease theory which cannot be reduced to the action of the elements and temperaments – the qualitative balance of hot and cold, moist and dry.

Fernel's definition of temperament, in the third book of his *Physiologia*, is based on Galen's, but describes the relationship of the four primary qualities with greater complexity and precision. Like Sylvius, he imagines an innumerable variety of 'latitudes', of temperament, with the most temperate temperament, *eucrasia*, at the centre of a huge set of co-ordinates. And following Galen, he relates the varieties of temperament to the body's simple or similar parts. The structural differences between the similar parts are the result of variations in their temperament; but not their actions, and here Fernel parts company with Galen and with more orthodox medical textbooks such as those of Montanus and Sylvius.

Function – even the functioning of the simple parts, and those most basic activities or faculties, like attraction and retention, which Galen associated with an organ's 'fibres' and attributed to 'nature' or *physis* – requires a soul, according to Fernel. This soul can be perceived only through its works, that is, the actions of a living body; hence its definition by Fernel as 'the principle and cause of function of a living body'.[14] In fact, we define the soul by the number of its actions, and this number is equal to the number of its faculties.

Why is this distinction between faculty and temperament necessary? Because, says Fernel, of the obvious difference between a dead body and a living one. The elemental structure, the temperamental balance of qualities are the same in the corpse as in the living man, but the function of the body is completely absent.[15] Therefore, function must derive from some extra-elemental and extra-temperamental source which in *De Abditis* he calls the total form, and in *Physiologia* the soul.

In *De Abditis Rerum Causis* he extends this argument, and also tells us why temperament is too limited a concept to be useful in explaining the function of a body and the action of disease. *De Abditis Rerum Causis* is a dialogue among three philosophers, two of whom, Philiatros (who always asks the right questions) and Brutus (who puts the contrary view, but is generally won over in the end) go to consult a third, the doctor-philosopher Eudoxus, who represents Fernel. The question on which they go to consult him is the Hippocratic one, 'that there is in disease something of the divine'. But their discussion ranges more widely; broadly speaking, the first book is devoted to natural philosophy, and the second book to medicine. Partway through book two, the discussion returns to the question with which Brutus and Philiatros began in the first place: the question of 'hidden causes' in disease, and of what Fernel calls 'diseases of the total substance'.

In the preface to book one, Fernel explains that he has deliberately chosen a dialogue form for the work because the subject of 'hidden causes' is 'full of contentions' and for that reason should be presented as a debate, with all shades of opinion represented.

Fernel's contention throughout the work, that 'there is much in philosophy outside the order of the elements', is made clearer if we look briefly at the presuppositions on which his medical philosophy is based. Philosophy, says Fernel, seeks after causes; even though the reasons it arrives at are probable ones only. In pursuing this search, the medical philosopher must go beyond the evidence of the senses, if his conclusions are to be more than superficial and incomplete. For the true beginnings of things are 'inward, hidden, and far removed from the senses': inaccessible to the eyes and ears, and attainable only by the mind.[16]

This rationalistic approach to how one attains truth has implications for the limitations which he places on temperamental medicine. For the elements are defined by the possession of certain sensible qualities, those of hot, cold, dry and moist. The heart of Eudoxus–Fernel's argument in *De Abditis* is that, just as a true scientific method must move beyond observation to reasoning based upon observation, so one must move beyond defining the properties of living things and medicines in terms of their elements and temperaments – their sensible qualities of heat and cold – and instead consider their soul or form, the true source of their powers, which is divine in origin.

What is more fundamental to medicine, and in particular to pathology, is Fernel's claim that temperament is not enough to allow us to completely explain the structures, much less the functions, of a living body. His argument, as he presents it in parallel in the *Medicina* and *De Abditis*, is based on three pieces of evidence:

1) Simply to discriminate between organs, we need to consider more than their temperament; for example, the lungs and heart are both temperamentally hot, but very different in their structure, and in particular in their density:

   For we distinguish many things, which although they have the same temperament have dissimilar shapes, and others which are similar in shape but differ in temperament; which is furthermore proved more fully and abundantly from medical opinions.[17]

2) Structure, and therefore elemental and temperamental heat, are present in inanimate objects, which were never alive, as well as in a corpse, in which life and activity are lost. There is something in a living man 'by which he is more excellent than a dead man', as Fernel puts it, and which is the cause of his life and activities.

3) This 'something' cannot be related to the temperament, since even those animals, such as snakes and salamanders, and plants, such as mandragora, which are temperamentally of a cold nature, still live. But since in them the elemental quality of cold dominates that of heat, they must live by virtue of a separate, vital heat, which is superior to the elements in its origins – in fact, divine – and which 'does not stink of the crasser nature of elemental fire'.[18]

This divine heat, which Fernel also calls the vital or innate heat, is a central, and unorthodox, part of Fernel's system of physiology, and thus of his pathology. By claiming that the efficient cause of vital actions lay in a heat whose origin was 'different from, and more excellent than that of the elements', Fernel introduced problems in his physiology and in his account of disease action which could not be solved by recourse to the system of medical spirits and humours derived from Galen. Elemental heat could quite naturally perform its actions through and by means of the elemental and temperamental composition of the body of which it was a part. But a celestial heat required a different, and in some sense 'nobler', base for its actions. It was for this reason that Fernel introduced the concept of the *spiritus*, which is intimately bound up with the innate heat in all its activities.

In book two of *De Abditis*, Fernel looks at the action of the innate heat and *spiritus* in relation to two medical questions. One is generation; the other is the cause of disease, in particular those diseases which he identifies with the total substance. It is the second of these questions which concerns us here.

Diseases of the total substance

In chapter eight of book two, 'That many functions and operations within us are hidden in their causes', Fernel gives us an important definition for the discussion which is to follow: in effect, he defines both 'divine' and 'occult' causes in nature with reference to the limitations of human reason:

Philiatros: What, then, do you consider as divine functions?
Eudoxus: Those which are above nature, and beyond the grasp of the human mind. Because they lead us to wonder, we are used to call them wonders; these wondrous functions are rightly called divine, because their cause and reason are hidden, secret and obscure, and cannot be demonstrated or rightly explained.[19]

In the remainder of the chapter, Eudoxus argues, as he had in book one, that the natural faculties – the natural functions of attraction, retention and expulsion – are effected by a 'certain power, more noble and divine than the elements'.[20]

Brutus, however, argues that, for the doctor as healer, the nature of the cause of disease or cure is irrelevant: does it really matter to the patient whether you attribute his cure to the primordial elements and their temperaments, or to 'diviner' causes? And he urges Eudoxus to return to the original subject of their enquiry: 'the "hidden" diseases which have something of the divine in them.'[21]

In chapter nine, Eudoxus accordingly turns to 'the vast field of medicine', to argue that the cause of disease does matter. In addition to temperament, there are, he says, two other causes of disease, and similarly of drug action: matter and form. Temperament is in fact the least notable of the three, and is subsidiary to the other two. Just as the health or disease of the similar parts inheres in these three principles, so there are, it follows, three genera of diseases of the similar parts: one material, one temperamental, and the third affecting the 'total substance' of the body.

It is the third of these which concerns us here, and which concerns Fernel, too, in most of the remainder of *De Abditis*.

While claiming these three categories of disease, in place of Galen's one, based on temperament, Fernel-Euxodus does his best to claim that he is basing his theory on Galenic authority, and indeed is only following the Leader. Philiatros and Brutus are predictably convinced. But, as Jacques Aubert sternly warns in his commentary on *De Abditis Rerum Causis*,[22] it seems fairly certain that Fernel's interpretation of Galenic authority in this case is Procrustean, if not plainly disingenuous. So here again we find Fernel in a minority – out on a limb, it would seem, of his own devising. What is the nature of this limb, and what is he doing there? Why introduce new causes of disease into an established system?

Fernel is trying, I think, to explain certain actions, and categorize certain particular diseases, which do not fit smoothly into the temperamental categories. He gives several examples of such actions. One is the 'occult' or 'hidden' power of the magnet; another is the alleged ability of the ostrich's stomach to digest iron, not by means of elemental heat or indwelling temperament, but from the nature of its total essence. Such powers are also to be found, according to Fernel, in less spectacular form, in the ability of the total substance of the parts of the human body to concoct food and perform a range of other functions. All of them, according to Fernel, are functions which depend on the total substance, soul, or form of the body, and not its balance of qualities.

A disease which acts by weakening these functions is a disease of the total substance. The notion of diseases of the total substance is necessary, says Fernel, because none of the standard causes of disease – repletion and inanition, obstruction, putrefaction – is adequate to explain either the variety of symptoms these diseases present, or their peculiarly violent and pernicious effect on the body.

Once again Fernel turns to Galen for corroboration: rather more plausibly this time, since the passage he cites, from *De Simplicium Medicamentorum Facultatibus*, (*On the Powers of Simple Medicines*) is a standard authority for discussion of action of the 'total substance', in the context of drug action. Drugs, says Galen, act by altering the body in some way; and this they do either qualitatively, for example, by warming, cooling, moistening or drying; or 'by their total substance, as do many deadly poisons, a number of *alexiteria* or amulets, all purges, and many drugs which act by attraction.' Fernel argues from this that 'if medicines affect us either by their qualities or by their total substance, they must change either the qualities or the total substance of our bodies.'[23] Diseases, similarly, can affect either.

In chapter eleven, he classifies diseases of the total substance into manifest and occult. Manifest diseases of the total substance are those which arise from 'simple putrefaction' and include 'simple putrid fevers, many ulcers, phthisis, scabies, pruritis and other similar afflictions.'[24]

Occult diseases of the total substance generally have an external cause. Fernel divides them broadly into poisonous, contagious and pestilential, and distinguishes between them, not on the basis of symptoms, but according to the way in which they are transmitted.

Pestilential diseases for the most part arise from the air, though they also contaminate by social contact. Contagious diseases, as the name suggests, 'are those which are first contracted by contacting and touching a particular external poison . . .'[25]

The care with which one must approach the use of words here is indicated by the list of contagious diseases which Fernel gives: stupor caused by a torpedo fish or opium; hydrophobia (rabies); the bite of scorpions or other venomous creatures. There are others which seem not to come from an external cause, and which attack by means of sexual contact; a group which includes lues venerea (syphilis) and elephantiasis. A number of manifest diseases of the total substance also arise from contact in the same way, among them phthisis, pruritis, scabies and leprosy; these, however, are not included in the contagious category, since they have no hint of the occult or malign nature which characterizes contagious diseases proper.

Venomous or poisonous diseases are of two types: those from poisons which are generated within the body and those which are taken in. The latter may be animal, vegetable or mineral; Fernel gives a long list, most of which we would recognize as poisonous substances. Examples of the former are *strangulatio uteri* or hysteria, arising from corrupt semen retained in the body; epilepsy; syncope, from corrupted blood transformed to a venomous nature; palpitation of the heart; and 'other obscure symptoms which poisonous humours are accustomed to introduce'.[26]

The essence of poison action is that it attacks, not just the heart (as usually claimed), but the total substance and faculty:

For in fact, we do not call it poison only because it always kills, or because it is dangerous to the principles of life and the heart, but because it either extinguishes or injures the total substance and its hidden faculties, and attacks their functioning by dark methods.[27]

In the next three chapters, Fernel discusses each of these categories of occult disease of the total substance in turn.

Pestilential epidemics arise 'from a poisonous impurity spread by the air' ('a venenato inquinamento aeri insperso prodeunt'). These are taken into the body with *spiritus*, and attack the heart in the classic manner of poisons. Their cause is not the excess of a prime quality – as evidenced by their appearance at the Hippocratically 'wrong' time of year, and by plagues which sweep the known world, taking in 'hot and cold regions, moist and dry, summer and winter'– but 'hidden and obscure'. It is not simply a corruption or putrefaction of the air, which is often put forward as a cause of epidemic disease. 'Healthy air' contains a spirit which sustains and protects all living things; made putrid or corrupt, it endangers all life in equal measure. True pestilences attack one species only, and in this are akin to poisons, which act specifically on the total substance of the species concerned. Therefore the cause is hidden, contrary to the total substance, and not flowing from the elements or their qualities.

'Where does it flow from then?' asks the persistent Brutus. From the heavens, replies Eudoxus: not from the motion of the prime mover, or of the sun, which produces the seasons of the year; but from 'certain mixtures of stars' ('a certa permistione siderum') which determine the character of the seasons and are why some summers are hotter and drier than others, some have flies and some do not. There are many genera of pestilence, and each has its own proper causal conjunction.

The true cause of pestilence, then, is 'a hidden and malign quality sent down from the heavens.'[28] The causes usually given – exhalations and vapours from stagnant and putrid pools, caves and cadavers; qualitative changes in the air brought about by storms – are preparatory or auxiliary, and help to explain why a pestilence has differing effects in different places; it is thus more serious in a place infected with putrid exhalations than in pure air, in summer than in winter, with south winds than with north; in summary, more serious in combination with endemic or epidemic factors than in starry isolation.

In chapters fourteen and fifteen, Fernel deals with contagious and poisonous diseases in similar detail. Contagious diseases, as we have seen, are the result of the action of certain poisons, and are contracted either by a bite which punctures the skin; or in a more tenuous form which can enter the body simply through contact with the skin. Poisonous diseases proper are the result of a poison which enters the body, for instance with food or drink or is produced within it; only the former are substances we would recognize as poisons.

Thus far, Fernel has shown himself methodical in classifying and identifying the category of diseases of the total substance. Their common factor is that they all act violently and in a way which threatens life. Fernel considers them all as 'poisons', which can be observed to be both violent and specific in their harmful effects. And he argues that they attack, not the

elemental or temperamental composition of the body, but its total substance or form.

He gives almost exactly the same account in the *Medicina*, and in book
one of the *Pathologia*, which deals with the causes of disease. Here again
there are three genera of disease, divided into manifest and occult, with the
latter category subdivided into poisonous, pestilential and contagious. He
gives a longer list of diseases, as one would expect; and adds a new list of
'lesser' diseases of the total substance, including a range of skin diseases and
'not a few others, emerged as novelties with new and unheard-of causes.'
When he comes, in later books, to discuss diseases individually, he again
chooses the same examples. Pestilential fevers, elephantiasis, syphilis,
hysteria – all are the effect of a 'poisonous and malign quality'.[29]

Those who dismiss *De Abditis* as a juvenile flight of fantasy cannot do so
with Fernel's work of maturity, the *Medicina*. Yet the message is the same
in both works. And if we look at the fuller selection of diseases which, in
the *Pathologia*, Fernel claims as arising from the total substance, we find
that they have several things in common. Often, they are newly identified
or diagnosed, or diseases, like hysteria and elephantiasis, whose diagnosis
was disputed or uncertain. Typically, they are difficult to cure, not
responding to conventional methods. And usually, they are spectacularly
violent and life-threatening in their action: highly visible, as it were.

The same pattern might be found in the list of diseases where Paracelsian
medicine made its biggest inroads: 'new' diseases, such as syphilis, and
intractable ones such as certain skin diseases, which did not fit neatly into
the patterns nor respond easily to the treatments laid down by the ancients.
Is Fernel responding, in his own more classical fashion, to the unsolved
problems which such diseases presented? A comparison between Paracelsian areas of success and those marked out by Fernel and others as outside
the scheme of traditional Galenic medicine might well be worth pursuing;
unfortunately, it lies outside the scope of this chapter.

The medical problem, for Galenist and Paracelsian alike, was not just
the cause of such diseases, but their effective treatment. But if occult
diseases occur, there must also be their contrary, occult remedies. For, says
Fernel in a statement of belief which recalls the medieval, and Paracelsian,
doctrine of correspondences, there is nothing in the universe of things
whose like, and whose opposite, is not produced in nature – it is thus a
challenge to our diligence to find it out.

But when he turns to the occult remedies for these occult diseases, he
again has to sidestep an inconvenient piece of Galenic authority, which was
too well known to be ignored. As well as the passage from *On the Actions
of Simple Medicines*, Galen refers to the action of the total substance also in
another work, *De Methodus Medendi* (*On the Method of Curing*) in discussing
medicines which operate by attraction. All of these remedies act 'by

contraries', but some are contrary in their quality (for example, a cold remedy treating a hot disease, or vice versa) and some in their total substance. Galen refers the reader to his 'book on medicines' for further details, and points out a distinction between the two types of medical action which was echoed in renaissance treatments of the topic:

Those which oppose by quality operate according to method. For those which oppose according to their total substance, there is no method, but everything is known from experience.[30]

Now, experience is for Galen a valid source of insight in medicine, and particularly in pharmacy; but when Brutus tackles Eudoxus by citing the passage above, Fernel shows himself sensitive to any suggestion that occult medicine is empiric medicine. He devotes a chapter to remedies 'above nature' and to so-called magical cures of occult diseases, and his message is clear. Divinely caused diseases can have divine cures, as in the healings by Christ and his disciples; but today's diseases are to be cured by doctors, not magicians. Magic, as it is practised, has no power over diseases of the total substance, or indeed over ordinary temperamental diseases either. Neither words, nor figures, nor characters have any effect whatsoever on disease.[31]

Fernel's tactic, in fact, is to make diseases of the total substance look as normal and methodical as possible, when discussing their treatment. The trick is, having insisted that the powers of the total substance are different from those of the elements and temperaments, and much superior, now to make them sound as much alike as possible.

Medicines which act temperamentally do so according to their opposing qualities? Very well, so must the powers of the total substance, for everything in nature has its like, and its opposite. And anything you can do, we can do better: 'If simple qualities are equipped with powers [for example to cure disease] the forms and substances of things must of necessity greatly exceed them in eminence' for they represent 'the whole thing, pure and simple'; the kernel of physiological action, as it were.[32]

In the principle of *similitudo* (which he introduces also in the third book of the *Physiologia* as an alternative to the powers of temperament) Fernel considers that he has found a general explanatory principle which takes in the actions of temperament and matter in disease, as well as those of the total substance. The principle recalls Hippocrates rather than Galen – for example, the description in *The Nature of the Child* of the differentiation of the foetus from seed and maternal blood, with like going to join like.[33] It also recalls contemporary theories of the action of the magnet and other 'occult' phenomena, which Fernel takes as types of the total substance, but which may not have been quite respectable in medical theory.

Fernel relates *similitudo* to a familiar bodily action: our nourishment by the food we eat. We are nourished by what is similar to us – which explains why all our sources of food were at one time themselves alive – and when we digest it, we assimilate it to ourselves. If all our food is alive, though, it is not true to say that all that is alive is our food. To nourish us, foods must contain 'the living heat which is suitable (*familiaris*) to us.' But not all sources of celestial heat and *spiritus* are friendly; some are 'entirely hostile and pestilential'. *Alimenta*, foods, and *deleteria*, poisonous substances which harm the total substance, are diametric opposites on the scale of *similitudo*; medicines are the midpoint.

All things in nature have their occult powers; but they are occult only because of our ignorance. We may not know the reason for the cures which we observe each day, but we have them firm in our experience, and we can use secondary indicators of a plant's powers, such as its colour and scent, as a guide. In many cases, all we are lacking is the words to describe powers which we can see; Philiatros tricks Brutus by describing a wonder 'seen in India' in terms which force even that sceptic to admit that its powers must have been occult; then confesses that he has simply been describing fire.[34]

In the final chapter, Eudoxus takes up Brutus's challenge ('Galen says in many places that powers which arise from the total substance are remote from method and reason,') head on. That, he tells his colleague, is an ignorant and stupid thing to say. Galen did not mean 'remote from all possible methods', but simply those based on his principle of heating, cooling, moistening and drying.

In fact, there is art and method in the cure of occult diseases; we have manifest *demonstrationes* of the occult powers of our remedies, even if we cannot explain how they work. Even observation and learning from experience requires a rational approach, says Eudoxus; and the doctor must first of all diagnose the cause of the disease, discriminating occult from manifest and even treating combinations of the two. And as with any other form of the art of medicine, the doctor's aim is the health of the patient, and the extinguishing and exterminating of 'all that is pernicious and poisonous.'[35]

How was this theory received by Fernel's contemporaries and successors? The third and final section of this chapter discusses a selection from this response, and tries to suggest why a theory of disease action put forward by one of the most sophisticated theoreticians of his day met with such a cool response.

The response to Fernel

This section of the chapter considers the response to Fernel's theory of diseases of the total substance from two groups of writers. First, and closest to Fernel, two medical writers, Jacques Aubert and Jean Riolan the Elder, who wrote commentaries on *De Abditis Rerum Causis*. Secondly, a more amorphous group of authors who wrote treatises on the theory of poison action and contagious diseases in the decades after the publication of Fernel's work, and who refer to or acknowledge a debt to him. Of this latter group, the two I shall be considering in most detail are Jacques Grevin and Julien Le Paulmier, or Palmarius, who wrote on poisons and contagious diseases respectively.

The 'Preface to the Reader' of Jacques Aubert's *Progymnasmata in . . . de Abditis Rerum . . . causis* (1579?) suggests that he was a devoted Fernelian. Following the almost obligatory praise of Fernel's learning, genius, and other 'near divine' qualities, Aubert announces that he will be following closely in his footsteps: 'there is nothing in this book, which is not true Fernel'.[36]

The first fourteen chapters of Aubert's commentary, which is arranged as a series of *quaestiones* drawn from the *Hidden Causes*, concern philosophical questions; but in chapter fifteen he turns to medicine, and almost immediately parts company with the master on the question of the three genera of disease. Like Bronzerius, he is careful to point out that Fernel's position on this point is a minority of one:

Indeed, all physicians, both ancient and more recent, excepting only Fernel . . . claim only one particular form of disease in the similar parts of our body, that is, simple or composite temperamental imbalance.[37]

Aubert thus questions Fernel's interpretation, arguing that what Fernel says in the *Hidden Causes* is inconsistent with the account in the *Medicina*. He disagrees, too, with Fernel's thesis that celestial heat is a working partner in all things that live; and actually presents Fernel's own argument in favour of the distinction between elemental and celestial heat, the wrong way around.

Fernel's action of the total substance is reduced to the 'properties of the total substance' in Aubert's account, and these in turn are identified with the primary elemental qualities, overturning Fernel's position completely Similarly, Aubert takes Fernel's manifest and occult diseases of the total substance and ascribes them to temperamental imbalance: scabies an excess of heat, phthisis of hot and dry, and so on.

In particular, he demolishes Fernel's argument that 'pestilential diseases are roused by the powers of the heavenly bodies, in contaminating the air'. This, say Aubert, is simply not reasonable: Aristotle, in *Generation of Animals*, book two, tells us that the powers of the heavens are beneficial, and generative; how can our 'first parent' corrupt or contaminate the air we breathe? The true causes of pestilence are rotting cadavers and the other 'auxiliary' causes mentioned by Fernel; not a 'poisonous quality'.

Hysteria, too, is not a disease of the total substance, but a cold and moist imbalance of the temperaments; and even when he does not suggest an alternative cause, Aubert refuses to accept Fernel's premise, or even the existence of diseases of the total substance.

Such a blanket refusal is not surprising: what makes it so is that the author is a professed disciple of Fernel, who claimed to be following where he led. Instead, what we seem to have is a man who has come up against a new idea, and spends his time trying to sweep it under the carpet, or convert it back into an old one. Aubert nowhere gives any indication that the action of the total substance was anything but a Fernelian aberration, despite its appearance in Galen and in discussions of medical theory by several contemporary medical writers – as Andrew Wear points out in his chapter.[38]

The case of Jean Riolan the Elder is somewhat similar. Riolan, a stalwart of the Paris faculty, produced a set of remarkably dry and pedantic comments on the books of the *Physiologia*, the *Therapeutics* and the *Hidden Causes*. His chapter-by-chapter commentary on *De Abditis Rerum Causis* appeared in several editions, and was evidently popular.[39] Riolan's commentary is a paraphrase, where Aubert's is a debate or dialogue; he is more reluctant to oppose Fernel directly, but instead he soft-pedals the 'occult' aspects of his pathology, and smoothes over Fernel's careful distinctions, such as that between pestilential and contagious diseases. The result is a rather bland and bloodless precis, with all the intelligence wrung out of it.

Riolan introduces Fernel's treatment of diseases of the total substance by considering the underlying question of whether the innate heat is truly divine, or actually elemental, but so perfectly tempered that it has won the description 'divine' as a kind of courtesy title. In his commentary *Ad Librum Fernelii de Spiritu et Calido Innato*, Riolan clearly leans towards the latter interpretation, though he stops short of coming down firmly against Fernel.[40]

A similar reluctance to take a clearly opposing stand is evident in the discussion of diseases of the total substance in his commentary on *De Abditis Rerum Causis*. Like Aubert and Bronzerius, he too makes Fernel's minority position clear in various ways. In his commentary on book two, chapter ten, he points out that the concept of diseases of the total substance was either unknown to or unmentioned by the ancients. Though they produced accurate descriptions of the diseases which Fernel places in this category they gave the cause as either temperamental imbalance or 'putrefaction'. Modern writers have, in general, followed their lead.

For example, Galen in book one of *On the Differences of Fevers* held that plague – the major occult disease Riolan discusses – had a manifest cause, *putredo* or putrefaction, arising from 'putrid' or 'corrupt' air with an excess of moisture. Modern writers have tended to agree. Fracastoro, for instance, followed the ancients in defining contagion as 'putrefaction which is transmitted from one to another'. If this is so, then all contagious diseases, says Riolan, must be 'putrid' in their origin and their effects. Fernel, of course, recognized the existence of 'putrefaction' as a cause of disease and gave it an auxiliary role in some cases, but distinguishes it firmly from the occult causes of disease which, in his view, were of a different and higher order.

It is not at all clear that Riolan is willing to accept this distinction. His paraphrase of Fernel's own arguments erodes the difference in subtle ways – for example, by using a word like *corrumpit*, corrupts, to describe the action of poisons of the total substance – a word with overtones of putrefaction, and one which Fernel avoids in favour of terms like *inquinatus*, contaminated or impure.

Some of Riolan's interpretations are more illuminating, however. He makes clear the link between generation and contagion which is implicit in the *Hidden Causes* – both for instance are the works of the *spiritus*, and they are discussed in the same part of the work. Riolan gives a definition of 'contagion' which makes the similarity even more explicit: 'we do not call a disease contagious unless the morbid excretion generated by the disease can generate in another.'[41] He also makes clear that all Fernel's occult diseases are in fact caused by poisons – though Riolan himself distinguishes, as Fernel did not, between the action of poisons proper, of the Borgia sort, and 'poisonous diseases' as Fernel defines them.

Finally, he is less sanguine than Fernel himself on the possibility of bringing occult phenomena into the circle of art and method. Art, after all, is about definitions, divisions, demonstrations:

And we cannot define, nor distinguish into clear categories, much less demonstrate specific properties, if we are truly ignorant of their causes.[42]

And this is the case with diseases of the total substance, whose cause is 'occult': as with the action of the magnet, we can only observe, not explain:

That the magnet draws iron, we have explored using the evidence of our senses; why it does so, we are ignorant: a kind of general and indefinite cause, namely sympathy or similitude of forms, is known to us, but we cannot define or clearly distinguish what the two forms have in common.[43]

All we can do is collect instances, work back from the effect towards the cause, – and treat diseases as successfully as we can. For Riolan, this is not an acceptable research programme: but Fernel, as we have seen, argued that this was exactly the way in which the doctor could attain a knowledge of the cause and cure of occult diseases, working not from *a priori* definitions but from distinctions based on observation.

Once again, we seem to see in Riolan someone wrestling with an unfamiliar set of ideas, and failing to find a purchase which will allow him to relate it to the system with which he is familiar and in which he was trained. There is, almost, a hint of betrayal in Aubert's and Riolan's attitude: how could the great Fernel have presented them with a piece of the medical jigsaw which does not fit the rest? One answer, I think, lies in the fact that Fernel himself straddled the worlds of medicine and natural philosophy, and moved easily from the relatively free speculation of the one to the pragmatism of the other. I suspect that the concept of diseases of the total substance is one which fits more happily into the theoretical world of natural philosophy; in applying it to medicine, with its emphasis on the practical aim of curing patients, Fernel appears to be offering his medical colleagues an explanatory tool for which, like Brutus, they can see no need.

We can test this theory by looking at a selection of treatises which are nearer the natural–philosophical end of the scale. A survey of other writers who dealt with the action of poisons or contagious diseases reveals two distinct camps. As a generalization, it seems that Italian writers preferred to avoid the total substance in their explanations, while French and Germans are more prone to follow Fernel.

What follows can only be a whistle-stop tour of the major arguments, related to Fernel's own account. Cesalpino, in his *Quaestionum Medicarum* (*Medical Questions*); Andrea Bacci, in *De Venenis et Antidotis . . .* of 1586 and Giuseppe Aromatari in his *Disputatio de Rabie Contagiosa* (Venice, 1625)[44] all opt for the action of qualities or putrefaction in the diseases they discuss. Bacci defines poison as 'the opposite of food' in its action – destroying, not nourishing – and relates the poisons he discusses to the humours of the body, which become imbalanced in their temperament and so 'putrid'.

Both Caesalpino and Aromatari also make clear the importance to them of a method of therapy that can be based on rational principles. Aromatari is particularly outspoken in condemning any willingness to take refuge in hidden powers and unknown qualities:

The duty of the doctor is to understand what the nature of this power of poisoning is; if he takes refuge in 'unknown poison' as a cause, he is no doctor, but clearly a layman . . . We seek a light, which will distinguish poison from poison, and demonstrate the root cause of each; we will sharpen our eyes to recognize its proper nature and location; so that we may fight, not at hazard, but with a clear and distinct method, and certain remedies . . .[45]

Aromatari's treatise is much later than the rest, and there is a Cartesian ring in his voice. More typical, perhaps, of the medical profession in the last quarter of the sixteenth century are writers of practical treatises like Laurent Joubert's *Medicinae Practicae*,[46] which appears to operate entirely on the basis of humoral medicine, but discusses the influence of the heavenly bodies on the total substance in its account of plague in a way which echoes Fernel; or Horatio Augenio, who wrote several books on protecting oneself from the plague.[47]

Augenio refers to Montanus, Fracastoro, Fernel and Joubert as modern authorities on the subject, and his discussion of the celestial causes of the plague both follows Fernel and reveals an indifference at the thought of unknown causes that would have made Aromatari grind his teeth. Plague arises, says Augenio, not from putrefaction of the air as some say; others, much more learned, attribute it to the planets, which introduce into the air

a kind of evil quality, secret, hidden and obscure to our senses, which therefore has no proper name, because we understand nothing of it except in general, for it is an occult and incomprehensible quality, known to us only from its horrible effects . . .[48]

One would expect a work on occult properties in medicine to be sympathetic to specific forms and diseases of the total substance, and both Antonio Lodovico's *De Occultis Proprietatibus* (1540) and Joannes Franciscus Ulm's two versions of a treatise on occult quality in disease, *De Iis quae in Medicina agunt ex Totius Substantiae Proprietate* (1576) and *De Occultis in Re Medica Proprietatibus* (1597) fulfil this expectation.[49] Ulm is interesting for several reasons. Both works are very similar, and both are organized around Galen's four categories of substances which 'act from the properties of the total substance' which Ulm identifies as foods, medicines, *deleteria* or poisons and *alexipharmaca* or antidotes. He devotes a book of his treatise to each, attributing such properties firmly to 'certain celestial powers' which are not elemental. He credits Avicenna with this opinion; and notes also the authority of the 'most elegant Fernel' in the *Hidden Causes*. Ulm indeed follows Fernel quite closely; an interesting feature of his account is the way in which he positively makes a virtue of the central role of *experientia* in understanding occult phenomena, and, indeed, manifest causes of disease as well. Medicine takes its beginning from the senses, and proves its reasons correct by what fits, or does not fit, with sense experience. Ulm's basic argument in favour of properties of the total substance is similar to Fernel's: without it, the difference between the action of bodies of similar temperament cannot be explained.[50]

Two French texts on poison and contagious diseases deserve a little more attention, as they were written by doctors who cite Fernel as an authority and in one case as 'praeceptor meum'. Jacques Grevin's *Deux livres de Venins* was printed in Anvers in 1568.[51] It is a naive and conventional work, often confused in its arguments, but adding a few details to the picture. Grevin divides occult disease into two categories, contagious, which he defines as spread by touch, but which also includes plague; and 'simply poisonous'. The poisons which cause both types of disease can act in one of three ways:

1) by a 'hidden power' which is based on a particular, occult mixture of the four elements;
2) by a temperamental imbalance in the prime qualities;
3) most dangerously, 'by a particular evil received from the influence of some celestial sign, as several have thought.'[52]

Julien Le Paulmier's *De Morbis Contagiosis* (1578) is even closer to

Fernel, and much more comprehensive in its theoretical treatment.[53] It deals with four diseases, syphilis or lues venerea, elephantiasis, rabies and pestilential fevers, all of which Fernel identified with an occult cause. All four – indeed, Le Paulmier seems to be saying, all diseases of any sort – inhere in the simple parts of the body. The details of his account follow Fernel closely; it is as though the *Pathology* had been rewritten to include all the theoretical detail of the *Hidden Causes*. Occult diseases, then, arise not from an imbalance in temperament, but from an attack on the substantial form. Like Riolan, Le Paulmier conflates Fernel's pestilential and contagious categories in practice, though in theory he divides diseases by their origin as Fernel had: from the air, by contact from something outside the body, and internal, in the form of poisonous food, drink or medicines. A disease like syphilis attacks in the classic manner of poisons, entering the body and changing not only the (especially vulnerable) spirituous parts, but also the humours and fleshy and solid parts as well to its own likeness.[54]

Can we see a pattern here? I think, as I have already suggested, that the fate of Fernel's doctrine of the diseases of the total substance depended upon the purpose, and the background, of the later writers who encountered it. Undoubtedly, it was a minority view, with a certain amount of Galenic authority against it. At best, it was a complex and unfamiliar theory, introducing new layers of facultative action which Galen had been able to do without. At worst – and this is an aspect which clearly made medical writers uneasy, despite Fernel's spirited defence – it cast those who accepted it loose on a sea of empiric medicine, weakened their defences against lay practitioners and meant that they had to start from scratch in piecing together the principles of action of diseases and the remedies which would benefit them. Theories based on the action of the temperaments existed for most of the diseases which Fernel classed as occult. Faced with the problem of discriminating between diseases which Galen had described in similar terms but which clearly were different, doctors could choose to multiply the types of temperament allowed, producing a mesh of latitudes which became almost unusable; or they could follow Fernel in identifying a new class of diseases with an entirely different method of operating.

Those who chose the latter route were, on the whole, those who had something to gain from the change: those whose speciality, for whatever reason, lay in the areas of disease action – poison and contagious diseases – which Fernel had spotlighted; those who were based at universities in parts of Europe – France and Germany in particular – where Fernel's reputation as an authority was especially high; those who were convinced by the 'elegance' of his arguments to abandon the web of temperamental causes in a genuine attempt to understand the action of this group of spectacularly dangerous diseases.

But the unfortunate fact is that, as with other aspects of Galenist medicine in the late sixteenth century, the theory of temperaments still had a lot to recommend it. Those who chose not to follow Fernel – and the sliver of evidence I have been able to examine suggests that they were the majority – had a proven and comprehensive method on their side, which could be applied to the action of any disease whatsoever, and which fitted neatly into the Aristotelian–Galenic system of natural philosophy in which they had been educated. It was a familiar method, of which they could have the rules, codified in banks of treatises and commentaries, at their finger-tips. It was a comfortable solution, and, besides, it gave them security from the claims of empirics, and a weapon in the battles against unlicensed practice which concerned many faculties, those of Paris and London in particular. Faced with such a choice, what established academic could afford to raise his eyes to Fernel's celestial regions, 'beyond the power of the elements'?

10

Fabricius and the 'Aristotle project' in anatomical teaching and research at Padua

ANDREW CUNNINGHAM

After J. H. Randall Jr's classic paper of 1940[1] and the work of other scholars since, which show late sixteenth-century Padua to have been a hot-bed of discussion and modification of Aristotelianism, to claim to have discovered that anatomy (or indeed any other discipline) at Padua was 'Aristotelian' at that period is like claiming to have invented the wheel. But my claim is in fact somewhat different. I want to maintain and illustrate the following case in this chapter: that at Padua in the second half of the sixteenth century there was a deliberate, sustained and successful attempt, under the leadership of Hieronymus Fabricius (1533–1619), to recreate *the research programme of Aristotle in anatomy*; that this consisted of an enterprise far more thorough-going than the adoption of particular Aristotelian categories or techniques; and that an appreciation of the nature of this 'Aristotle project' (as I call it) will provide us with a far better and more authentic understanding of what Fabricius and his followers were doing and why they did it. In particular it should lead us to reconsider whether the anatomical research in this school was primarily an attempt to resolve long-standing 'problems' in anatomy, or not.

In order to admit the possibility that such a comprehensive 'Aristotle project' might have existed at all in late sixteenth-century anatomy, we have first to concede that the history of anatomical investigation in this period is not a monolithic whole. We do in fact tend to see it in this way usually, and we are fond of identifying those people in the past who made what we term 'significant contributions' to it. I want to urge, by contrast, that we develop a willingness to recognize that people at different times and places might actually have been doing *different* things when they explored and discussed anatomy. My colleague Roger French has been engaged on a characterization of the anatomical work of Berengario da Carpi in this light, and it is becoming clear that what Berengario was doing in the first couple of decades of the sixteenth century was something different from what Vesalius was to be doing some twenty years later.[2]

What I want to maintain here is that certain people after Vesalius – though working perhaps in Padua, working even in the shadow of what Vesalius had done – began to do something different again in anatomy from what Vesalius had been doing. The nature of their anatomical research was different.

If we are prepared to concede this possibility, then we may also be persuaded to look in a different light on that supposed age-old quarrel between Aristotle and Galen, purportedly carried out in dutiful fashion over the centuries by their respective followers. For when I talk about the 'Aristotle project' I am not referring merely to a continuation of this venerable quarrel (if such it had been); nor am I talking about the differences in the doctrines of Aristotle and Galen which might be brought into discussion when a given topic was being explored. Instead I am talking about a commitment to *a particular type of research*.

Well, what was the 'Aristotle project'? It might be tempting to assume that anyone engaging on a project describable in this way, would follow the sorts of activities that we normally interpret Aristotle as having been engaged on. So we might expect an 'Aristotle project' in the late sixteenth century to have been a matter of taxonomy and comparative anatomy, for this is how we most often teach or write about Aristotle the 'biologist': as taxonomist *manqué* and as the 'father of comparative anatomy'. But these are not the directions in which I want to go in portraying the 'Aristotle project'. For my purposes here, what matters is what particular sixteenth-century anatomists thought Aristotle had been doing: how they read him. And if they were actually reading his works as *programmatic* for their own anatomical research (as I am claiming), then they were definitely looking at him for purposes different to ours, and thus seeing something different in his writings.

Fortunately a reading of Aristotle's 'biological' writings which offers some useful pointers to how he might have been read as a model *researcher* into nature, has been offered in a superb paper by Professor D. M. Balme.[3] To briefly resume Balme's argument: Aristotle has much discussion on the criteria for a classificatory system; and he criticizes the use of a dichotomous system when applied to animals because it will always fail. Three major works by Aristotle survive which are on 'biological' themes: *History of Animals*, *Parts of Animals* and *Generation of Animals*. Can Aristotle's theory be reconciled with his practice in these works? Balme argues that if we assume that these books are contributions towards a taxonomy, then the answer is no. For Aristotle was not actually making a classification of animals. What then was he doing with all his apparently random groupings of animal differentiae in his discussions? His discussions (according to Balme)

show how differentiae are essentially associated or divergent, and this is the real use that Aristotle makes of them in *Parts of Animals* and *Generation of Animals*. In his arguments about causes there, he appeals largely to the interrelationship of differentiae which appear to belong together. He seeks the significant, causal grouping of differentiae . . . His method in fact is what he briefly describes at *Posterior Analytics* II, 98a, 14–19: by looking for the characteristics which are regularly associated we may detect their cause . . .

Aristotle's purpose in *Parts of Animals* and *Generation of Animals* is made clear: to find the 'causes' of animals' parts, and of their generation and growth. In doing so, it seems that an important part of his method is to look for significant differentiae and combinations of differentiae; he constantly groups and regroups them to focus on particular problems.

And in what might look like an incoherent jumble of observations in *History of Animals* too, Aristotle

does state his purpose: 'first to grasp the differentiae and attributes that belong to all animals; then to discover their causes' (HA I 491a 9).

For anyone who might have seen himself as a practising Aristotelian anatomical investigator, this sort of reading of Aristotle's own activity is much more likely than our customary view of Aristotle. It provides the elements of a programme of research. For what Aristotle has to say about such 'causes' of parts and of processes (such as generation) is manifestly incomplete; and further investigation along the same lines would soon reveal that Aristotle's conclusions are often contentious. Neither of these facts need necessarily undermine the validity of following such a programme. Indeed they could well serve to reinforce the acceptability of both the method and the programme: after all, a research programme has to feel reasonably open-ended in order to be worth taking up.

For researchers who are committed Aristotelians, this sort of enquiry into *causes* is the very stuff of philosophical investigation, and it provides the material for *scientia*-status statements and conclusions about why the world is the way it is. It is precisely the work of the Natural Philosopher. Aristotle had provided an impassioned argument that the bodies of animals (including man) are a legitimate area of study (I am referring to that celebrated passage in *Parts of Animals* I 5, 644b–645a), he had provided examples of the method at work, of topics appropriate for investigation (such as generation), of the terms in which the answers should be given, and (best of all perhaps) he had left the enquiry unfinished.

In addition we have to recognize that any explanation that Aristotle offered had to be true of all apparent exceptions too: the explanation (or 'cause') of the presence and function of a given part or organ in one creature had to be one which also covered its possible different incidence, or even its total absence, in another creature. What Aristotle does in practice is to specify either what other part or organ fulfils an analogous role in the other creature, or what particular features of that animal make the part or organ in question different in its incidence, or even unnecessary. The reasons for such particular occurrences or absences lie, for Aristotle, in one or more of four aspects of the creature in question:

1. its life
2. its activities
3. its habits
4. its (other) parts.[4]

This then is what I have in mind when I talk of the 'Aristotle project': an open-ended research programme on animals, devoted to the acquisition of true causal knowledge (*scientia*), on certain kinds of topic (not research 'problems'), such as parts, organs and processes, and employing a thought-through and consistent methodology and epistemology, a suitable technical vocabulary, and the like. And when I talk of such an 'Aristotle project' being practised in the late sixteenth century, I am referring to a deliberate and self-conscious attempt to model new anatomical research on this kind of view of Aristotle's own practice. What I have to do now is show that anyone actually followed such a programme in the late sixteenth century. Let us turn therefore to Fabricius, whom I consider to be the central figure in the practice of this kind of anatomy.

When looking at Fabricius I have the inestimable advantage of being able to build on the splendid work of H. B. Adelmann, who has edited and translated two of Fabricius' writings.[5] Adelmann in his introduction points out quite rightly that

We must turn to the philosophy of Aristotle for a key to the proper understanding of the rationale of Fabricius' treatises on embryology. Its essence is contained in Aristotle's dictum that "wisdom is knowledge about certain principles and causes" . . .

Nevertheless, Adelmann does not in fact portray what Fabricius is doing as being a piece of Aristotelian research; instead he tends to see every page as revealing a 'conflict between observation and authority': for 'his [Fabricius'] difficulty came when he attempted to adjust the evidence of his senses to the doctrinal pattern or framework of the times'. In other words, for Adelmann, Fabricius is a diligent, even occasionally inspired, empiricist and observer, struggling to throw off the shackles of authority, Aristotle and Galen.

In portraying Fabricius' teaching and research, I intend to work from his published writings. So it is necessary for me first to establish that his writings do indeed substantially represent both his teaching and his research. To do this I need to make an important point about his teaching, and the relationship that his writings bear to it.

For most of his career Fabricius was Lecturer on Surgery and Professor of Anatomy at Padua (1565–1613); from 1600 he had the title of Professor Supraordinarius in anatomy. Throughout his career, in these roles, his responsibility was to act as a teacher of anatomy by dissection, lecturing and demonstration, not just to limit himself to surgical matters.[6] In these positions Fabricius was personally one of the centres of world anatomy for half a century. He constructed an astonishing piece of equipment to facilitate his work: the famous anatomical theatre at Padua (finished in 1594), the first permanent structure of its kind, and which fortunately can still be seen and experienced today. Now, when students came, from all over Europe, to hear Fabricius lecture, what most of them wanted and expected was a concise account and demonstration of the human body, to which they could relate the human physiology, the pathology and the therapeutics they were also learning. They wanted this because they were training to be practising physicians. But what Fabricius gave them (when he could be persuaded to lecture at all) was often something different: whenever he could get away with it, Fabricius taught topics of his *research* programme. The records of the students of the German Nation reveal this conflict of interests quite clearly. Listen to this plaint of 1590:

He promises, but to no purpose . . . He has already spent two months on the exposition and description of the bones of the head. Having been brought on to the muscles he has completed three, devoting one hour to each muscle. There are so many muscles that, proceeding in this way, two years will not suffice. When then will he deal with the viscera? In addition, everything is treated confusedly and in a disorderly way: once he discussed the detached arm, going on after many days to discuss the foot. I don't see how anyone can learn the sequence and connection of the whole from looking at these.[7]

What might seem confused and disorderly to the student, wanting one thing ('the sequence and connection of the whole' in the human body), might well be highly organized and systematic to the teacher – if he was actually doing something else. Indeed Fabricius retorted angrily to the above complaint 'You came to prescribe to *me* the sequence – something you do not understand?' The Paduan medical student was caught in a bind: Fabricius was one of the world's foremost anatomists, at the world's most famous medical school; but when students arrived there they found either that he did not teach at all, or that he taught something other than what most of them felt they needed.[8]

In his late sixties Fabricius started publishing, and although he did not live to complete it, his programme for publication is quite clear. He wanted to write a *Theatrum totius Animalis Fabricae*, a Theatre of the whole animal fabric. This curious choice of title for his intended great work was an exquisite touch. For the book was meant to be a 'theatre' of anatomy in the same way as the physical building he had created was a theatre of anatomy: both of them were places to exhibit and display his teaching to an international audience.[9] Just as he had designed the physical building to give the best view to the maximum number of people, so too he was writing the book in order to reach the widest readership (even issuing it cheaply in parts), and designing it to give the best view to its readers.[10] He did this by employing a text systematically arranged to provide the most accessible exposition, together with an unrivalled range of illustrations executed to the very highest standards. But the book was not a substitute for the physical theatre. Rather it was a summation of the work that had gone on for over forty years in that theatre and in its makeshift predecessors. The book was to contain 'the whole anatomic business', that business of research and teaching to which Fabricius had devoted a lifetime. So the book was intended to cover the whole range of topics which Fabricius had taught and investigated. The lines along which this second Theatre was designed are still readily visible, for despite his late start Fabricius did manage to publish several items which were intended as contributions toward it. This publishing programme is precisely Fabricius' report on his research programme: what we see in the works he published is a sizeable fraction of his report, in the way he wanted it presented, of more than forty years of his research.

So, since Fabricius' publishing enterprise was a recording of his research (and preferred teaching[11]) activities over all these years, it is legitimate for us to look at all the publications in the way that he himself intended: as a series of items which were destined to make up a single large volume.[12] Indeed it is misleading for us to look at them as individual self-contained publications, because we are likely to miss the point of them if we do so. Thus, although they were issued over a long period (from 1600 to 1621) it is not essential for us to look at the works sequentially in order to allow for any major changes in Fabricius' views or intentions from 1600 until his death in 1619. There may indeed be a significance in the sequence in which the items were published, but there is no difference in his overall intentions and aims in the works themselves. Fabricius was filling his declining years 'writing-up' his research; he was no longer developing intellectually to any degree. Hence what I intend to do is to look at the prefatory material of all the individual items to discover Fabricius talking about his single large enterprise; the points that emerge will give us an idea of what he intended, of what issues he was pursuing, and in what categories. To satisfy the demands of chronology I will, however, treat the items in chronological order of publication (with one exception[13]). I shall also be offering some examples of his work: of what his *answers* look like. I hope thus to show the 'Aristotle project' in practice in the hands of its greatest sixteenth-century exponent.

The questions we shall be asking throughout this exploration are: what is Fabricius' concept of the nature of the anatomical enterprise, and of the rôle of the practising anatomist? what sort of questions does the proper anatomist ask? how does he investigate his material? what is the nature of this material? what does an anatomical answer look like? and so on.

We come then to the first works which Fabricius published, and they consisted of three individual studies, on the eye, the larynx and the ear, issued together in 1600 under a common title-page. From Fabricius' point of view this was an opportunity for him to thank and honour three men who had helped advance his career: hence he wrote three separate dedications, one to each item, all of which have the same date. I shall treat these three dedications as one large dedication divided into three.

In the dedication to the treatise *On the Eye*, Fabricius says he wanted to be useful to the world of learning, so he is (at last) publishing on anatomy (*de re Anatomica*). There is room for a contribution from him, even though many ancients and moderns have written about this matter. Many of the writings of the ancients have, after all, perished; and those which survive, such as the works of Aristotle and Galen, are of such a kind that it is obvious that many things escaped their attention, and many matters misled them. And after teaching the subject for forty years Fabricius cannot agree that the moderns have supplanted the ancients. Only one modern has a claim to have done so, and that is Vesalius. Yet even his work has serious limitations: it is devoted to attacking one man, Galen, more than is justified; it is obscurely written. It is not as complete as people think, Fabricius says, as the subsequent work of Columbus, Fallopius, Eustachius, Iasolinus, the Bologna anatomists, and of Fabricius himself and others shows. But more than this, Vesalius' work is particularly inadequate because he 'both rambles on rather generally sometimes, and also spreads himself too much in all the parts; yet he does not include all the matters which pertain to the Anatomic business, pursuing virtually dissection alone – scarce touching the actions and utilities of the organs'. So Fabricius is upbraiding Vesalius for having dealt with only one facet of the task of the anatomist: something so patently incomplete can hardly claim to be a full account of anatomy. And even on the issue of illustrations, Fabricius judges Vesalius' work to have been inadequate:

Now, if you look at his illustrations, Vesalius only gave forty eight, and those not large enough. We give more than three hundred, and those in royal-paper [that is, of large size]. And what about the fact that our illustrations are far superior in quality and perfection? As in those pictures of Vesalius which we have also diligently portrayed: we have added many things, everywhere in their natural size, and what is no less important, depicted them also in their natural colour. Furthermore, we have wanted all the pictures to be pairs: one coloured, one not; so that by this means educated men of any standard might be able more readily to profit from this useful (unless I mistake) brainchild of ours.

The exposition of his motives and intentions continues in Fabricius' dedication to *On the Larynx*. When learned men come to commit their thoughts to writing they adopt a certain way and order (*viam et rationem*) so that the things themselves (*res ipsae*) which have been grasped in the writer's mind should be clear to the understanding (*perspicuitatem habere*) by being the more distinctly related, and also so that the sequence (*ordo*) followed in the relation should assist the memory of the reader. What method (*methodus*) should Fabricius adopt for reporting his anatomic researches? He has decided that the best way would be to give (1) the *dissection* and *historia* of the part in question (this is the account to which, in his view, Vesalius had limited himself). Then should come (2) the *action* of the part, and (3) finally its *uses* or utilities. In this way the 'total knowledge' of the organs (*notitia organorum tota*) will be shown. Parallels to this procedure can (Fabricius says) be found in the respective coverage of particular books by Aristotle and Galen.[14]

> Moreover, lest anyone by chance imprudently neglects these parts [of anatomy], or imprudently denies that they are of such great importance, I can assert this truly: that they are of such consequence that the person who knows these exactly (*exacte*) can claim unhesitatingly that he has now learnt the whole anatomic business and that he is master of it (which whole anatomic business, in my view, is nothing less than the true and solid basis of the whole of Medicine, and the ultimate perfection and consummation of natural philosophy).

Turning, finally, to that part of his exposition which provides the dedication to *On the Ear*, we find Fabricius explaining why he is writing separate treatises. He claims to be following the procedure (*via*) of that great Artist 'whose works were at once both seen and approved'. For this artist thought it best not to show a statue as a whole, but first to let the parts be seen separately (such as a leg, an arm, the head), so that the necessary corrections could be made. He adopted this approach so that 'after every part had been judged sufficient and gradually approved one at a time, the whole work, made up from these parts subsequently joined and fixed together, might suddenly come into existence, in which nothing could now be criticised'. Fabricius is adopting this same approach in this his *Theatre*: offering a treatise at a time for the criticisms of learned people, just as it had been his practice for many years to ask his most celebrated colleagues 'admitted to my theatre' at Padua to use their 'lynx eyes' to assess and judge his findings.

In this three-fold dedication Fabricius has so far revealed quite a lot about his aims and intentions, and revealed also that these treatises represent some of the fruit of forty years of research. To summarize: a proper anatomical account must cover three areas: (i) dissection/*historia* (ii) action and (iii) uses/utilities. It should *display* the parts properly, which in the context of a book means ample illustration. He has said that anatomy in its fullness is the basis of medicine *and* the ultimate perfection of Natural Philosophy. And of course he has put forward these treatises as being an example of such proper anatomy.[15]

But more can be discovered about Fabricius' activity by inspecting the fruit itself. We may start with the title-page. Here the treatises are described as being about vision, speech and hearing: in other words, about physiological actions or activities. Each treatise however actually deals with an organ. This is not an error or oversight in titling; rather, it reveals something very important about Fabricius' attitude. It reveals that Fabricius takes it for granted that a full account of *organs* (their dissection/*historia* plus their actions plus their *uses*/utilities) comprises a full account of physiological *function*. There is no distinction here between merely structural anatomy on the one hand and physiology on the other. Proper anatomy *is* physiology: the equivalence is built into the methodology. It is also built into the etymology: a proper account of *organs* is a proper account of their role as entities which *do* something (*organa*).

Secondly we may note (from the very fact that he undertakes it) that Fabricius regards such research as possible, as important, and as necessary: physiological knowledge *can* be progressively developed and refined by more rigorous, more systematic, more detailed 'anatomic' research. Neither the ancients nor the moderns have said it all yet. (So much for the dead hands of Aristotle and Galen on research.)

Thirdly we need to note a most significant absence here. Nowhere in this lengthy three-part dedication has Fabricius talked about *human* anatomy as such. This ought to surprise us, for we would expect (as a very minimum) that someone whose job it was to teach the anatomy of the human body would have it as his central interest. It most certainly was the central interest of Vesalius, for instance. But this is not Fabricius' theme. Instead he has talked about a *Theatre of the whole ANIMAL fabric*. The organs and parts of a range of animals are indeed portrayed in his illustrations; others are mentioned in the text. So, if it was not human anatomy which was the focus of Fabricius' research, then was it perhaps 'comparative anatomy' on which he was engaged? It would be nice to think so, and F. J. Cole, the historian of comparative anatomy, claims that this was indeed the case: that Fabricius was in all his works comparing the parts of animals amongst themselves (vertebrates with vertebrates for instance), and sometimes also comparing the parts of man with those of other animals.[16] But closer inspection reveals that this is not the case either. Fabricius just is not interested in 'comparative' findings. He just is not offering accounts of given organs or parts which compare the form, structure and function of the organs or parts in different creatures; nor is he offering accounts of human organs or parts elucidated by comparison with those of other creatures. No, his enterprise is quite different.

What he is in fact offering are accounts of '*the* eye', of '*the* larynx', of '*the* ear'. His account of organs deals with the norm, with what can be said securely about eyes-in-general, or larynxes-as-a-whole: about their structure, their function and their *causes*, about how they are, and about why they are the way they are. His statements are ones which have the status of *scientia*: universally true explanatory accounts of the causes of phenomena. The knowledge which equips him to make these statements of general validity is of course built up from a wide acquaintance with the bodies of many different creatures. (He has in fact been making inductions, though this is not all that he has been doing.) As a result of such work, Fabricius feels confident that the general account he offers is indeed true of all creatures, or of all eyes (for instance) in all creatures.

Except – one should add – for the exceptions: for those which depart from the norm. For the general run of eyes one causal account is sufficient, being built up from the particular instances, and comprehending what they have in common. But for those which depart from the norm a *particular* account is necessary, to give the causal grounds for whatever particular difference is observed to obtain. It is on these occasions that Fabricius mentions the anatomical peculiarities of particular creatures: where they follow the norm they do not need to be specifically mentioned. (Hence we are hardly doing Fabricius justice if we assume he was acquainted only with the anatomy of the creatures he actually mentions.) One of the animals whose anatomy sometimes differs in some way from the norm, is, of course, man.

We do not have a suitable term to express this characterization of anatomical activity. 'Anatomy' is not broad enough and, without qualification, it makes us think exclusively or primarily of human anatomy. 'Comparative anatomy' we have seen carries the wrong emphasis. This is why I have chosen for the moment to call it the 'Aristotle project'. But in time we shall come across a term which does successfully embrace this activity, and it will be a term sanctioned by Fabricius himself.

It might seem that the very next work Fabricius published gives the lie to this conclusion that he is not particularly concerned with human anatomy as such. For in 1603 Fabricius published *On Speech* [*locutio*] *and its instruments*, a topic 'which it seems appropriate to deal with after the instrument of the voice'; and here Fabricius explicitly says that speech is the characteristic feature which distinguishes man from other animals: it is the means by which the concepts of the mind are expressed. And the work does indeed deal only with man. But it was published as one of a pair of treatises,[17] and the other is *On the Vocal Communication* [*loquela*] *of Brutes*, and this in turn deals with the comparable, but more limited, activity in animals. 'Brutes' is the term Fabricius uses for 'animals' when he does not mean to include man among them. It is of course entirely appropriate for Fabricius to have separated these two treatments, since man is, as he says, the only animal which does have speech (it is a peculiarity, a *difference*) and it is the feature which so completely differentiates him from other creatures. But only in this trivial respect has Fabricius departed from the enterprise he was undertaking in the three earlier treatises. His scope of enquiry is still in fact *all* animals.

Fabricius felt he was breaking new ground here. He considered it incumbent on him to specify that his treatment of human speech would be exclusively anatomical:

Anyone can infer from these [considerations] that grammatical and childish matters (as I might say) are not to be expected from me – though I have been expert for a long time in the pronunciation and formation of letters. For in the first place, I will bring forward the *natural* causes of all things; then, I will not depart even a finger's breadth from anatomy; and lastly, I will cite virtually no author(ity) besides Hippocrates, Aristotle and Galen.

As the marginal note (of the edition I have used) says: 'The Anatomist ought not to expound this topic [speech] in the Grammatical mode, but in the Philosophic one'.

Similarly, in writing on the vocal communication of brutes, Fabricius offers a justification for its study, representing it as an important part of philosophy proper. His introduction deserves quotation in full as it so clearly places this subject in the arena of philosophical enquiry:

Do not think that a useless subject is being proposed to you, dear Readers, when I decide to deal with the vocal communication of brutes. For this is nothing else than Philosophy, which investigates the natures of animals. Aristotle wrote much on this theme, and produced more books than about any other part of Natural Philosophy; therefore just as it is very useful to read the books *On Physics*, and to listen to their commentators, so it is rewarding to deal with the vocal communication of brutes. Indeed it is perhaps rather preferable to contemplate (*contemplari*) this and with it the whole *historia* and nature of animals, and then the volumes written on this subject, than to read the books of the rest of Natural Philosophy. For the books which have been written *On Physics*, and *On the Heavens* and *On Generation* [*and Corruption*] merely contemplate the first principles of Natural Philosophy and the elements; but those *On Animals*[18] examine and reach the conclusions and intended and perfected end. The former books embrace universals; the latter, particulars. The former reveal philosophy shapeless, the latter fully-formed. The former demonstrate just the roots of Philosophy, the latter demonstrate also the branches. And just as in the branches are produced the leaves, flowers and fruits, which are more useful, more pleasing and more perfect than the roots; so the aspect which investigates the nature of animals is much more excellent than the other parts of Philosophy: more perfected by the flowers and fruits, and more splendid.

I believe that the vocal communication of brutes should be added to this part [of Natural Philosophy]; six heads are drawn up on this topic:

Firstly: whether the vocal communication of brutes may be granted to exist, and what it is or what kind of thing it is.

Secondly: in what way the vocal communication of man resembles and in what way it differs from that of other animals; and [the resemblances and differences of the vocal communication] of other animals among themselves.

Thirdly: what might be the utility of the vocal communication of the other animals.

Fourthly: in how many ways animals show their mental states among themselves.

Fifthly: how the vocal communication of brutes may be understood or perceived by men.

Sixthly: what is the instrument of speech in brute animals, and what is the principal part in it; and how sounds are formed by brutes.

From the introductory material Fabricius presents for these two works, then, we can detect more about his enterprise. Again he is taking a physiological activity, and subjecting it to anatomical scrutiny in order to reach its 'causes'. Equally he is concerned with doing this for the class of animals as a whole (that is, brutes plus man). But he has now made it quite clear that he sees anatomy as a legitimate and important part of Philosophy – the enquiry after causes – and not as an area of knowledge valuable merely for its medical applications. Indeed this is for him the central component of Natural Philosophy. What is more, anatomy deals with the particulars of the world; it deals with natural philosophy in action as it were, with its conclusions and intended and perfected end (*conclusiones finemque consummatum et optatum*): it is an appropriate topic for the true philosopher. The masters of this *anatomic* enquiry are Hippocrates, Aristotle and Galen; they are the only authorities to whom the proper anatomist need have regard. But when it comes to the *natural philosophy* of which this anatomy is a branch, then Aristotle is the only authority who needs to be taken into account, either for its principles or for its intended end. So we have two important things here: anatomy is part of natural philosophy; and natural philosophy is as Aristotle has laid it down. But by actually extending the scope of anatomic enquiry into speech and the vocal communication of brutes, Fabricius is also demonstrating that the Aristotelian investigation of natural philosophy is capable of being extended into new areas. It is not a set of discrete problems; it is, much more, a programme of research.

In the same year as these two works appeared (1603), Fabricius also put into print an account of a discovery he had made as long ago as 1574: *On the little Doors in the Veins.*[19] It is clear that he had discovered these first in the veins of a human corpse he was dissecting: the demonstration of the veins in the human subject was, after all, one of his teaching duties. The illustrations that he provided for this work are confined exclusively to the body of man. Does this work therefore represent a departure from Fabricius' enquiry into the *animal* fabric? Is it an instance of a piece of purely man-centred anatomical investigation? I think not, even though this is how we customarily read it. (Our customary readings are of little use here, however, for we customarily read *ostiolum* as 'valve', which makes nonsense of Fabricius' exposition.) For if we read it in the light of Fabricius' publishing programme, as dealt with so far, we can see that this treatise is indeed of a piece with the other works. Fabricius himself says that it is part of his larger work on the fabric of the whole animal: it is indeed (he says) an example of the format in which he wants the other parts of the *Theatre* to be printed. As it has long been a central text for historians of physiology, *On the little Doors* deserves a more extended discussion here, in the course of which it should be possible to demonstrate how Fabricius treats his discovery as an integral part of his enquiry into the *animal* fabric.

No-one could claim that this short treatise is written in a way which is as systematic as the other treatises we have been discussing (unless it is perhaps constructed on some formal pattern unknown to me). Moreover its topic is somewhat different, for the *ostiola* are not single discrete bounded organs (like the eye, larynx and ear), since they are distributed throughout the body. Nevertheless an analysis of the presentation that Fabricius adopts shows that he does deal with these *ostiola* in a way directly comparable to that in which he had treated the discrete organs in the earlier treatises. What then is he doing? Fabricius refers to his discovery as *res nova inventa*, a 'new-discovered thing', and a 'thing' (*res*) for him is a phenomenon or object with a real material existence. He takes it for granted that it is the role of the natural philosopher to give an account of why such 'things themselves' (*res ipsae*) in the real world are the way they are, and fill the role they do: in other words, to investigate their causes. So this is what he does. It is not enough for him merely to report on the existence of these little structures: as an anatomist it is his role to *explain* them, for nothing less is a proper anatomical account in his eyes. The account he gives of them is as rigorous as anything else in his writings. But (naturally enough) the causes which Fabricius ascribes to the *ostiola* are generated from his underlying understanding of physiology.

So Fabricius quite naturally starts from the understanding that the veins are a system for distributing nutriment to the whole body, nutritive blood continually moving out unidirectionally in the veins to the parts, from the vena cava. The arteries by contrast contain blood with a vivifying role, and are based on the heart, and in them 'a flux and reflux of the blood constantly takes place'. Nevertheless, though the two systems have distinct functions, they both contain blood, and both exist to distribute essentials to the parts: they are both 'canals' of the blood. It is entirely appropriate therefore that they have similar (but not identical) structures. What Fabricius has discovered, in these *ostiola*, are membranes which occur only in the veins, and only in some of them at that. His causal explanation therefore has to be able to account for why there are no *ostiola* in the arteries (why they are not needed), even though the function and structure of the arteries is comparable to that of the veins; and also to account for why the *ostiola* exist in some veins but not others: what role do they fulfil where they are present, and what are the conditions which make them unnecessary where they are absent? His account of the *purpose* of the *ostiola* must be one which answers all these questions in the same terms. And while Fabricius does indeed discuss the occurrence of these *osticla* in the body of man – where he had in fact first discovered them – his account nevertheless is still of the membranes as they occur in *animals*, with man as a special (or typical) case. Let me offer a simple tabulation of some of Fabricius' prose to bring out some of these points.

Definition: What I am referring to by this name ('little doors'): delicate membranes in the cavity of veins, occurring singly or in pairs, mostly in the limb veins; opening upwards, and having a form like a node in a twig.

Overall purpose: To *delay* the blood, in the interest of the proper distribution and assimilation of nourishment throughout the body.

The *ostiola* are necessary in order
    (a) to ensure that the 'upper' limbs receive adequate nourishment;
    (b) to prevent permanent swelling in the extreme ends of limbs.

No anatomist has discovered them hitherto. Why not? Maybe because
    (a) since the veins are intended for the free flow of blood, anatomists would not expect to find *ostiola* in them;
    (b) they do not occur in arteries;
    (c) they do not occur in all veins (for example the vena cava, the jugulars, the 'outer' veins).

Why arteries do not require them :
    [Arteries have a different role: (a) although they contain blood, the arteries are not concerned with nutrition;]
    [Arteries have a different structure:] (b) their thick walls are unlikely to suffer distension;
    [Arterial blood has a different movement:] (c) in arteries there is constant flux and reflux, rather than predominantly one-way flow.

It was necessary to retard the flow of blood to ensure appropriate delay for aliment to be assimilated. This is shown (observationally) by the *construction* of the *ostiola*.

Why small veins do not need them:
    (a) they contain only a small amount of blood 'and all that suffices for them' for purposes of local nutrition;
    (b) their needs are met by the action of the *ostiola* in the larger veins.

Another need for the *ostiola* in the limbs (where they mostly occur):
    The frequent local motion which is characteristic of the limbs creates local heat; this would naturally draw more blood to the limbs, hence creating
    (a) undernourishment of the principal parts;
    (b) rupture of the limb veins;

. . . either of which was going to be very pernicious to the whole animal (*toti animali*), given it was essential that the principal parts such as the liver, heart, lungs and brain should always abound most copiously with blood. It was for this reason, I believe, that the vena cava (where it passes through the trunk of the body) and similarly the jugulars, should have been quite destitute of *ostiola*. For it was requisite that the brain, heart, lungs, liver and kidneys – which procure the conservation of the whole animal (*totius animalis*) – should abound with nourishment, and it was essential that it should not be detained in them even for a moment, both in the interests of replacing lost substance, and of producing the vital and animal spirits whereby life is conserved for animals (*animalibus*).

But if you observe *ostiola* at the beginning of the jugular veins in man, you may say that they have been placed there to detain the blood, so that in the declined position of the head it should not flood into the brain like a river and be accumulated there more than is appropriate.

Enough material has now been presented from this little work for us to see the nature of Fabricius' account. He deals with the *ostiola* as phenomena of the whole animal (*totius animalis*), giving a *historia* of them (number, form, site, distance, and so on), an account of their action, and of their use. And his account is at all points a *general* one. The last passage quoted is of particular interest, for here Fabricius gives the general case on the incidence of the *ostiola* in the jugulars, based on observation: that the jugulars are devoid of *ostiola*; and he gives the general reason for it: that here the blood must suffer no delay since the brain, as one of the principal organs, needs an unchecked supply of fresh nourishment. He then deals with an apparent exception, the case of man, where *ostiola* may be seen in the jugulars. This exception is resolved by relating it to the particular characteristics of the life of this animal. The *general* reason for the presence of *ostiola* (even here) still holds good: *ad sanguinem detinendum*. But man usually carries his head upright, and the supply of nourishment to his brain is suitably catered for in that position. So, when man bends his head, a rush of blood would occur to the brain: hence the (exceptional) presence of *ostiola* in the jugulars of man, fulfilling a function necessary for the life of this particular animal.

Thus, even in a treatise clearly first inspired by his having discovered the *ostiola* in a human subject, and a treatise illustrated exclusively by pictures of the *ostiola* in man, it can be seen that Fabricius is still dealing with the incidence of the *ostiola* in *all animals*, of which man is but one instance. For him to treat matters in this way was virtually second nature to him, since the investigation of the whole animal fabric was the subject-matter, goal and point of all his research.

The case is the same with a further area of Fabricius' research project, when he reported in 1604 on *The Formed Foetus*.[20] As with *On the little Doors*, it is very easy for us to misread the nature and purpose of this work. It is normally treated as an incident in, or 'contribution to', the history of embryology. And it may not be going too far to suggest that we normally see this sort of anatomical work as contributory to an investigation of *human* embryology; it is as if Fabricius uses the chick and other creatures because he cannot get hold of human material. Or, to put it in a more positive way, we normally regard Fabricius as performing research in 'comparative embryology', primarily to the end of refining knowledge about human embryology. It will be obvious by now that I believe all these assumptions are wrong. What Fabricius was doing was something different.

For Fabricius' topic of research here is not 'embryology', but *generation*, a topic defined in a way we no longer recognize among modern research disciplines. Again, his topic is not 'comparative embryology' (or 'comparative' anything else either), but the generation *of animals* – that is, of brutes plus man. We know that this is the case because Fabricius says so. Firstly, he says that his topic is generation: the text begins –

We are dividing our treatise (*tractatus*) on the matters which pertain to generation conveniently into three parts. The first deals with the generation of semen and its instruments. The second contemplates (*contemplatur*) the nature and faculties of the semen once produced, that is the procreation and formation of the foetus. The third deals with the foetus once formed, that is the care which is due to the foetus as long as it is contained in the uterus, after it has once been fully formed. Now discussion will begin about this last part.

Thus, from Fabricius' own words we know that he was engaged on a study of 'the matters which pertain to generation'; that he was dividing the content of one *tractatus* into three parts; and that this is the last of these (although the first to be published). He does not define any of the parts of the *tractatus* as pertaining to 'embryology'. Instead he has taken *one process* (generation) and, in the interests of convenient presentation, divided it into three stages. It might even be maintained that he has divided the process effectively into three organs: (i) the semen and its instruments; (ii) the uterus, and the egg as another uterus; and (iii) the parts which sustain the foetus once formed (which, though not organs were, Fabricius argues,[21] provided for the sake of the foetus and hence of *its* action).

On the second question, whether this was the generation *of animals*, we can again turn to Fabricius' own words, in the dedication of this work to the count of Arona. And although, in this context, the first mention of the subject of the book may sound somewhat startling, we need to listen to how Fabricius continues.

I am offering you the principles (*principia*) and rudiments of human life. Not only of human life but also of the life of most living creatures (*animantium*) – or at least of those which depart from the common pattern (*ratio*) of the others. How can anything more important, more abstruse, or more marvellous than this be spoken of or thought up? They say that the emperor Nero himself, highly captivated with wonder at this thing (*res*), wanted to look inside the cadaver of his dead mother, and contemplate that first home of man from which he himself had come forth. Nor is this surprising, for if there is anything diligent in the whole of nature, if there is anything provident, anything careful, God the creator of nature seems to have collected them all in forming, nourishing and conserving the foetus. Hence the Prophet breaks forth in these words: "I will praise thee o Lord, for I am wonderfully made". The delicate and fragile embryo originates in the confines of the maternal uterus, as if without sense, without motion, without thought, without deliberation, and what is more without that common enjoyment of light and air which we enjoy; and yet it is nourished, it grows, it is looked after.

But it is also possible to contemplate (*intueri*) an admirable wisdom in varying [this pattern]. All animals, which have been set up under diverse shapes, could not all be sketched and formed on one pattern (*ratio*). Moreover, to virtually all brute creatures – who have a rather brief destined period of life, and are [useful] for the food and clothing of man, and who fall prey to one another – it was necessary to allow the capacity of bringing forth multiple foetuses, lest a species of them be extinguished. And among these some meet the need by bearing two foetuses, some five, some eight, some more, some less, according either to the requirements (*usus*) of man or as their shorter or longer life demanded. Nature excelled in this matter, by arranging most suitably for the conservation and generation of each animal, so that whoever looks carefully into the matter may detect nothing which is not admirable, nothing not divine.

Truly *ta chalepa ta kala*, 'Difficult things are beautiful', as the saying goes: no little difficulty attends the eminence of this issue (*tractatio*), which difficulty is also increased by the fact that few of the ancients and none at all of the moderns have addressed themselves to this topic. Why this has happened I do not know, since indeed it is unworthy that such great marvels of nature should lie hidden from us. We shall reveal them with as much brevity as we can, and so effect it both by the placing of the illustrations and by the plan of exposition (*ratio dicendi*), that anyone henceforth may be able by himself to understand and contemplate (*contemplari*) those first beginnings of the life of every animal. In this way we shall both follow and expound that great interpreter of nature, Aristotle, who first and alone inquired into these mysteries; and if anything at times escaped him, we shall point it out.

The above passage does, I hope, firmly show that the scope of Fabricius' inquiry into generation covers all animals; he appreciates, but is undaunted by, the breadth of the enterprise. It should also be clear where it is that Fabricius looks for his model: to Aristotle. And he sees Aristotle as his *only* predecessor in this enquiry. The 'generation' of animals is of course a quintessentially Aristotelian theme, being the subject of one of his own books. Nothing could better demonstrate the way in which Fabricius identifies his enquiry with that of Aristotle, than that he has taken up an identical project. But the point I now want to stress is that the identification is not simply with Aristotle's topic (generation), nor with its extension (*all* animals), but that it also involves the detailed way the topic is investigated *and* the nature of the answers, both of which were also expressly modelled on Aristotle's work. Fabricius is deliberately picking-up anatomical investigation at the point where he believed Aristotle had dropped it, and pursuing it in precisely the way he believed Aristotle had pursued it. Fabricius' books *On the Formed Foetus* and *On the Formation of the Egg and the Chick* are attempts to continue and amplify Aristotle's own work on that Aristotelian theme of generation. It is part of Fabricius' active devotion to the resuscitation of the 'Aristotle project'.

It may be appropriate to give a couple of instances from *On the Formed Foetus* of 1604 and the posthumous *On the Formation of the Egg and the Chick*, of the detailed way in which Fabricius' inquiry is Aristotelian through and through.

For the first instance we can adapt a tabulation made by Adelmann, covering part of the chapter on the *historia* of the 'fleshy substance' or placenta. Fabricius writes:

In the first place a certain fleshy substance may be seen in virtually all viviparous animals, spread and poured on the internal surface of the uterus, applied to the ends of the vessels stretching to the uterus. In colour, softness, laxity, rarity [of texture], thickness, it is similar in almost all animals; but in magnitude, position, figure, number, it is considerably dissimilar; and it is by no means to be reckoned among the investments of the foetus.

Fabricius then turns to these aspects in which the incidence of the 'fleshy substance' is dissimilar in different creatures. We can use this section to uncover how Fabricius generates the content of his *historia*, and what he does with the information he then possesses.

We can see that the first stage of Fabricius' procedure is to build a full *historia* of the thing he is investigating, which on this occasion is the 'fleshy substance': that is, a full account from observation and dissection of everything noteworthy about the object, about its matter and form. It will be noted, in the passage above, that the ways in which Fabricius assessed 'dissimilarity' was according to number, figure, magnitude and site. These are, of course, among the *categories* of Aristotle's logic, and they had first been drawn up to give an exhaustive list of all the kinds of being that there are. When applied to anatomy, such categories embrace the totality of the *form* of any organ (as well as its matter). Fabricius has generated his *historia* by using just such categories. So he had asked a series of questions of each 'fleshy substance' he had investigated in every kind of animal available to him, including what number? what figure? what magnitude? what site? The systematic asking of such questions had produced a series of accounts of the 'fleshy substance' in its actual material manifestations in all creatures – of all the ways in which the 'fleshy substance' actually has being in nature.

But whatever its precise incidence in any animal, what makes each and every 'fleshy substance' a 'fleshy substance', is its possession of the *form* of 'fleshy substance' imposed on the appropriate matter: each and every 'fleshy substance' actually existing in nature is a 'fleshy substance' precisely because it is a material instance of this one general form. This general 'form' is itself the cause of why each of these 'fleshy substances' is a 'fleshy substance'. This brings us to the second stage of Fabricius' procedure (finding the similarities). For Fabricius' series of separate accounts provide him with the data from which to now make an induction, and thus to reach the *general* 'form' of the 'fleshy substance', the form of which the particular material ones are instances. The similarities in its incidence in the different animals reveal what are the essential characteristics of the form of the 'fleshy substance'.

Still in pursuit of a full *historia* of the 'fleshy substance' in general, Fabricius' third stage of procedure is to distinguish and group the *dissimilarities* in the incidence of the 'fleshy substance' in different creatures. In the first place Fabricius has found that it is not present in all animals; and this is a dissimilarity in the category of substance (does it exist in all animals or not?). Then come dissimilarities in the categories of number, figure (or form), site and size. To make this third stage of distinguishing and grouping of the dissimilarities clearer, I have rendered Fabricius' remarks into a dichotomous table (Table 1) (something which he does not do).

All this is still just the *historia*, the recorded account of what can be seen by observation, helped by dissection. By the time Fabricius finishes his treatment of the 'fleshy substance' he will have been able to offer reasons (causes) why these aspects of dissimilarity fall into these groupings.

Following his usual sequence of exposition, in part II Fabricius comes to deal with the *action* of the 'fleshy substance' and its *use*. Now, the problem he has here with the 'fleshy substance' (and indeed with all the parts dealt with in this treatise) is that it has no 'action' by Fabricius' criteria; that is to say, it does not carry out some unique and public rôle contributing to and indispensable to the effective functioning of the whole animal.[22] However, the 'fleshy substance' does, he argues, have an action with respect to (*gratia*) the *foetus*. Hence a usefulness can in fact be determined for it.

Fabricius starts his discussion of the *use* of the 'fleshy substance' by opposing the opinion of Arantius that in the human uterus the placenta has the function of a liver, purifying the blood from the mother before it enters the foetus. In the course of opposing this he raises several arguments from anatomy, which lead him to point to the existence and special characteristics of the 'anastomoses' between the uterus and the 'fleshy substance'. Hence, when he has finished demolishing Arantius, there is (he says) only one matter left to investigate: the mode or *ratio* of the union of the uterus and the 'fleshy substance', and its usefulness. Although anastomoses are involved, they are obviously not like the usual tight joins of the mouth of one vessel to that of another: for it is known that at birth the 'fleshy substance' peels away from the uterus without rupture. Hence

Nature therefore placed the fleshy substance at the end of the vessels, so that like glue it might preserve the connection of these vessels up to the time of birth. And this is the first and chief usefulness of this fleshy mass . . . We may say . . . that the special goal of usefulness in forming it was the protection and defence of the vessels.

The general *use* or *cause* of the fleshy substance has now been found: the general reason why it exists, and why it is as it is. This cause has been derived (or, more strictly, induced) from the visual, anatomical evidence of the *historia*. The second use it has, which Fabricius attributes without comment to Aristotle, is to serve as a storehouse of sanguineous aliment for the foetus.

Table 1. *Distinguishing and grouping dissimilarities of 'fleshy substance'*

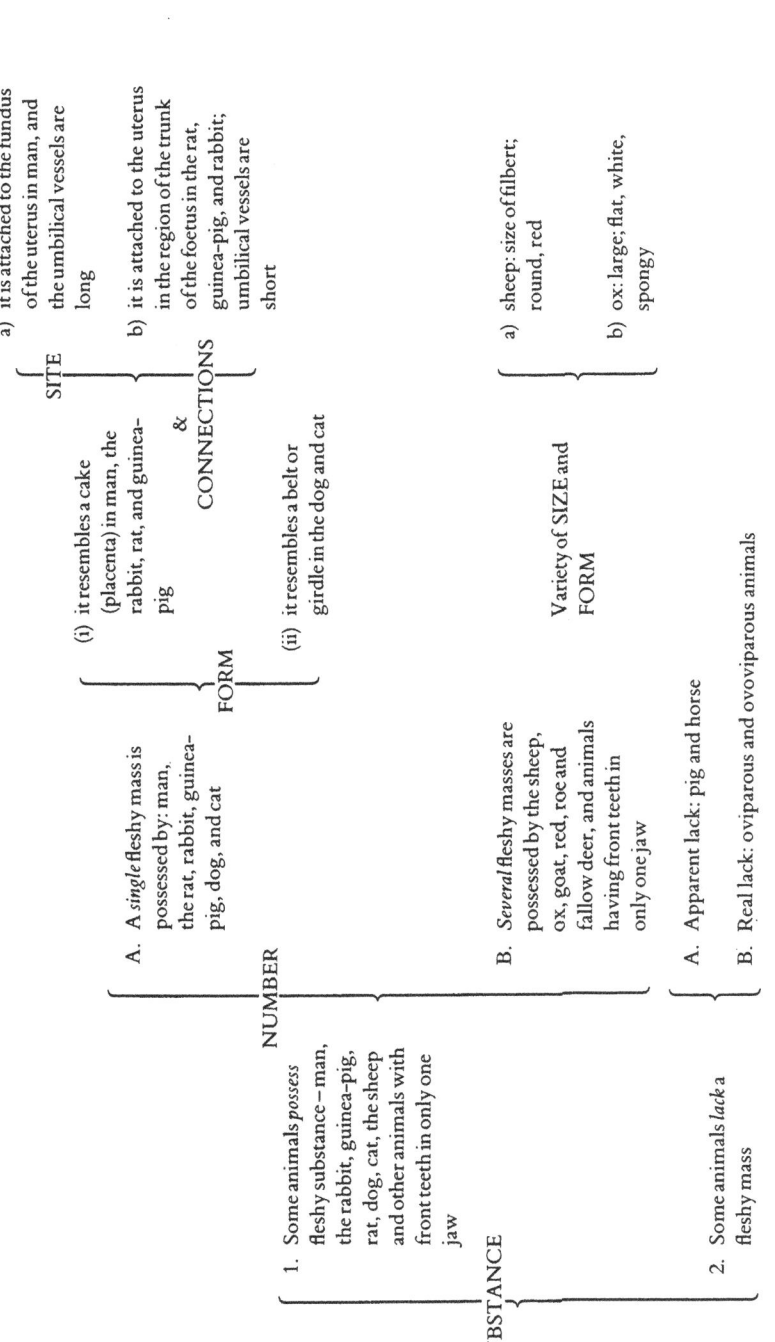

SUBSTANCE

1. Some animals *possess* fleshy substance – man, the rabbit, guinea-pig, rat, dog, cat, the sheep and other animals with front teeth in only one jaw

    NUMBER

    A. A *single* fleshy mass is possessed by: man, the rat, rabbit, guinea-pig, dog, and cat

        FORM

        (i) it resembles a cake (placenta) in man, the rabbit, rat, and guinea-pig

            SITE & CONNECTIONS

            a) it is attached to the fundus of the uterus in man, and the umbilical vessels are long

            b) it is attached to the uterus in the region of the trunk of the foetus in the rat, guinea-pig, and rabbit; umbilical vessels are short

        (ii) it resembles a belt or girdle in the dog and cat

    B. *Several* fleshy masses are possessed by the sheep, ox, goat, red, roe and fallow deer, and animals having front teeth in only one jaw

        Variety of SIZE and FORM

        a) sheep: size of filbert; round, red

        b) ox: large; flat, white, spongy

2. Some animals *lack* a fleshy mass

    A. Apparent lack: pig and horse

    B. Real lack: oviparous and ovoviparous animals

Finally Fabricius now sets out to *demonstrate* how the parts and attributes of the 'fleshy substance' (as determined during the *historia*) are suitable for these uses. For this purpose he turns again to the categories: he seeks to demonstrate (now using deductive argument) how the number, size, connections, quality of the 'fleshy substance' and its attachments are eminently suitable to (and indeed demand) the two usefulnesses he has established. The tenderness of the uterine vessels, the weight of the foetus, the movements of the mother, all demand that the 'fleshy substance' be soft in *quality* – which it is. For it to serve as a storehouse of sanguineous aliment (the minor use) it needs to be lax and rare in texture (*quality*) – which it is. In order to attract blood from all the parts of the uterus there needs to be a large *number* of 'placentulae' – which there is. To be safe from all injuries, it should be round in *form* – which it is. And to fit with the veins of the uterus, to allow blood to descend to the foetus by its own weight, to be clear of the residues, to avoid being compressed by the foetus, and to give sufficient room for the foetus, the 'fleshy substance' needs a *situation* high in the uterus – which it has.

The demonstration so far has dealt with what was similar in the incidence of the 'fleshy substance' in all animals which possess it. Now, finally, Fabricius turns back to the task of explaining the *particularity* of the incidence of the 'fleshy substance' in particular creatures: turns back, that is, to the cases where the incidence was *dissimilar*, and to showing how they are nevertheless cases of the general uses he has established for it. And we have seen him write that 'in magnitude, position, figure, number, it is considerably dissimilar'. It is to these issues that he now turns, in order to complete his account:

Before I put an end to this thing (*res*), it is worthwhile to enquire why this fleshy mass is single in some [creatures], such as man and dogs, multiple in others, such as sheep, the ox, goats; and again, why in some it resembles a large cake, as in man, or little cakes, as in the sheep, the ox, goats, or a broad belt or girdle or band surrounding the trunk of the body, as in dogs and cats; and finally why it is present in some, absent in others.

These questions are respectively about the categories of number, form, substance.

In what terms are these questions to be answered by Fabricius? By specifying what *other* particular feature(s) of the creature in question determine(s) that the 'fleshy substance' will have this particular incidence in it. The range of headings under which such particular features can be sought are one or more of the following (and only of the following):

the life; the activities; the habits; the (other) parts

of the particular creature. Fabricius' own sentiment is as follows:

This diversity [of incidence] – although it has been explored by no-one – yet I believe that it comes (unless I mistake) from the diversity both of the uterus and of the foetus: of the uterus insofar as it either has horns or is destitute of them; of the foetus insofar as one or several foetuses are procreated in the uterus.

In other words, Fabricius is putting the diversity of incidence down to variation in *other parts* of the animal (the uterus), or to the fecundity of the animal (the foetus) – which itself is determined by the animal's use for man or its falling prey to other creatures[23] – that is, to its *life*. The several pages which Fabricius devotes to spelling out how this double diversity affects the incidence of the 'fleshy substance' in various creatures can be conveniently read in Adelmann's translation.

These, then, are the components of Fabricius' full answer (insofar as he can find one for this part):

(1) a *historia*: generated from the observation and dissection of the organ in question in all animals, by asking a particular series of categorical questions; and an induction from this data to reach the *general* form or *historia* of the organ;

(2) an investigation of the *action* of the part;

(3) an induction to discover the *use* or *cause* why it is as it is; and finally

(4) a demonstration of the validity of this cause, and an explanation for the dissimilarities in the incidence of the part in question.

Then the account is complete: as far as his research has allowed him, he has acquired *scientia* about the 'fleshy mass', for he knows about its *causes*, both in general and in its many particular incidences. But it cannot be stressed too much that the object of study here, which is subjected to this procedure, is a part or organ, *not* a particular creature, nor a part *in* a particular creature. In our instance it was the 'fleshy substance', not 'the "fleshy substance" in man' or any other particular animal. And, in the context of this book on *The Formed Foetus*, the 'fleshy substance' was being studied in order to understand a common process, one applicable to all animals, the process of *generation*. The result obviously throws light on what we might call 'human embryology', but the enterprise is not about it.

Finally in this section we can look briefly at a passage from *On the Formation of the Egg and the Chick* (1621), which may further illustrate the manner of accounting for the *peculiarity* of incidence, this time of an activity. Fabricius has been expounding the utility of the action of the uterus (that is, the 'usefulness' of egg-laying), and now turns[24] to explaining why (*cuius gratia*) the formation of the foetus is effected via eggs in birds and some other animals. There are five different reasons why various creatures do so, and such creatures fall into five groups with respect to this activity. Now I tabulate his prose.

1. *Birds:* They lay eggs because they *fly.*
   A living foetus inside them would impede their flying, which is 'the special action of birds'.

[Confirmatory reason:] The rest of their anatomy shows they have no other
internal parts which might flap around and impede their flying either.

Apparent *exception* to this explanation:

the bat: it flies yet bears live young.

The apparent exception is *solved*:

'It is solved from Aristotle, because the bat is partly a flying animal and a
biped, partly a terrestrial quadruped, or it should rather be said it has both
natures deficient, since just as it is a maimed biped, so it is a mutilated
quadruped, although it has teeth.'

2. *Serpents:* They lay eggs because they *crawl*

A foetus growing inside would be injured by their form of locomotion.

Apparent *exceptions* to this explanation:

the viper: it produces both eggs and living foetuses, and bears them within
itself;

cartilaginous fishes: they do likewise.

3. *Turtles:* They lay eggs because of their *body structure*.

A foetus could not grow inside them, because the hard and rigid carapace
would restrict it.

4. *Fish:* They lay eggs because (a) they *cannot copulate properly* –

thus, because the male has to sprinkle the foetuses with semen outside the
body, they have to be produced as eggs;

and (b) because fish *must produce many offspring* for which there would not be
enough room inside the parent's body.

Apparent *exception* to this explanation:

the dogfish: it is a fish yet is both oviparous and viviparous.

The apparent exception is *solved:* because the dogfish is cartilaginous, cold and
humid. Hence it must produce a soft egg; this would perish if laid outside the
body.

5. *Ants* and creatures with very small bodies.

They lay eggs (a) because they are *small*, and could not produce sufficient
nourishment for live foetuses;

and (b) because they produce *many young*.

Each of the reasons Fabricius has given to explain egg-laying is particular to each group. And each cause has respect to either the *other parts* of the
creatures, or their *habits*, *life*, or *activities* (flying, crawling, mode of
copulation). But what of the exceptions which Fabricius himself mentions?
The two exceptions that he 'solves' are both solved in the same way. The
bat is shown to have *two natures* (it is partly a flying animal and a biped, and
partly a terrestrial quadruped) and it is deficient in both (*utram naturam
mancam habet*). It is neither fully in one group nor the other; therefore it
cannot be expected to have the foetus-producing characteristics of either
one group. The dogfish also has a curious set of characteristics, being at the
same time cartilaginous, cold and humid (though I confess to ignorance
about the precise dual nature of these characteristics). Such 'sharing in both
sides' is exactly the sort of explanation that Balme has shown that Aristotle

was using when seeking the significant, causal grouping of differentiae.[25] The exceptions are explained *by virtue of* 'sharing in both sides'.

Some ten years passed between *On the Formed Foetus* (1604) and Fabricius' next publication.[26] Fabricius was now in his eighties. We can move somewhat more quickly through these works of his oldest age, for they each and all continue to conform precisely to the pattern we have established for his earlier writings. But the physical format of the works was somewhat different: they generally lack dedications or prefaces; none of them have illustrations (except for the posthumous *On the Formation of the Egg and the Chick*); and the first publication was in quarto. Thus the format has changed, although the intentions are still the same.

If we glance briefly at *Two books on Respiration and its Instruments* of 1615, we are still on familiar territory. Fabricius here again takes a physiological activity for treatment. Again it is a theme on which Aristotle had written a treatise. Again, like that of Aristotle, the treatise deals with respiration as a phenomenon common to all animals. And this time Fabricius follows Aristotle quite precisely, which leads him to change his normal order of presentation. For Aristotle had opened his own treatise *On Respiration* by exploring the question why this phenomenon happens in living creatures, and Fabricius does likewise (that is, he deals with 'use' before *historia* and 'actions'). Recognizing that respiration is the most critical activity for the life of all animals, Fabricius concludes that 'the greatest and most principal usefulness of respiration is the conservation of the innate heat; and the minor usefulness is the nourishing of the animal spirit', both of which happen in the heart. It is therefore to the heart that respiration is most *utilis*. Thus Fabricius is not strictly dealing with an organ in this treatise, for the lungs do not have this role: he sees the thoracic muscles as the main instruments of respiration, while he sees the lungs as mere passive containers without an action of their own. As might by now be expected, Fabricius' treatment of respiration is of it as an activity of all animals. To go no further than the opening words of book II:

With the use of respiration now explored, it is also easy to understand why, amongst animals, some of them respire, and some lack respiration; further, why some satisfy their need for respiration in the air, others in water; while with regard to these [water-creatures], some fill the *usus* of respiration with a thorax and lungs, others achieve it without lungs, and others in yet another way . . .

In 1618, the last year of his life, Fabricius issued three treatises: *On the Local Motion of Animals, as a Whole; A Treatise on the Gullet, Stomach, Intestines;* and *On the Coverings of Animals.* The title pages celebrate him as 'Supraordinarius of Anatomy at Padua University now for fifty years'. I will take it for granted that I no longer have to prove or to show that each of these works, like all the earlier ones, constitutes a continuation of the

'Aristotle project' in theme and treatment. I will instead concentrate simply on a couple of passages from them in which Fabricius points to a critical distinction between his own approach to anatomy and that of other anatomists.

The first of these comes from *On the Local Motion of Animals*, at a point where Fabricius has been discussing the muscles of the leg.

> You will perhaps be surprised, Reader, that I did not describe the muscles like Vesalius did throughout his writings, and Galen did in the book *On Anatomical Procedures*; they described them with regard to their sequence or convenient dissection, since indeed they merely wanted to put before our eyes and display the dissection of them, as one follows another and is contiguous and connected. But we, whose aim is to teach by means of (*per*) what pertains to the muscles – their actions and uses – have, in dealing with them, appropriately led you in a different order, one which leads us certainly to a knowledge (*notitia*) of the occurrences of the muscles and joints. For if anyone should seek a simple dissection, and number them in this way: first, second, third, and so on, he would get confusion rather than useful[27] knowledge of the muscles. But when we search for the *causes* of what pertains to the muscles, then we are seeking their *use*, and we commit the number of them to memory more exactly (*exactius*).
> [p. 82].

Fabricius has here claimed that going about things in his way actually provides one with a more appropriate and a 'more exact' account even of something as apparently straightforward as the number of the muscles! In particular he has here distinguished his enterprise from that of Vesalius, and from that of Galen in *On Anatomical Procedures*: he has in effect taken his own work out of the tradition into which we usually put it.

What Fabricius meant by knowing something 'more exactly' (*exactius*) will be elucidated in our consideration of one last passage from his writings. It comes from the opening sentences of *A Treatise on the Gullet, Stomach, Intestines*. His theme, Fabricius says, is the stomach; but various other parts are connected to it in a series of organs:

> Therefore we are beginning a consideration (*tractionem*) of the stomach, intestines, gullet, omentum, and the muscles of the anus and abdomen. We must deal with these *pros akribeian*, not *pros tēn opsin*, to use Aristotle's words: that is, *exactly and most diligently*, not just *for the eye alone* and by a so-called 'popular' anatomy. And thus we shall explore, according to my custom, three matters about each organ, viz. the *historia* or structure or anatomy; then the *action* of the organ; in the third place its *usefulnesses*.

The words of Aristotle to which he is alluding come from his *On Respiration*, and may be translated as follows:

> How the position of the heart relates to the lungs, must be investigated with the eye (*pros tēn opsin*) from dissections, but with exactness (*pros akribeian*) from *historiai*. (478b 1–2)[28].

The key to the distinction Fabricius is making in the above two passages and in his citation of Aristotle, lies in another passage from Aristotle's writings. It is a passage which indeed holds the key to virtually every feature of Fabricius' anatomical enterprise. The passage in question is Aristotle's main statement of his own programme of investigation into animals, and it comes from early in his *Historia Animalium*. After citing various general ways in which animals differ (some are aquatic, others are terrestrial; some are viviparous, others are oviparous, and so on) Aristotle wrote:

> So these things – about which we shall speak later with exactness (*di'akribeias*) – have now been said in this manner in outline as a foretaste about all such things; all must be inspected (*theōrēteon*) so that first we might grasp (*labōmen*) the recorded differentiae and the attributes. After this we must attempt to discover (*heurein*) the causes (*aitiai*) of them. For the method (*methodos*) must be followed thus in accordance with nature, since the recorded *historia* [is] about the particular: for demonstration (*apodeixis*) must be about the particulars and from them; out of them it obviously arises.
> (491a 7–14).

Not only does this short passage contain the distinction Fabricius employed above, between *exactness* and *visual inspection*, but it also contains the whole programme which we have seen him pursuing in all his work. In this passage Aristotle announces his goal: the discovery of *causes*. He calls his procedure for arriving at these causes a *method*, and specifies how it is to be achieved. First one *inspects* closely the variety of the different parts, organs, arrangement of their bodies, and ways of living of all animals: this visual inspection produces a *historia*, a record of the attributes and differentiae of animals. (For Fabricius this comprehends all the things that can be seen by dissecting and anatomy: the structure or *fabrica*.) Then, secondly, one generates or derives the underlying common *cause* – the universal nature – which accounts for a given phenomenon. Finally, one *demonstrates* the validity and applicability of this universal cause in its particular occurrences: in those very same particular instances from which both the *historia* and the *cause* had been generated. What makes the account 'exact and most diligent' is the very fact that a *complete* causal answer has been arrived at and then demonstrated. It needs to be noted that the Greek term used by Aristotle, the Latin term used by Fabricius, and the English term 'exact' (in a now obsolete usage) all have the sense of 'perfected, consummate, finished', as well as 'rigorous, precise'.

Aristotle's method is a three-stage procedure (*historia*–cause–demonstration), each stage of which Fabricius' account fulfils. But Fabricius, as we have repeatedly seen, gives an account which actually has four stages. As he never tires of saying, a proper *account* – one which reaches causes – alone requires three stages:

  (i)   a *historia*
  (ii) an inquiry into *actions,* and
  (iii) a specification of *usefulnesses.*

Demonstration would therefore make a fourth stage. The *historia* stage is precisely the same as that of Aristotle; while the *usefulnesses* stage is the equivalent of Aristotle's final stage of *causes.* For his second stage (*actions*), and his reformulation of the third stage (causes = usefulnesses) Fabricius was heir to the anatomists after Aristotle. The early Alexandrians had reportedly made *actions* the focus of their inquiry; while it was Galen who insisted that this needed to be completed with a critical third stage, that of *usefulnesses* (this is what *On the Usefulness of the Parts* is about). Fabricius says [29] that Galen is his source for these.

    Even though Galen's name has now been brought in to our discussion alongside that of Aristotle, it would be wrong to see any 'contradiction' here in Fabricius' anatomical endeavour. For, from one perspective, Galen's innovation here had consisted simply of a spelling-out of the hidden necessary stages which lay between Aristotle's *historia* and *aitiai.* Certainly this is how Fabricius treats it. And, in the work where he introduced these features Galen had portrayed himself as doing *philosophy* just like Aristotle;[30] hence he may be seen as simply elaborating on the requisite mental operations needed to fulfil Aristotle's own objectives. So the fact that Fabricius uses terms originated by Galen does not make his enterprise any less the 'Aristotle project'.

    But for someone pursuing the 'Aristotle project', like Fabricius, it needs to be remarked that Galen's anatomy had more than one aspect. Obviously *On the Usefulness of the Parts* was 'exact'[31] in its procedure, and its status was as part of the philosophical inquiry. But (as we have seen) *On Anatomical Procedures* did not fit into the same category for Fabricius: it was more limited, simply a *historia,* less 'exact'; it was for the eye alone. It simply did not go far enough to be considered a full, philosophical, piece of anatomy. (Nor, of course, had Galen intended it to be the same kind of work as *On the Usefulness of the Parts.*) Likewise with the work of Vesalius which, even according to its own title, was simply a *fabrica.*

    The term for his own enterprise which Fabricius himself sanctioned was, thus, 'exact anatomy', and it embraced everything we have portrayed under the name of the 'Aristotle project'. Fabricius' most famous pupil, William Harvey, was to use yet another term for it, which he employed for the title of his earliest surviving work: '*Universal Anatomy*'.[32] But whatever the title we use for it, the distinctive defining characteristics of this anatomical enterprise are, I trust, now clear.

    Leaving aside many of the aspects that I have discussed during this paper, it is perhaps worthwhile to return to the issue of how Fabricius found topics for inquiry. We recall that he wrote works on *generation* (*On the Formed Foetus*, and *On the Formation of the Egg and the Chick*); there was *On the Local Motion of Animals* and *On Respiration* too. All of these processes are topics on which Aristotle himself had written a treatise; in each case Fabricius claims that Aristotle was the only person who had explored them before. So some of Fabricius' topics of inquiry, his research subjects, are *precisely* the same as those of Aristotle. And I have argued that in the other works, Fabricius takes *organs in all animals* as his theme, which again is faithful to Aristotle's own way of demarcating issues for inquiry. All the topics that Fabricius chose were, as he said, intended to build into a study of 'the fabric of the whole animal': not of particular species of animal, and not of man alone either. This reveals something positive about how Fabricius chose (or naturally found) topics for research: he simply followed Aristotle's way of conceiving them. It also reveals something negative: Fabricius did *not* start research from the existence of some current (or even some eternal) anatomical/physiological 'problem'. 'Problem-solving' was not, in itself, his way of finding things to work on.

It has been quite irrelevant to my inquiry whether Fabricius was right or wrong in his findings, whether he 'missed' things which were supposedly staring him in the face, or whether his findings were inferior or superior to those of any other investigator. What has been important for my purposes was discovering what he was doing, and therefore why his writings are the way they are. For if we can appreciate this, we might be able to recognize that some things were not in fact 'staring him in the face' after all; that, by the criteria of what he was actually doing, his answers were competent answers to *his* questions; that his work represented a serious piece of research into nature using tools that he had every reason to believe were the best tools for generating knowledge of a proper kind.

In lieu of a summary of my argument, I will just make two final points. First, everything I have said in trying to define the 'Aristotle project' in the late sixteenth century carries an implicit contrast with other anatomical research projects being contemporaneously pursued by other anatomists. I believe such other, equally distinctive and equally definable, projects did indeed exist in the late sixteenth century, though their characterization must wait until another occasion. But it is obvious that they were separated from the 'Aristotle project' in at least two major ways: they were centrally concerned with just one animal (man), and they were not Philosophy as Fabricius understood it.

And finally I want to suggest again that if we can begin to recognize that 'anatomy' was not just one monolithic activity in which all sixteenth-century anatomists were participating, and to which they can be considered to have been 'contributing', then we will (I believe) enable ourselves to gain a better understanding of what given anatomists were actually looking for, how they created topics on which to do research, and why they saw what they did out there in 'the things themselves'.

11

Disputation and description in the renaissance pulse controversy

JEROME J. BYLEBYL

Among the more widely discussed issues in renaissance medicine were several questions about the movements of the heart and arteries. These have been of interest to historians chiefly for their bearing on the work of William Harvey,[1] and at the end of my discussion I shall note some additional Harveian implications of these disputes. However, my principal aim will be to consider these issues in their sixteenth-century context, especially as exemplars of the diverse methodological strands – dialectical, authoritarian, textual, observational, and experimental – that helped make up the fabric of renaissance physiology.

The origin of these questions can be traced back to ancient sectarian controversies, which in turn gave rise to standard topics for disputation in the medical schools of late medieval Europe.[2] This dialectical tradition continued throughout the sixteenth century and beyond, but our period also witnessed the emergence of new approaches and trends. Important among these was the medical humanists' emphasis on textual scholarship which, in the early sixteenth century, had a marked impact on the pulse debates.[3] This quest for textual purity was inseparable from the movement toward Galenic orthodoxy that was so predominant in sixteenth-century medicine, but there nevertheless continued to be some diversity of opinion on the pulse controversies. For one thing, the very breakdown of earlier compromises between Aristotelian and Galenic physiological doctrines provoked a few Aristotelians into more stridently anti-Galenic positions on the heartbeat and pulse than they might otherwise have taken.[4] Furthermore, the very study of Galen's own discussions of these matters brought with it both understanding and the beginnings of acceptance of some of the other ancient doctrines that he opposed. And yet another consequence of textual scholarship was the availability of Galen's instructions for studying the movements of the heart and arteries in live animals, leading to the renewal of such investigations. Thus although the debates were chiefly dominated by dialectical, authoritarian, and textual considerations, they provide a prime example in which these approaches coexisted, and interacted, with a nascent experimental tradition.

In addition to reflecting these diverse doctrinal and methodological strands, the pulse controversies are also of interest because they cut across several academic disciplines, including physiology, anatomy, natural philosophy, and medical sphygmoscopy. In this chapter I shall not deal in a systematic way with the latter two contexts, but it will be useful to begin with a brief overview of the relationship between the other two disciplines involved, namely anatomy and physiology.

These terms are now virtually synonymous with 'structure' and 'function,' respectively, but this is a modern conception that will serve only to mislead if one attempts to apply it to the sixteenth century.[5] Traditional medical physiology had long held a central place in the curriculum, and as Nancy Siraisi has shown, in the sixteenth century it was still frequently taught through a commentary on the first *fen* of the *Canon* of Avicenna, whose major topics included elements, temperaments, humours, parts, faculties, and functions.[6] Thus the discussion of function was only one part of physiological doctrine, which also included a survey of the constituent principles of the body as well as a descriptive account of its parts or organs. However, the survey of the parts of the body was also the central task of the teacher of anatomy, and to further complicate matters he too was expected to discuss the functions and uses of the organs as well as their structures.[7] Thus there was a large overlap in the subject matter of anatomy and physiology, and the long persistence of this anomaly was perhaps due in part to the fact that anatomy was often taught by academic surgeons, whereas physiology was quintessentially a physician's subject.

In principle the two subjects might also be distinguished by their methods, in that medical physiology was a scholastic discipline, avowedly based upon commentary and disputation, whereas anatomical teaching was closely linked with the dissection of the human body, and thus had an empirical foundation. However, even here the line cannot be drawn with any clarity, as is well illustrated by Roger French's account of Berengario da Carpi (*c.* 1460–1530) in this volume.[8] Thus Berengario had a clear notion that the central core of anatomical teaching is knowledge of the human body derived from sense perception, but he sought to combine this with an alternative conception in which the subject matter was defined by the text of Mondino. Berengario therefore considered it his duty to give a complete exposition of the text, including the evaluation of a wide range of other authorities, even if this often diverted him from the straightforward description of the body's parts and functions.

Unlike Berengario, the immediately following generation of anatomists had access to the full range of Galen's original anatomical writings.[9] The availability of these works further magnified Galen's unique authority on anatomical matters, but it also provided a precedent for trying to follow the first of Berengario's inclinations, namely to equate anatomical doctrine with what can be reliably learned through observation, rather than with everything that has previously been written on the subject. Thus anatomists not only could but should ignore such authors as had no original observations to report, and should also try to avoid those topics and modes of argument that would lead them away from observation and description.[10]

But at the same time, the renewed study of Galen also reinforced the belief of anatomists that the functions no less than the structures of the organs can be learned through observation, and should therefore remain within the purview of anatomy.[11] Thus throughout the *Fabrica* Andreas Vesalius (1514–64) routinely followed his accounts of morphology with often lengthy functional analyses of the structures, and he concluded the book with a separate chapter on vivisection, which he presented as the method for investigating function *par excellence*:[12]

> Just as the dissection of the dead accurately teaches the number, position, shape, proper substance, and composition of each part, so also the dissection of a live animal sometimes clearly shows the function itself [*functionem ipsam manifesto ostendit*], and sometimes conveniently reveals evidence from which the function can be inferred.

However, even while Vesalius wrote, another leading authority was propounding a rather different view of the role of sense perception and anatomy in relation to knowledge of function. The author was Jean Fernel (1497–1558), whose *Physiologia*, first published in 1542, represented an effort to reform the teaching of traditional physiology comparable to that of Vesalius in anatomy.[13] Fernel was also concerned to escape from the scholastic legacy of unresolved questions, as we learn from his disciple Plancy:[14]

> He was the first, so far as I know, to drive out of the Schools those futile mystifications, the stigmata of an uncultured age, in the form of questionaries, blatant, nasty, and couched in barbarian language, inextricable labyrinths of quibbling and sophistry, whereby things, clear enough in themselves, became wrapt in blinding obscurity. [In the *Physiologia*] he expounded this natural part of medicine fully, and none the less tersely, in Latin.

The *Physiologia* is not entirely lacking in formal, pro and con argumentation, but by and large Fernel did proceed by a straightforward, systematic exposition of his own views, frequently ignoring the multiplicity of conflicting opinions that might exist on any given topic.

Fernel also reformed the overall organization of physiological doctrine, and for our purposes the most important change was to move the survey of the parts of the body from fourth to first place.[15] He held that the students ought to have a course of dissections as a prelude to a course of lectures on physiology, so that it was appropriate to begin his text of physiology with a fairly substantial 'description of the parts of the human body.'[16] However, he also appealed to a more fundamental methodological distinction: anatomy is, quintessentially, an empirical science, to be grasped only through observation; but the rest of physiology is, just as inevitably, a speculative science which derives its conclusions from rational contemplation.[17] Therefore to place anatomy before physiology is to follow the proper order from the seen to the unseen, from the empirical to the rational.

Most anatomists would probably have agreed with Fernel's equation of their subject with empiricism, but unlike the anatomists, Fernel tended to think of anatomy as being limited to morphological knowledge, in contrast to the functions and uses of the parts, which belong rather to the rational, contemplative part of physiology.[18] Indeed, he stated that the relationship of anatomy to the rest of physiology is similar to that between geography and history – it provides indispensable knowledge of the places where the bodily functions take place, but he does not expect it to reveal the functions themselves.[19] Accordingly, in the preface to the second book of the *Physiologia*, his earlier note of praise for anatomy is succeeded by one of condescension.[20] The physician who attempts to practise based only upon anatomical knowledge will find himself mired 'in perpetual obscurity', with 'dense night and clouds before his eyes.' However, it is far otherwise with those physicians who are not content with the 'rude contemplation' of what is obvious to the senses, but who gradually penetrate more deeply into the underlying causes of things, which can be grasped by reason alone.

Thus Fernel promises true insights into the body's hidden causes and functions through rational contemplation, whereas Vesalius proposes to make the functions themselves manifest to the senses through animal vivisection. It will come as no surprise that neither author and neither approach swept disagreement and uncertainty from the scene. Fernel eventually did become a major authority in his own right, but his text did not completely displace Avicenna as the basis for physiological teaching, and his own doctrines often provoked as much controversy as consensus. On the other hand, while the morphological aspects of anatomy did consolidate into an evolving and expanding consensus during the course of the sixteenth century, this was not the case with the functional aspects. On the contrary, the anatomists became increasingly disunited in their functional doctrines, as an earlier Galenic consensus gave way to a proliferation of idiosyncratic points of view.

Symptomatic of this disharmony was the survival within anatomy of the scholastic *quaestiones* and *disputationes*, which were so well adapted to the review of controverted issues, if not to their resolution. A striking, and late, example of this wedding of anatomy and scholasticism is the *Historia*

Anatomica (1600) by Andreas Laurentius (1558–1609).[21] In naming his book, Laurentius took on the mantle of the observational, descriptive ideal shared by all anatomists, but it turns out that the avowed 'histories' or descriptions of the individual organs are each followed by lengthy 'controversies,' touching mostly on matters of function. These are essentially scholastic *quaestiones*, in which arguments drawn from reason and authority overshadow any efforts at empirical resolution, and in his preface Laurentius made an explicit distinction between these two components: 'first I describe the history of each part; . . . then I append all the anatomical controversies, in the manner of commentaries.'[22] Thus he may be commenting on his own text rather than that of Mondino, but eighty years after Berengario there is still a very sizable part of anatomical doctrine, focused primarily on the bodily functions, that has resisted incorporation into the neutral, descriptive core of the discipline.

Among the dozens of controversies included in Laurentius's text are a series of four having to do with the movements of the heart and arteries, beginning with one called, simply, *De Motu Cordis*. William Harvey would allude to this discussion near the beginning of his own very different *De Motu Cordis*, and Laurentius for his part was writing within a long line of works bearing this title that began in the thirteenth century.[23] The central issue in these traditional questions was the underlying cause of the movement of the heart, including Galen's view and two different Aristotelian positions. Galen attributed the heart's active movements to a part of the soul called the 'vital faculty', and also ascribed to these movements the important purpose of ventilating the innate heat.[24] This contrasts with the view in Aristotle's *De Respiratione*, that the movements of the heart are merely the passive results of the concoction and ebullition of the blood contained within its ventricles.[25] However, *De Respiratione* had not been available to Averroës, the influential interpreter of Aristotle,[26] so that he directed his efforts toward showing that the movements of the heart are caused by the Aristotelian vegetative soul, rather than by the Galenic vital faculty, whose existence he denied.[27] In the medieval West *De Respiratione* was available, but in the absence of support from Averroës, and in the light of a medical tradition solidly committed to the notion of active pulsation, the ebullition theory garnered little support.

There was also another aspect to the traditional discussions *de motu cordis* that was even more heavily influenced by textual considerations. In book three of *De Anima* Aristotle briefly outlined the principles governing the local movements of animals, and chose the ball-and-socket joint to exemplify his points.[28] But the medieval translators did not understand the relevant technical term, '*gigglymos*,' and rendered it as 'circular motion [*motus girativus, circulatio*].'[29] It came further to be assumed that the whole passage referred specifically to the heart, so that the medieval doctors then faced the challenge of finding some sense in which the heartbeat might be regarded as a species of circular motion.[30] For example, in the early fifteenth century Nicolò Falcucci (d.c. 1412) proposed that:[31]

Just as in spherical motion there is to be found a middle point around which the mobile revolution [*circulatio*] takes place, so also in the dilatative and constrictive motion of the heart there is to be found a middle point from which the motion begins in dilatation and to which it reduces in constriction. And as the heavenly bodies by their spherical motion flow into the inferior regions, and by flowing in regulate and preserve, so the heart by its dilatative and constrictive motion flows in over all the members, and by flowing in regulates, governs, and preserves.

In addition to these questions *de motu cordis*, the medieval doctors were also concerned with the more concrete issue of whether the heart and arteries dilate and contract simultaneously or in alternation, a controversy that began with Herophilus and Erasistratus in the third century BC.[32] According to Herophilus, the heart both moves itself and communicates to the arteries the power of active pulsation, with the result that they dilate and contract simultaneously with the heart, and assist it in ventilating the body's innate heat. But according to Erasistratus, the arteries are moved passively, and in alternation with the heart: when the heart dilates, its left ventricle sucks in air from the lungs through the pulmonary veins; when it contracts it forcefully expels the air into the arteries. The arteries are distended by the impulsion of air, but as the air in turn flows out of them at the periphery, they return to their contracted state.

Galen's support of the Herophilean position was consistent with his general hostility toward Erasistratus's mechanistic explanations, but he also sought to refute the Erasistratean theory on specific factual grounds. One objection was that there ought to be some perceptible lag in a mechanically transmitted pulse, whereas all of the arteries seem to move simultaneously, regardless of their distance from the heart.[33] The Erasistrateans apparently maintained that any lag would be barely noticeable, but even they seem to have assumed that such rapid and smooth transmission would be possible only if the arteries are ordinarily free of blood.[34] Therefore by proving that the arteries do naturally contain blood Galen could further undermine the Erasistratean theory.[35] In addition, Galen claimed to derive conclusive evidence of an active pulsific faculty from his procedure for inserting a tube into an artery in a live animal.[36] By tying a ligature around the part of the artery containing the tube, one could, in effect, ligate the wall of the artery without interrupting the flow of its contents. Galen asserted that when this is done, the artery immediately ceases pulsating distal to the ligature, thus showing that the pulse is transmitted through the arterial walls (by an immaterial faculty) and not through the lumen (by impelled spirits).

Galen also held that the simple issue of coordination could be resolved by exposing the heart and a length of artery in a live animal, and then establishing their movements in relation to each other. But since it was clear from external palpation that the dilatation of the arteries coincides with the beat of the heart, one could also settle the question *in vivo* by determining whether the heart strikes the chest (and makes its beat) when it dilates or when it contracts. In *On Anatomical Procedures* Galen outlined two alternative procedures to permit such determinations.[37] In one of these, the sternum would be carefully removed without collapsing the lungs, thereby providing prolonged but limited access to the beating heart. In the other, the whole ventral thoracic wall would be reflected upward, giving much greater access to the heart, but only for a short interval before suffocation. However, while Galen indicated elsewhere that the arteries dilate and contract simultaneously with the heart,[38] in this passage he left the question open, perhaps revealing some underlying uncertainty.

Galen could avoid reaching a conclusion in *On Anatomical Procedures* because there his avowed aim was to provide only a protocol for such investigations, rather than a detailed description of what he had observed or concluded from them. The distinction between protocol and description will be a useful one in the discussion that follows, although I do not wish to suggest that these categories are mutually exclusive ones. In fact, the passage in *On Anatomical Procedures* concludes with a striking description of the dying heart:[39]

> Brief movements of both ventricles will be separated by long periods of quiet, and the dilatation of the right ventricle according to its own nature will become evident, especially when [the ventricles] approach the point of immobility. First both of them cease moving near the apex, then the part next to that, and so on, until only the bases are left moving. And when even these cease, there appears a brief and indistinct motion at long intervals in the auricles.

But this underscores, by way of contrast, that the main thrust of the preceding passage was to outline methods and issues for prospective observations, not to capture the results of such observations in a full written description.

In the early fourteenth century, when these ancient debates were resumed, neither *On Anatomical Procedures*, nor Galen's other accounts of the demonstration of blood in the arteries and of the tube-in-artery experiment, were available in Western Europe. Various other works were known in which he simply asserted that the heart and arteries move simultaneously, but this was not the only opinion that was available. There exists an anonymous Greek *Compendium of the Pulses* whose author maintained that the arteries dilate when the heart contracts, and vice versa, and a Latin version of this treatise was known during the later middle ages under the name of Galen.[40] Thus there appeared to be two opposing Galenic opinions, and out of this quirk of textual transmission there arose lengthy discussions of the question. The author of the *Compendium* did not, however, state clearly that the diastole of the arteries is actually caused mechanically by the heart's impulsion of spirit, so that the debates turned chiefly on the question of chronological coordination.

The author of the *Compendium Pulsuum* did make it clear that he was opposing common opinion in defending alternation.[41] Because the heartbeat and pulse are perceived simultaneously, he noted, most people suppose that the heart and arteries dilate and contract at the same time. This view is wrong, however, because in fact the heart makes its beat when it contracts and is emptied, as can be learned from 'anatomy'. He then explained the structural relations of heart, lungs, pericardium, and sternum, and continued:[42]

Thus it happens that when [the heart] draws spirit from the lung, and is completely filled, it moves back laterally and is separated considerably from the sternum. But when it contracts again, and is emptied and returns to its natural shape, it leaps up to the sternum and makes its beat. And thus it is in contraction that it makes its pulse.

It is not clear whether the author claimed to have observed the heart *in vivo*, or simply to have deduced the course of its movements from the structural relations, but the medieval doctors took his statements to be an authoritative description of what had actually been observed to occur. The issue was taken up by Pietro d'Abano (1230–1315?), in the eightieth *differentia* of his *Conciliator*, 'Whether or not the arteries are dilated at the same time as the heart is dilated and constricted when it is constricted.'[43] After briefly outlining some of the arguments pro and con, he quoted (authentic) Galenic passages which seem to indicate that the heart and arteries dilate and contract simultaneously, but then noted that in the *Compendium Pulsuum* Galen upheld the opposite view. Pietro explained this discrepancy by regarding the first position as merely introductory and probable, but not demonstrative and true: 'for nothing prevents something false from being more probable than something true.'[44]

Pietro therefore defended the view that the heart and arteries dilate and contract in alternation.[45] His defence consists primarily of two parts, of which the first is simply the quotation, at length, of the account of the heartbeat and pulse from the *Compendium Pulsuum*, which is thus allowed to stand in its own defence. It appears that it was the ostensible character of this passage as description from 'anatomy' that made Pietro feel that this was justified. But although the facts in this instance seemed to be beyond dispute, this hardly brought an end to Pietro's disputation, for he went on to a lengthy logical demonstration of why the arteries *ought* to dilate when the heart contracts, and vice versa. Thus, when the heart contracts, it expels material, but if the arteries were constricted at the same time, there would not be sufficient space into which the heart might expel, indeed the arteries would be seeking to expel into the heart at that time. Furthermore, in *On the Natural Faculties* Galen showed that whenever one part of the body expels something, another attracts it. This principle is also illustrated by the auricles of the heart, 'for they follow the motion of the heart in an opposite way, for when the heart is dilated they are constricted, and vice versa.' And finally:[46]

Art is the imitator of nature. In art it also happens that when one device expels something another takes it up, and so on, until the artifice accomplishes its appointed end . . . Therefore when the heart is dilated the arteries are constricted, and when it is constricted they are dilated.

In accepting this position from the *Compendium Pulsuum*, Pietro d'Abano was followed by his younger contemporary Pietro Torrigiano (*c.* 1270–*c.* 1350),[47] who also linked it with a mechanistic explanation of the movements of heart and arteries based on Aristotle's ebullition theory.[48] According to Torrigiano, the heartbeat is not caused by the soul or by any faculty of the soul; rather, the dilatation of the heart is simply the consequence of the vaporization of blood under the influence of heat. If this continued unabated it would lead to the rupture of the heart, but this is prevented by the return of the heart to its natural shape, with a consequent expulsion of spirits. At this time the arteries dilate, but Torrigiano made it clear that their dilatation could not result simply from the impulsion of spirits, because the latter could not distend all of the arteries at the same instant.[49] Instead, the principal cause of the arterial pulse is the innate heat which, unlike vaporous spirits, can indeed pass out from the heart to the periphery instantaneously, 'in the manner of a ray'. This heat then vaporizes the blood that is already contained in the arteries to cause simultaneous dilatation of them all, followed by their contraction, as they return to their natural shape. Torrigiano went on to try to show that his explanation of the heartbeat and pulse was fully compatible with the general assumption that these movements are purposeful ones which ventilate the innate heat.[50] Thus, even though the dilatation of heart and arteries is caused by the expansion of their contents, it nevertheless creates enough of a vacuum to draw cool air into them. This air ventilates the innate heat and also contributes to contraction by provoking in the heart and arteries 'a certain natural flight (*fuga*)', with consequent expulsion of heated air and smoky wastes.

Torrigiano's version of the ebullition theory was widely discussed from the fourteenth to the seventeenth century, but the reaction was almost uniformly negative. Typical was the objection of Jacopo da Forlì (d. 1413 or 14), that the heart is the most important part of the body, making it inconceivable that its motions should be violent, rather than proceeding from the soul.[51] Furthermore, Jacopo pointed out that if the heart and arteries dilate precisely because of the swelling of their contents, then the latter will always fill whatever space is available, leaving no void to draw in additional·air. Besides, Torrigiano himself invokes a natural recoiling of the heart and arteries to explain contraction, but what does this amount to if not a faculty, and why then does he not admit that a faculty is involved in dilatation as well?

But while Jacopo rejected Torrigiano's ebullition theory, the combination of 'Galen's' observations and Pietro d'Abano's arguments convinced him that the arteries must dilate when the heart contracts.[52] This position was also endorsed by most other leading medical teachers of the fourteenth and fifteenth centuries, including Nicolò Falcucci, Ugo Benzi (1376–1439), and Michele Savonarola (1384?–1462?).[53] Thus Gabrielle Falloppia was justified in remarking around the middle of the sixteenth century that 'almost everyone up until our time [*omnes fere usque ad nostra tempera*]' was of the opinion that when the heart contracts, the arteries dilate, and vice versa.[54]

As Falloppia implies, by his time the earlier consensus had been displaced by a decided shift toward the view that the heart and arteries dilate and contract at the same time. This was largely a result of textual scholarship, which showed that the *Compendium Pulsuum* was not an authentic Galenic treatise after all, but reflected the very Erasistratean doctrines that Galen had argued so forcefully against. In all genuine works, Galen maintained that the heart and arteries dilate and contract at the same time, and this then became the orthodox position.

An excellent example of the textual approach to the pulse controversy occurs in the *Medical Letters* of G. B. Teodosi (1475–1538), a professor of medicine at Bologna.[55] He began by noting that the discussion arose from the apparent conflict between the view in Galen's *De Pulsibus ad Tyrones* that the heart and arteries move in the same way, and the opinion of Pietro d'Abano and other 'recent physicians' that the arteries dilate when the heart contracts.[56] He identified the *Compendium Pulsuum* as the source of the latter position, and after pointing out that this book is most likely spurious, he proceeded to an extensive review of the authentic literature to ascertain Galen's true opinion in the matter. He quoted at length from *On Anatomical Procedures*, where Galen described techniques for studying the question *in vivo*, and correctly pointed out that in this place Galen left the issue in doubt. But Teodosi then cited various other passages in which Galen maintained that the arteries dilate and contract actively and simultaneously with the heart.

Teodosi then turned to the late medieval view, which he regarded largely as a product of faulty scholarship.[57] First of all, Pietro d'Abano and others placed altogether too much emphasis on the exchange of materials between heart and arteries, failing to realize that in Galen's view (which Teodosi documented extensively) the arteries carry on exchanges with many parts other than the heart, so that it is not really so crucial to work out a neat mechanical relationship between heartbeat and pulse. Second, they have been misled by the *Compendium*, which clearly could not have been written by Galen, as Teodosi again sought to demonstrate at length.[58] Thus Teodosi assumed that the aim of the discussion was to understand correctly and to follow Galen's position, and this the medieval doctors had failed to do.

A similar approach was taken by Leone Rogano (d. 1558) in his commentary on Galen's *De Pulsibus ad Tyrones* (1556). The bulk of this work dealt with medical sphygmoscopy, but Rogano devoted the first seventy pages to the cause of the pulse and its relationship to the heartbeat. The views of Pietro d'Abano and Torrigiano provided the occasion for this review,[59] but Rogano worked back from this medieval phase to a full consideration of the ancient disputes as well. In particular, he gave quite a good account of Erasistratus's theory and of Galen's refutations of it, including the demonstration of a pulsific faculty by the tube-in-artery experiment and the arguments that the presence of blood in the arteries blocks the orderly transmission of a mechanical pulse, and that in any case a mechanical pulse ought to be transmitted in the form of a wave.[60] Moreover, Rogano not only quoted Galen's directions for vivisectional studies, he also implied that he had used them himself to confirm that the heart and arteries dilate and contract at the same time.[61] And he also extended the use of vivisection to refute the ebullition theory:[62]

> If you open the thorax of a live animal and cut out its heart, you will see it move for a time, even if its ventricles have been incised so that all the blood contained in them is evacuated. Therefore the pulse is not caused by the fervor of the blood, or its conversion to spirit, but by a faculty which, because it is inherent to the heart, can survive for a certain space of time.

Teodosi and Rogano are but two examples of the widespread swing of opinion that occurred during the sixteenth century, but although the discrediting of the *Compendium Pulsuum* may have removed the chief source of the earlier consensus, no amount of textual scholarship could destroy the inherent plausibility of Pietro d'Abano's arguments in support of alternation. In fact, among those who continued to agree with these arguments were none other than Jean Fernel and Andreas Vesalius, although there are some interesting differences in their approaches and the ultimate results of their inquiries.

In the *Physiologia*, Fernel was quite forthright on the question of coordination between heartbeat and pulse:[63]

> The heart in diastole sucks prepared air from the lungs into the left ventricle through the pulmonary veins . . . In systole it pours forth the now perfected vital spirit from the left ventricle into the aorta and into the smaller arteries, at which time it is necessary for all of them to dilate. Therefore, although their movement corresponds to the beat of the heart with regard to size, speed, and frequency, so that by touching them it is possible to infer the movement of the heart, the arteries

are nevertheless dilated in the systole of the heart, and constricted in its diastole. For they are dilated when the heart impels the spirits into them.

Fernel's approach exhibits the general characteristics of his reform of physiological doctrine, as discussed above. Note that he makes no appeal to either observation or authority, nor does he even acknowledge the possibility that the heart and arteries might dilate and contract at the same time. He simply declares that the arteries must dilate at the time when the heart contracts and expels spirits and blood into them. He is, however, careful to maintain that the movements of heart and arteries are similar in all other respects, thereby preserving the basis of medical sphygmoscopy, and he went on to make clear that the mechanical impulse alone could not account for the instantaneity of the transmission – there must be a pulsific faculty in the walls of the arteries as well.[64]

Fernel thus relies on a logical argument, whose correctness is dogmatically asserted, to resolve the issue of coordination, but this hardly proved adequate to the task. In fact, in his commentary on the relevant passage in the *Physiologia*, Jean Riolan, *père* (1538?–1605), simply declared that the heart and arteries dilate and contract at the same time, citing various passages in Galen to support his contention.[65] Thus Galen's authority trumps Fernel's reason – and Fernel's authority.

In contrast, Vesalius looked to vivisection to confirm the alternation of movements, but with even more problematic results. It was noted above that he included in the *Fabrica* a chapter on vivisection, although the nature of this chapter reveals something of the limitations of the method as then practised. Its title – 'Some points regarding the dissection of live animals [*De vivorum sectione nonnulla*]'[66] – proclaims its selective character, as does the fact that it amounts to only some five of the 663 folio pages in the *Fabrica*. Furthermore, while in the rest of the book Vesalius strove to provide as comprehensive a description as possible of the anatomy of the dead, the vivisection chapter is only a series of protocols, interspersed with brief, fragmentary descriptions of the relevant phenomena. And finally, there was the gap between the promise of functions being 'clearly revealed' in vivisection, and the actual difficulties that such investigations might entail – a gap that was especially notable in Vesalius's efforts to resolve the pulse controversy.

Vesalius's first published references to this issue predated the *Fabrica* by several years. In his revised edition of Guenter's *Anatomical Institutes* (1538) he hinted at the idea that the arteries ought to dilate when the heart contracts and expels into them, and added, 'sense also indicates this obscurely [*obscure*] in the dissection of live animals.'[67] The following year, in his *Letter on Venesection*, he expressed himself more clearly in both respects:[68]

For by many arguments the motion of the heart and arteries appeared to me to be clearly opposed and contrary. For when the heart contracts, it pours spirit into the great artery and blood into the pulmonary artery, and this motion of the heart is systole . . . But when the arteries are dilated, we believe that they . . . are filled by that spirit from the heart . . . Thus it remains that the motions of the heart and arteries are contrary and opposed. In some manner [*aliquo pacto*] this can be tested in the dissection of live animals, if the artery lying on the sacrum is grasped in one hand, while the entire uninjured heart is held by the other.

The technique of exposing the heart and a remote artery was described by Galen in *On Anatomical Procedures*, but it will be noted that the main burden still rests on the logical argument – vivisectional observations are said to confirm this only '*aliquo pacto*.'

If Vesalius showed some increase in confidence between 1538 and 1539, by 1540 he had retreated to a posture of agnosticism. In an anatomical demonstration conducted at Bologna that year, he carried out the procedure of exposing the heart and a remote artery, and asked the students to feel the two in order determine the relationship between their movements. According to our informant:[69]

Some students asked Vesalius what the true fact about these movements was, whether the arteries followed the movement of the heart, or whether they had a movement different from the heart. Vesalius answered: "I do not want to give you my opinion, please feel for yourselves with your own hands and trust them."

This seems an admirable pedagogical principle, except that the crowding of the students prevented anyone from making a determination of his own. And in view of Vesalius's earlier diffidence, one might suspect that he did not trust his own hands to the extent of taking a strong stand.

By the time of the *Fabrica* Vesalius had significantly improved upon Galen's techniques for studying the living heart by combining the more radical opening of the thorax with the periodic reinflation of the lungs to prevent suffocation.[70] This made the movement of the heart more accessible to observation, and, in particular, made it possible to compare the heart directly with the aortic trunk, rather than with a remote artery. But with what result? The most definite thing that Vesalius had to report in this regard was: 'Nothing will strike you more clearly than the rhythm of the pulses of the heart and arteries.'[71] The observation may have been clear to Vesalius, but it is not clear what this statement is supposed to mean. Perhaps Vesalius meant to affirm only that the heart and arteries obviously beat at the same time and with the same rhythm, leaving open the question of their dilatation and contraction. But it is also possible that he now meant to affirm that the heart and arteries do indeed dilate and contract at the same time, because statements made elsewhere in the *Fabrica* strongly suggest that he took the (actual) contraction of the heart to be its dilatation.[72] In any event, the protocol format of the vivisection chapter gave Vesalius the option of being so unforthcoming about the substantive issue as distinct from the methods of investigation.

Another sixteenth-century anatomist who tried his hand at unravelling the movements of the heart *in vivo* was Realdo Colombo (*c.* 1515–59). In his *De Re Anatomica* Colombo also included a separate chapter on vivisection that takes the form of a series of protocols, though here too some of the stipulations of things to be observed actually amount to brief descriptions of what he had observed. Thus when the thorax is laid open in a live animal, one can see 'the motion of the heart, how it is enlarged and constricted.' Colombo continued:[73]

> If you want, you will also see the nature of the arterial motion in vivisection, and whether it is the same or opposite to the motion of the heart. For you will find that when the heart is dilated the arteries are contracted, while in the contraction of the heart they are dilated. But you will notice that when the heart is drawn upward and appears to swell, then it is constricted [*tunc constringitur*], but when it stretches out, it turns downward as if relaxed. And at that time the heart is said to be quiescent. And the contraction of the heart occurs at the time stated [*estque tunc cordis systole*], because it can receive [materials] more easily and with less labour, but when it transmits there is need of greater strength. Nor should you make light of this, for you will find not a few who think for certain that the heart is dilated when it is in truth contracted.

Thus Colombo begins with the longstanding issue of coordination between heart and arteries, but he is quickly drawn on to a new issue, that of the intrinsic nature of the heart's movements. Instead of construing these, as was commonly done, as active diastole and active systole separated by brief intervals of quiet, he refers to an active 'drawing upward' followed by a 'turning downward', which must be at least relatively passive because it is also said to be a period of relaxation or quiescence. He indicates that appearances are somewhat confusing as to which of these phases is contraction, and which dilatation – when the heart is drawn upward 'it appears to swell,' but it is in truth undergoing contraction. He buttresses this conclusion by an important theoretical argument: the heart 'can receive [materials] more easily and with less labour, but when it transmits there is need of greater strength.'

Although Colombo was quite clear on the basic point that the arteries dilate when the heart contracts, and vice versa, his further – and much more novel – views about the character of the heart's movements embody a significant ambiguity. The phrase *estque tunc cordis systole* would seem most naturally to refer to the immediately preceding description of the relaxation of the heart, but such a construction would confuse the meaning of the whole passage, since both movements of the heart would then be identified as contraction, or systole. Colombo was quite aware that the terms are synonymous,[74] and on the assumption that he did not mean to contradict himself, I take the *estque tunc cordis systole* to refer back to the earlier (and somewhat parallel) *tunc constringitur* – having previously asserted that the drawing up of the heart is its contraction, he now gives a reason for this designation.[75] However, this is not the most obvious interpretation of his statement, so that some of his readers were left in doubt as to exactly what he meant to affirm by it.[76] And one might also note that the extreme brevity of the passage left it vulnerable to being so compromised by a single accident of wording.

One close contemporary who did understand Colombo was Volcher Coiter (1534–76), whose own observations on the heartbeat, published in 1572, were the culmination of sixteenth-century efforts to investigate the phenomenon in live animals. His discussion was part of a collection of 'Anatomical Observations', and was entitled, *De cordis motu, diastole, systole, et quiete.*[77] It differs radically from the traditional theoretical discussions *de motu cordis*, but it also departs significantly from earlier vivisectional accounts in that it is decidedly not a protocol for prospective observations, but a detailed description of those things which Coiter had personally observed. Only in the opening sentence does he mention procedural details, noting that to best observe the movement of the heart, one should choose animals that are 'lively [*vivida*],' such as are 'nearly all amphibians, cats, lizards, snakes, and, among the fishes, the eel, the pike, and so on.' Coiter then proceeds for several paragraphs to describe what he had observed in one particular experimental subject, namely a young cat. His account of the movements of the auricles will give some idea of the flavour of the whole:[78]

> In diastole, the auricles are seen to be inflated like bladders, and when they were distended they took on a red colour, pausing slightly before exerting themselves to contract . . . Just as in diastole they become red and distended because of the repletion with blood and spirits, so in systole they become white, they collapse becoming flaccid and wrinkled, and by the force of the heart they are drawn somewhat toward its base.

Coiter went on to describe the diastole, the quiet, and the systole of the ventricles, and toward the end related how he had excised the heart and found that it continued to beat for a time, even when further cuts were made into its ventricles.

Despite its empirical character, Coiter's discussion was dominated by an important presupposition, namely that when the auricles contract, the ventricles ought to dilate to receive what has been impelled into them. Chiefly for this reason, he took to be ventricular diastole that more vigorous movement that closely coincides with the obvious contraction of the auricles. Thus when he came to consider Colombo's view that the more strenuous movement of the heart is its contraction, Coiter said that he would be inclined to accept it, but for the fact that it would upset the sequence between auricles and ventricles that he had previously established. Accordingly, 'the arteries are seen to make their diastole and systole at the same time as the heart.'[79]

During the last part of the sixteenth century, references to the observation of the heart *in vivo* were not uncommon. For example, Costanzo Varoli (1543–75) reported:[80]

> If you studiously explore the movement of the heart in the vivisection of a dog or some other brute, it will clearly be seen that there are four motions, distinct in time and place, of which two are proper to the auricles, and two to the ventricles.

However, such descriptions tended to be rather perfunctory, and the level of detail achieved by Coiter was not to be matched until the 1610s, when anatomists such as Riolan, *fils*, and Harvey took up the question more or less where Colombo and Coiter had left off. Furthermore, vivisectional reports about the coordination issue continued to cancel each other out. For example, according to Caspar Bauhin (1560–1624):[81]

> The dissection of a live animal will teach anyone that when the heart contracts, blood is poured forth from the left ventricle into the aorta, whence it seems necessary for the aorta to dilate; but when the heart dilates the aorta contracts.

But to M. J. Flacius observation showed with equal certainty that the heart and arteries move simultaneously, while Johann Jessen's observations left him up in the air on the question.[82] And even Bauhin later reversed himself, to state that vivisection shows the heart and arteries dilating and contracting simultaneously.[83] Girolamo Capivacci was another contemporary who at various times upheld both sides in the coordination dispute, and this vacillation by individual authors fairly reflects a general division of opinion on this question by the end of the sixteenth century.[84]

But regardless of which side they took on the issue of coordination, most authors were quite clear in affirming that the arteries move actively, by the pulsific faculty supplied by the heart. We have seen that Fernel was careful to make this stipulation in endorsing alternation of movements, and Vesalius also seems never to have questioned that the arteries move actively. Indeed, in his vivisection chapter he even reported the successful repetition of Galen's tube-in-artery experiment.[85] And this experiment and the apparent instantaneity of transmission continued to be cited on into the seventeenth century as the two main proofs of the pulsific faculty.

Nevertheless, during the second half of the sixteenth century one begins to find glimmerings of support for various mechanistic explanations of the arterial pulse, including the Erasistratean impulsion theory. We have seen that Colombo emphasized the vigour with which the heart contracts and expels materials into the arteries, and possibly he meant to affirm that this impulsion is the actual cause of their dilatation when he stated, 'The artery is moved not *per se*, but by the spirit [*Arteria non per se sed a spiritu movetur*].'[86] The idea that the arteries are moved 'by the spirit' is certainly reminiscent of the Erasistratean theory, but the statement occurs only as a brief marginal heading, whose corresponding statement in the main text is even more ambiguous, namely that the artery is moved 'on account of the spirit [*propter spiritus*].'

J. C. Scaliger (1484–1558) expressed himself somewhat more clearly in support of the impulsion theory. Writing in 1557, he concluded that the movement of the heart is caused by the soul, that is, represents active motion, but then continued:[87]

> The soul which, I have said, is the mover of the heart: someone will ask me whether the arteries are also moved by the same. I do not think so. For when an artery is ligated, the lower part does not move, though it is by no means dead. Consequently, the dilatation of the arteries results from the contraction of the heart, because of the impulsion of spirits; and it is clear that [the arteries] subside as a result of the dilatation of the heart.

A similar view was proposed by Louis Duret (1527–86), a Parisian physician:[88]

> Through the systole of the heart is produced the diastole of the arteries, because they are filled and dilated. And contrariwise, the systole of the arteries is produced by the diastole of the heart.

It will be noted that Scaliger and Duret both state that the heart not only causes the dilatation of the arteries by its contraction, but also causes the arteries to contract by its dilatation, presumably by sucking the spirit back out of them.

Such back and forth movement was a prominent feature of a mechanical pulse theory discussed at some length by Falloppia (1523–62) in his *Lectures on the Similar Parts*, but in this case the impelled material was assumed to be blood rather than spirit. Falloppia associated this theory with the name of Erasistratus, though he appears to attribute the specific version of it under discussion to an unnamed person, possibly a contemporary. The opinion in question was that the heart alternately expels blood into the arteries when it contracts, and sucks it back out of them when it dilates. Thus:[89]

> When the arteries are moved, they are moved *per accidens*, and when the heart is contracted the arteries are dilated, but when the heart is dilated the arteries collapse as the blood is recalled to the heart, which is shown by the example of the inflated glove [*quod patet exemplo chirothecae inflatae*]. And this opinion is of such weight that there are even some in our own time who believe that it is true.

Erasistratus is known to have compared the pulse to the inflation of sacks or bladders, but this seems to be the first time that the example of the glove was used in this connection. In another version of Falloppia's lectures the wording is rather different:[90]

> Erasistratus and others (as is attributed to them) want the arteries to have motion not from themselves, but from the heart. Thus when the blood flows out the arteries are dilated, but when [the blood] flows back to the heart they are contracted, and the motion of the arteries is the accession and recession of the blood. For when the heart expels the blood, the diastole [of the arteries] takes place, but when it sucks it back the systole [of the arteries] occurs.

Thus the theory seems to entail the movement of the same limited portion of blood back and forth between the heart and arteries.

According to Falloppia, the proponents of this theory of flux and reflux gave various arguments to support their view, among them the following:[91]

> You will observe that whenever an artery is punctured the blood spurts forth when it is dilated, but when it is contracted it either does not spurt forth, or hardly does so. This would not happen, unless because the blood undergoes a flux and reflux. Does not Galen suppose that the contraction of the arteries makes for an expulsion of smoky wastes? Therefore it is a sign that when the artery is dilated, it is filled; when it is evacuated, it is constricted.

The spurting of blood from cut arteries had long been discussed in connection with the cause of their pulse, but the anonymous author seems to have raised an important new point, namely that if the arteries do indeed dilate and contract actively, then the more vigorous spurting of blood ought to occur during their systole, and not, as actually happens, during their diastole.

In rejecting this theory in favour of the Galenic pulsific faculty, Falloppia offered the usual objection that if the pulse is caused mechanically, then it ought to pass out through the arteries over a perceptible interval of time, 'for blood cannot pass in an instant out to the fingertips'.[92] In addition, he cited Galen's tube-in-artery experiment to show that the pulse is indeed caused by a faculty, rather than by impelled blood. Besides these standard arguments, Falloppia pointed out, with reference to the specific theory under discussion, that the aortic valve effectively prevents the return of blood to the heart, thereby vitiating the causal mechanism proposed for arterial systole.[93] And as for the evidence of the blood spurting from cut arteries, Falloppia argued that the blood 'leaps' during arterial diastole because it has freer passage, whereas in systole the opening of the artery is narrowed and the flow of blood consequently impeded.[94]

In addition to this updated version of the Erasistratean impulsion theory, Falloppia also argued at some length against Torrigiano's version of the ebullition theory, but before long the latter position would also re-emerge in more contemporary guise. The major protagonist was Andrea Cesalpino (1519–1603) who, in 1571, became perhaps the first Aristotelian since Torrigiano to mount an all-out defence of the ebullition theory in opposition to an active pulsific faculty in either heart or arteries.[95]

In doing so, Cesalpino also made significant changes in the theory. Thus, whereas Torrigiano had integrated the ebullition theory with the prevailing view that the heart and arteries dilate and contract in alternation, Cesalpino assumed with many of *his* contemporaries that the heart and arteries dilate and contract at the same time.[96] Furthermore, whereas Torrigiano had conceded that a simple mechanical pulse could not be transmitted instantly, Cesalpino met the argument head on: it is true that material could not actually flow the whole length of the arterial system in an instant, but the arteries constitute, as it were, a single continuous vessel whose cavity remains full even in the contracted state; consequently, when more material is added to any part of the system, the whole will dilate at the same time.[97] Cesalpino's was also a purer version of the ebullition theory in that he did not introduce any auxiliary factors besides heating and condensation to account for the movements of heart and arteries. And where Torrigiano had tried to show that a pulse caused by ebullition could nevertheless result in inhalation and exhalation by both heart and arteries, Cesalpino uncompromisingly rejected the whole idea that heartbeat or pulse serve any such ventilating function, or indeed that there is any movement of external air into either the heart or arteries.[98] There is nothing but alternating ebullition and condensation of the blood, with consequent dilatation and contraction of heart and arteries.

Cesalpino's efforts marked the beginning of a resurgence of the ebullition theory, culminating in its endorsement by Descartes and other seventeenth-century mechanical philosophers. It would, however, be misleading to suggest that Cesalpino's views in this regard had much of an impact on his contemporaries and immediate successors, for not only did medical opinion long remain solidly with Galen, but most authors continued to direct their refutations of the ebullition theory at Torrigiano, without even mentioning Cesalpino.[99] And more generally, the dominant impression conveyed by the many discussions of the pulse controversy that continued to appear in the late sixteen and early seventeenth centuries is that most authors were, both substantively and methodologically, stuck in the ruts that had been successively dug by the scholastics of the fourteenth and fifteenth centuries, and by the humanists of the early sixteenth. For example, Ercole Sassonia (1551–1603) devoted about a dozen pages near the beginning of his *De Pulsibus* (1603) to our group of controversies.[100] It is not at all remarkable that a Paduan professor of this period should follow Galen on these matters, but it is rather striking that he should still find it necessary to write at length about the spuriousness of the *Compendium Pulsuum*, as well as to refute Pietro d'Abano and Torrigiano, as if these matters could never be laid to rest once and for all.

Similarly, in his *Historia Anatomica* (1600) Andreas Laurentius devoted some nine folios to the following series of *quaestiones*:[101]

> De motu cordis.
> Quomodo moveatur cor, & an in sua systole aut diastole percutiat pectus.
> A qua vi moveantur arteriae.
> An dilatato corde dilatentur arteriae, aut contra, dilatato corde constrin-
> gantur arteriae.

As was noted above, the first question '*De motu cordis*' was the traditional dispute about the underlying cause of the heartbeat, in which he was chiefly concerned to uphold Galen's vital faculty. The second question of whether the heart strikes the chest in systole or diastole had long been a subsidiary issue in the coordination dispute, but Laurentius also gives it the broader title '*Quomodo moveatur cor*', and in the opening words related it, by way of contrast, to the preceding question '*De motu cordis:*' 'Previously, I would seem to have illuminated that most obscure issue of the cause of the heart's movement, and now I will proceed to explicate the mode and plan of that movement as I have learned it from *autopsia*.'[102] Thus Laurentius appears to acknowledge that one might try to describe how the heart moves, as distinct from explaining what causes it to move, atlhough the discussion that follows is actually based almost entirely on *auctoritates* and *rationes* rather than on Laurentius's own observations. Much the same is true of the third question, 'By what power the arteries are moved', in which he was concerned with defending Galen's inflowing pulsific faculty against Erasistratean impulsion and Torrigiano's ebullition. And the fourth of these questions is of course our old coordination dispute, in which Laurentius defended simultaneity almost exclusively on dialectical grounds.

We have seen that Laurentius sharply distinguished these and dozens of other *quaestiones* from the purely descriptive portions of his text, but his younger contemporary Jean Riolan, *fils*, (1580–1657) chastized him for the very idea of loading a supposed work on anatomy with such 'doubts and controverted questions': 'In these there is nothing worthy of note, for philosophical questions, as matters of logic, can be argued and defended on both sides.'[103] Riolan's point would seem to be that the realm of anatomy is ideally one of absolute truth or falsehood, as determined by observation, so that Laurentius has let down the side by resorting so routinely to purely logical, pro and con argumentation to resolve disagreements.

Elsewhere in the same work Riolan presented his own very different account of the movements of the heart and arteries, based upon observations in live animals – the first such extended account to be published since that of Coiter fifty years previously.[104] However, while Riolan did manage to sustain a strongly empirical tone through most of this account, he accomplished this chiefly by stitching together a series of observational statements drawn from perhaps a half-dozen earlier authors.[105] Riolan's own modifications and additions are interspersed among these, but he did not really transcend his literary sources to give an overall coherence to the account. Furthermore, he modelled his presentation on the protocol chapters of Vesalius and Colombo, so that on any given point he still had the option of shifting the burden to the reader to provide the full details. For example, on the issue of coordination he stated that 'when the heart is constricted and expels, the arteries are dilated in order to receive', and added, 'you will perceive this clearly if you grasp the heart and the aorta at the same time.'[106] But he did not provide any fresh circumstantial details such as might have given this long-familiar proposition a new measure of empirical credibility.

Even before Riolan published this account, his contemporary William Harvey (1578–1657) had written out his own conclusions drawn from the investigation of the heart *in vivo*, in his anatomical lecture notes of 1616.[107] Although he took inspiration from most of the same sources as Riolan, Harvey's approach and conclusions differ markedly from the latter's. For one thing, he had gone well beyond his sources to record a considerable wealth of fresh observational detail about the beating heart. Furthermore, his account is decidedly not a random collection of observations, but a highly coherent effort to reach some fundamental new insights into the nature and purpose of the movements of the heart and arteries. But if Harvey's ambitions were much larger, he was at the same time more diffident concerning his results – where Riolan assures the reader that he will be able to perceive the relationship between cardiac systole and arterial diastole 'clearly [*manifeste*]', Harvey emphasizes the great difficulty of discerning when the heart is dilating and when contracting, even after prolonged study.[108] Accordingly, for all its observational richness, Harvey's presentation is also much more overtly logical than Riolan's – the observations had to be organized into a coherent argument in order to yield definite conclusions that elude simple, direct sense perception.[109]

Finally, Harvey's approach is also more scholarly than Riolan's, in that it recapitulates in a more comprehensive way what his predecessors had had to say on these matters. Thus among the ideas, observations, and methods mentioned by Harvey we find, from Aristotle, the ebullition theory; from Erasistratus, the impulsion theory; from Galen, the description of the movements of the dying heart, the tube-in-artery experiment, and the inflowing pulsific faculty; from Pietro d'Abano, the argument that the heart could not very well transmit materials to the arteries if they were to dilate and contract at the same time; from Vesalius, the technique of pulmonary insufflation; from Colombo, his whole account of the movement of the heart, and the argument that the heart must exert more strength to transmit materials than to receive them; from Coiter, the notation of colour change in the contracting auricles, and the incision of the cardiac ventricles; and from Falloppia, the differential spurting of blood from severed arteries, and the model of the inflated glove.[110] Thus one could regard Harvey's oldest surviving account of the movements of the heart as an exquisite synthesis of the logical, the scholarly, and the observational approaches to these questions that had prevailed among various of his predecessors.

However, when Harvey eventually came to publish these conclusions in the first part of *De Motu Cordis*, he seems to have made a deliberate effort to remove much of the scholarly and logical scaffolding, and to present the material largely as a matter of observation and description.[111] His self-consciousness in this regard probably derived from the literary model that he chose, for by his own avowal the first part of *De Motu Cordis* was patterned on Hieronymus Fabricius's series of anatomical monographs on individual organs, which Andrew Cunningham discusses in this volume.[112] These all began with a purely descriptive '*historia*' or '*dissectio*' of the organ in question, and as I have noted elsewhere, Harvey's chapters on the movement of the heart correspond to the Fabrician *historia*, but with the important difference that they seek to capture in words the organ's observed movements rather than its observed structures.[113] This descriptive intent is made clear by the titles of the three relevant chapters:[114]

Ex vivorum dissectione, qualis sit Cordis motus
Arteriarum motus qualis ex vivorum dissectione
Motus cordis & auricularum qualis ex vivorum dissectione

The tone is likewise established by the opening words of the first of these chapters:[115]

In the first place, in the hearts of all animals that are still alive, when the thorax is opened and the pericardium dissected, it is possible to observe that the heart sometimes moves, and is sometimes at rest.

Thus, as regards the movements of the heart, Harvey is not about to argue a thesis nor to evaluate previous theories and observations. He proposes simply to take the reader by the hand and to tell him, clearly and authoritatively, what he has observed in the beating hearts of live animals.

These opening lines also reflect another characteristic feature of the Fabrician *historia* to which Cunningham calls attention, namely their universal character, in that Fabricius sought to describe a given organ as it appears in the whole range of animal species. We have seen that Coiter was Harvey's one significant predecessor in making the movement of the heart the object of sustained written description, but Coiter had sought to describe the movements of the heart of one particular cat, whereas Harvey proposes to describe these movements 'in all living animals'. His account does indeed fulfil this broadly comparative ambition, but this only underscores its character as a very artful fiction – dozens of observations made on many different occasions have been woven into a 'description' of a universal heartbeat common to all animals.

The publication of *De Motu Cordis* did not immediately silence all opposing views about the heartbeat and pulse, but eventually the treatise did succeed in transferring many of these issues out of the realm of controversy and into that of anatomical consensus, and for this Harvey's skill at communicating his findings was as important as their inherent validity. His achievement seems all the greater if one turns back just a few decades to the late sixteenth century, and sees how durable was the scholastic tradition of institutionalized disagreement on these and so many other issues. During the course of the century figures such as Pietro d'Abano and Torrigiano may have suffered considerable abuse at the hands of the medical humanists, but they continued to have a pronounced influence both on the agenda and on the methods of medical controversy.

However, one must also give the medical humanists their due since on these as on countless other questions they also had a palpable impact on the prevailing climate of opinion through their efforts to recover Galen's authentic doctrines. Their emphasis on textual scholarship and Galenic orthodoxy may not strike a very sympathetic chord with many modern observers, but it must be recognized as a major accomplishment to have established a much more reliable corpus of Galen's writings, and to have achieved a more profound grasp of their contents. Furthermore, the return to Galen was also inseparable from some of the other trends that we have noted in the pulse controversy. First, even in the process of refuting the views of Erasistratus and others, Galen preserved them and thus allowed for their rebirth in later ages. Aristotle, of course, could speak directly to posterity through his own writings, but even here the emergence of a triumphant and uncompromising Galenism in the first half of the sixteenth century was probably a necessary precondition for the marked, if somewhat diffuse, Aristotelian revival that gathered force in some medical circles toward the end of the century.

Finally, Galen's writings, including some that had not been previously available, conveyed to sixteenth-century anatomists the clear conviction that the body's internal functions, no less than its structures, can be the direct objects of empirical research and description, and they also preserved a repertory of vivisectional techniques with which to pursue such a programme. Indeed, the closing words of Galen's account of the vivisectional study of the heart could serve as the motto for the similar efforts of Vesalius, Colombo, Coiter – and Harvey: 'For it is not our present business to investigate causes [*tas aitias*], but only those things which are apparent in dissections [*mona ta phainomena kata tas anatomas*].'[116]

12

Academicism versus empiricism in practical medicine in sixteenth-century Spain with regard to morisco practitioners

LUIS GARCÍA-BALLESTER

In this chapter I intend to examine the relationship between empiricism and academicism in Spanish practical medicine in the sixteenth century. In particular I shall concentrate on certain aspects of the relationship between academic (or university-based) medicine and the remnants of Arab medicine which still existed in Spain.

In sixteenth-century Spain medieval Arab medicine was still practised by a large part of the so-called morisco population.[1] This was mainly composed of Muslims who had stayed in Spain after the Christian conquests of the thirteenth to fifteenth centuries and who were all forced to convert to Christianity at the beginning of the sixteenth century. In spite of this compulsory conversion they retained their identity as a separate culture. This culture, as Islamic, came into open conflict with the dominant Christian majority which then attempted to suppress it in the name of supposed national unity. The conflict continued, however, and became one of the most serious problems in Spain in the later sixteenth and early seventeenth centuries. The Christians could only solve the problem by deporting the moriscos to other parts of Spain or finally by exiling them. In contrast to the moriscos, those who had always been Christians, without any conversion either from the Islamic or from the Jewish faith, were called 'Old Christians'.

I propose that medicine cannot be divorced from the political, religious and economic forces which form social groupings. Therefore morisco medicine, in all its aspects, was an integral part of the general process of the moriscos' alienation and final suppression.

Arab medicine, both as a medical science (Arabicized Galenism) and a practical system used by the Muslim or converted minority, broke down between the thirteenth and seventeenth centuries.[2] This dissolution was complex, for it was not the result of one change nor did it follow any set pattern. In fact, Arabicized Galenism was in a state of crisis throughout the sixteenth century.

However, we should not forget that this medicine and its practice were only small parts of the social scene in Spain between the thirteenth and seventeenth centuries. In Spain at that time, as in the rest of Europe, the proportion of doctors in the population was the same as in modern day Ethiopia or some of the most depressed areas of Vietnam. In Barcelona, for example, in the fourteenth and fifteenth centuries there were on average only one and a half to two doctors for every ten thousand inhabitants, whilst the figure in Valencia in the first third of the sixteenth century varied between five and seven doctors per ten thousand inhabitants.[3] If this was the situation in urban areas then we can only assume that in the country the figure was much lower. Unfortunately there is not any solid documentary proof of this. So what, then, was the medical service given to the Muslim, and later morisco, population? A population, that is, which in the Kingdom of Valencia in the sixteenth century comprised a third of the total population and in Granada almost half. And what actually was the medicine practised by the moriscos? I hope to answer these questions in this chapter.

Valencia was conquered by the Christians in the thirteenth century and Granada at the end of the fifteenth. Before the conquests, because of socio-economic and socio-medical conditions, the majority of the people in these areas received medical aid based on empiricism and non-academic belief and they were served by 'professional' practitioners. This situation continued after the Christian conquests. However, the influence of empiricism and belief on Muslim and morisco medicine was greatly increased by the general disintegration of Islamic culture and the gradual social alienation of Muslims and moriscos. Some examples of these beliefs were the use of scapulars (religious images worn over clothes), religious texts on the pregnant womb, spells, certain forms of judicial astrology, the occult, and others. Simultaneously the image of the professional doctor diminished, giving way to a flowery and picturesque world of quacks. This is not to say that the quacks would not have existed alongside scientific medicine, and together with these empirical practitioners would have been practitioners whose knowledge could be assessed against an academic 'corpus' of learning. Thus the population as a whole could have benefited from the dialectic between 'academic medicine' and 'empirical medical knowledge'. Actually in Christian Spain the majority of the Muslim, and later morisco, population was served only by doctors with empirical knowledge.

Morisco culture suffered by the disappearance of academically trained doctors, even though it favoured the scholastic model in medical science which was typical of the Christian majority. The morisco population was denied access to academic medicine, not for intellectual or academic reasons, but because the moriscos were of 'another caste'. Thus the dominance of empiricism in morisco medicine is another symptom of cultural confrontation.[4]

A general characteristic of the moriscos in the sixteenth century was their tight grip on the surviving Islamic culture of the Muslim population. Medicine, as an integral part of culture, gives us evidence for these strong links with Islam. By looking at archives and sixteenth-century Inquisition cases, we can see that in the morisco society of the mid-sixteenth century Muslim teachers (*alfaquí*) continued to play the versatile and diverse role they had always done in Arabic culture.[5] Their functions included working in the Civil Service, religious duties, and teaching both arts and sciences. Their work was confined to their own community. However, their professional standing changed from that of doctor to quack for many reasons. Their medicine was pulled away from its relationship with natural science; they were often reduced to the conditions of peasants; subject to all kinds of social, political and religious pressures. Academic teaching and academically trained scientists disappeared. Even the Old Christian high society and the Court tolerated and accepted quack doctors. However, while fulfilling an important role at the heart of the community they also came into open conflict with academic medicine.

The cultural solidarity amongst the moriscos of which I wrote earlier was not in fact common to all the regions where the moriscos suffered cultural oppression. There were appreciable differences between the moriscos in, for example, Granada, the Kingdom of Valencia and the Kingdom of Aragon. In Aragon the Castilian language replaced Arabic as the means of communication, even in religion and amongst heads of communities.[6] As we know, language plays a vital part in the cultural unity of a group. For example the cultural disintegration of the moriscos in Castile and Aragon before the expulsion of moriscos from Granada in the 1570s was so great that Arabic remained solely as a ritual and holy tongue – fragmentary and completely meaningless to those who used it.[7]

Andrés Laguna's Castilian translation of *Materia Medica* by Dioscorides became one of the morisco healers' source texts.[8] The morisco healers personified the mixture of Christian and Arab cultures; the former because they spoke Castilian and read medical texts written in Castilian and also in Latin, the latter because Arab medicine was passed on by an oral tradition. Moreover, because they could not read and write Arabic they had no access to texts from their own culture. The texts were in any case very difficult to obtain outside certain libraries in the second half of the sixteenth century. We shall also see that this contact with academic Christian medical science occurred frequently in an area which falls between empiricism and academic science: that is clinical therapy.

Muslim medicine finally disintegrated when it changed into healing which drew on both beliefs outside academic medicine and on empiricism. For this we have proof from Valencia, Aragon, Granada and Castile.

Among the Muslim and morisco minority the move from scientific to folk medicine was due to social changes which were taking place throughout the middle ages and which culminated in the sixteenth century. The healer, who counterbalanced the scientifically trained doctor, owed his social respectability to a complex series of socio-scientific and socio-economic reasons. Among these was the lack of a medical service by academic medicine to large sectors of the population; discrimination between rich and poor in treatment (both Christian and morisco); failures in academic medicine; the existence of chronic and incurable diseases, and the cultural vacuum following repressive measures.

Before we go any further, we must deal with a semantic problem: the concept of 'doctor' and 'surgeon' and what they both meant to the people and those with academic training in the sixteenth century. Unfortunately it has not been very thoroughly investigated.

Leaving the morisco with a university degree to one side, we refer here to the morisco who had picked up a certain knowledge on the fringes of mainstream academia and was practising it in a community (both morisco and Old Christian) which accepted him as having healing knowledge and techniques.

The morisco healer was the continuation of the school of Moorish medicine of the late middle ages. The Moorish scientific system was born of the Greco-Arab paradigm and upheld an open academic system which passed on knowledge freely. To say that the morisco doctor was a continuation of this system, however, does not mean that he preserved it. The evolution of the Moorish to the morisco doctor was more a degeneration than a progression, owing to a number of external factors. So great was the change that the links between the two forms of medicine virtually disappeared. Surprisingly enough it took only two or three generations to dismantle a type of medicine that had been alive and well, although stronger in teaching than in innovation, in the last decades of the fifteenth century. For example in 1494 the Muslim minority in Aragon was vigorous enough socially and academically to retain autonomous medical teaching and practice along Arab cultural lines. This teaching took place in the *madrasa* or Islamic university of Saragossa. The language used was Arabic.[9]

Both extremes of sixteenth-century Spanish society (disregarding the minority of intellectuals) were slow to recognize the change from Moorish to morisco medicine. Moriscos who were merely healers were still called 'doctors' and 'surgeons' in the sixteenth century, as their predecessors had been in the last third of the fifteenth century: it does not help here to draw clear lines between 'the middle ages' and 'the renaissance' or 'modern age' as if a narrow straight had been crossed and a new continent entered.

Things began to change in the last third of the sixteenth century. The reason for this was Philip II's creation of a bureaucracy which was felt at all social levels. We should bear in mind that the social relevance of a professional is closely linked to the creation and effectiveness of a bureaucracy, or rather to a radical and rigid separation of social strata. This tendency was very strong in fifteenth- and sixteenth-century Spain – possibly as a balance to the upward surge of classes in a young, developing society. What in fact happened was that the concept of 'doctor' came to be seen as being on the top rung of a ladder above the Latin surgeon, the barber-bloodletter and finally above the quacks, who were outside any legal category yet very widespread.

Nevertheless it should be said that despite the solidity of the medical profession in Spain during the sixteenth century, and particularly at its end, the categories within the profession were not fixed as they are today. There were still traces of that early medieval overlapping I referred to earlier. For example the morisco healer was called a 'doctor' or 'surgeon' by both the people and the Inquisition Tribunal, whereas today we would have no hesitation in calling him a quack. Today academic medicine and the social standing of its practitioners are such that nobody would refer to a quack (even though he might mend fractures and cure illness) as a 'doctor' or a 'surgeon', even in the least advanced parts of Spain. This lack of definition is important when we try to explain the prestige enjoyed by the morisco healer among the Christian aristocracy and the commercial bourgeoisie in Madrid or Valencia and the absence of social prejudice when it came to consulting one. The only clear case that I have found of censure against a morisco healer was that by Daza Chacón (1510–96), a leading figure in Spanish surgery during the renaissance, and some of his colleagues from the court.[10] Their reasons for censure were entirely academic, based on the methodology which related medicine to natural philosophy and which separated the academic healer from the empirical healer. Outside small academic circles the words used for these empirical healers were 'doctor' or 'surgeon', even though they had no qualification or licence to practise.

This last point is very important for realizing that we should not apply twentieth-century assumptions to sixteenth-century Spain. We must remember that a university degree did not have the same rôle as today. Our contemporary university degree came into being during the nineteenth century in line with the bourgeois mentality which produced it. Thus in the first half of the sixteenth century the presence or absence of a medical degree was not the vital factor in acceptance or rejection of the medical practices of healers or magicians. The reasons were more complex. A good example of the exchange of ideas in the first half of the sixteenth century is personified by the converted Jew, Andrés Laguna (*c.* 1510–59) who was a student at the Sorbonne, was connected with the University of Alcalá, was the Emperor's doctor, and was a leading figure in the movement towards medical humanism.[11] Laguna was not averse to consulting wizards and healers, learning from them, applying their remedies, noting their results and even going to them himself when he himself needed attention for a serious illness. From his point of view as an academic (and with the material available) he studied the healers' remedies, and with respect, not contempt. In one of these studies he identified some herbs which 'a little old German woman . . . who looked like a witch' had given him as being henbane (*Hyoscamus niger*) and then went on to describe its effects. In another case he studied the hallucinogenic properties of 'a certain green ointment' used by two wizards in Metz.[12] He used it in experiments on a patient and found that it contained 'extremely cold and soporific herbs, which were hemlock nightshade (*Atropa belladonna*), henbane and mandrake'.[13]

Morisco healers were never labelled as 'wizards' or 'enchanters' (as Laguna had described the healers of Lorena) by their academic Christian 'colleagues'. The social prestige of the morisco healer together with his deep integration into Old Christian society, was in sharp contrast to the growing alienation of the majority of moriscos. Not that the morisco healers did not have any problems with already established doctors who were protecting their established practices.

What is surprising, though, is the limited use made by Christian society (and therefore also by the morisco population) of the doctors who had academic training – those doctors who also claimed a monopoly over science and medical practice. As it was, people had no qualms about consulting morisco doctors, knowing full well that they had neither university degrees nor licences to practise. Not only did they consult the morisco doctor but they were also quite happy to talk about it publicly. The church tried to stop this use of morisco doctors right up to the end of the sixteenth century with prohibition after prohibition. The church's concern shows just how far the morisco doctor (meaning healer) had become integrated into society.

From what I have written I hope I have given some idea of some medically-related aspects of Spanish society in the sixteenth century.[14] It is a very complicated topic, but the major points of background to my theme I hope have been covered.

To continue, I would like to take five topics as the basis for an examination of the relationship between academic practitioners with their rational medicine and morisco healers with their empirical or non-empirical medicine.

The five topics are these:

1. Academic science's attack on empiricism using a so-called rational methodology.

2. The failure of the academic world and society to recognize medicine and its practice as signs of a living cultural group. In this case the group is morisco.
3. The refusal of academic medicine to assimilate the morisco culture peacefully. Moriscos were barred from medical faculties.
4. The identification of the morisco social group as a causal factor (that is aetiological factor) of 'social pathology'.
5. The designation of areas common to morisco empiricism and academic science.

First, in the last twenty years certain historians of medicine and technology have looked at attitudes to practical techniques in the sixteenth century. Paolo Rossi[15] and López Piñero[16] have analysed European thinkers' new appreciation of techniques in the sixteenth century. This appreciation was to be one of the most important factors of change in the new era. Practical technique was represented in medicine principally by surgery, the importance of, and interest in which, had been increasing all through the early middle ages within academic circles, having come to Spain from Italy. In Spain this new interest went hand in hand with the high reputation of surgeons.[17] One of these surgeons was Dionisio Daza Chacón, who practised in Emperor Charles I's army. He proclaimed, changing the title of the well known work of Galen, that 'the good surgeon is the true doctor'. One of Daza's aims was to emphasize the worth of scientifically-based technique over mere empirical practice. Accordingly he was at great pains to emphasize the importance of the university-trained surgeon.

When the Valencian morisco Pinterete was summoned to treat Charles, the son of Philip II and heir to the throne, Daza took the opportunity to attack the empirical nature of morisco doctors' treatment. Daza was quite categorical:

Many times it was proposed that we doctors should cure his highness with the ointments of Pinterete, moor from the Kingdom of Valencia; there are two ointments – one white . . . another black . . . Most of us have rejected these ointments, first because we did not know their composition and it was not proper to use them without knowing what was in them, and secondly because it did not seem rational that the same medicaments were always used, whatever the time, and on all ages and patients.[18]

In spite of all this, the morisco healers' ointments were used on the prince and so Daza had to give an explanation. In his explanation he denounced the rôle of mere belief, which went more or less hand in hand with folk medicine, by saying: 'More in view of the faith which many had in those ointments . . . .'.[19]

I suspect that these same reasons were used by Luis Collado (*c.* 1520–89), professor at the medical faculty of Valencia (incidentally the person who introduced the anatomy of Vesalius to Spain),[20] when he had violent exchanges with the morisco doctor Jerónimo Pachet.

Let us see how these events are recorded in the Inquisitorial summary:

Item, this man (Pachet) also cured one Bautista Tridi eight or nine years ago, with the help of the devil. Tridi was being attended by doctor Collado and doctor Ardevol (Jaime Ardevol), and he had a diseased liver, a weak stomach, almost completely destroyed, and his intestines full of vapour, he was very sick, almost dead, and though the physicians visited him they gave him no medicines. So they sent for this man, and when he had come he argued with Collado and Ardevol, for they were dismissed immediately. *He understood the disease from experience*, but as it was in such an acute phase *and he did not understood the use of medicines*, he consulted with his 'familiar' (that is to say, he used the devil), and he showed him the medicines inside and outside. And the man was cured within two or three days. He was well paid, and he took both fame and money from the case, the other physicians hated him.[21]

In 1580 Pachet was tried by the Inquisition for practising the Islamic religion.

Second, the sixteenth century saw the gradual collapse of Muslim and Christian ability to live side by side. Due to the peculiar circumstances of the time and the nature of the two cultures involved, this break transcended merely religious or personal levels. It also brought out socio-economic and political conflicts.[22] Nevertheless, for neither the Old Christians nor the moriscos (converted from Islam) was religion a secondary factor. The introduction of the Inquisition at the end of the fifteenth century was to affect certain minorities greatly. Particularly affected were the Jews who had converted to Christianity and were more or less integrated into society, and also the moriscos who more by force than choice had embraced the Christian faith and recognized its baptism. For these people accusations of heresy loomed large.

Also, as Muslim theologians and institutional religion lost influence and control, popular morisco religious belief, which in Islam was very rich, had become flamboyant and superstitious. In the religious–theological field, then, there was the same process of disintegration that we saw in the medical field.

One of the most interesting aspects of this popular flamboyance was the belief in devils, with its roots in neo-platonic Islam. Along with their continued Mohammedanism after official conversion, this belief in devils and in their invocation was what brought morisco 'doctors' and 'surgeons' before the Inquisition. Here we see, once again, medicine as one of the manifestations of a living culture, in this case of the morisco community. All this, along with the diligence and detail of the Inquisition, has allowed us to penetrate the complex world of morisco beliefs and practices related to medicine. We can also examine, with solid evidence, its confrontation with academic science. Even though the richness of this world of belief is only partially expressed by documents, some of the books written in Spanish with Arabic characters (*aljamiado*) by morisco communities in Aragon (which Ribera studied and of which he translated large parts) have been crucial in getting a fairly accurate picture of popular morisco medical practices.[23]

The existence of these Inquisitorial trials against morisco doctors and surgeons raises a series of doctrinal and practical problems. We might ask why they were tried, and why invocation of demons was considered heretical. And what were the reasons for the Inquisition's persecution of the barbers and surgeons who performed circumcisions (*retajadores*), and of surgeons and midwives in general.

The crimes for which the moriscos were brought before the Holy Office were usually the following:

1. Crimes against the faith; accusations of Muslim practices and beliefs.
2. Crimes of superstition (witchcraft, sorcery and magic).
3. Offences against morality (for example sodomy and hermaphroditism).
4. Political crimes (alleged alliances with the Turks, Berber pirates and others).[24]

Almost all the cases against doctors seem to have fallen into the second category, allegations of being in league with the devil; whilst the proceedings against the surgeons who performed circumcisions fall into the first category.

The question of invoking demons was what worried the Inquisition officers more than anything else about morisco doctors. They considered it a very real possibility and a punishable one. However, diabolic belief meant quite different things to the inquisitor and the morisco. Both accepted its reality, yet each saw it from a different cultural point of view.[25] The inquisitor's view sprang from a scholastic conception of devil-pacts and invocation whereas the morisco's belief was based on his belief in semitic spiritualism and Alexandrine neoplatonism. They spoke a different language. Leaving aside the cases of deceit or mental illness which could have existed, the four or five trials which have been found (and the material provided by Ribera) leave no shadow of a doubt of the genuine belief in devils on both sides.

The entire universe, to a morisco, was not something static and lifeless, it was like a dynamic kingdom ruled by Allah's governors, or spirits of all sizes. These spirits ruled everything. It was necessary, therefore, to be on good terms with them, which meant knowing the words which pleased them, their categories, and the way to treat them. Knowing these things allowed the moriscos to call up spirits to protect them from illness, forecast serious illness, know about far-off events, and so on. Many spirits or demons had left signs by which they could be summoned by those who knew them. The signs varied a great deal: a drawn palm leaf, an iron, a figure drawn in saffron on spun cloth, etc. Each had to be combined with the necessary spell. There were, however, evil spirits which had to be cast out since they brought illness and bad luck.[26]

The invocation of demons was a common practice amongst morisco doctors. It was completely in keeping with the belief which ran through their whole society. It was also completely real for the Inquisitors. In the trial of the wretched morisco healer Román Ramirez (who worked in Aragon and Castile) we can see how the two worlds crossed. The public prosecutor said:

And crime followed crime, by evil means and with the aim of enrichment, curing illness, he has been and still is in league with the devil, with whose help and advice in the month of June 1594, he cast an evil spell on a woman of Tajaguerce, near the city of Soria. This woman whose name was Ana Sanz, had married one Bartolomé de Ortega. On their wedding night he caused her to lose menstrual blood with many fits of melancholy which cut her desire to share her husband's bed. He also caused her a feeling of rejecting holy things and other outward signs of being possessed, loss of sanity and memory in such a way as not to recognize her parents nor remember their names.

[The woman's relatives called the doctor] and when the woman saw the accused her condition worsened, she fainted and fell down. He treated her with the aromatic oil of juniper, made her rise, though not without great pain.

So that he could communicate with and treat the demon within her, the accused gave the woman certain powders in an egg . . . And since on that occasion they gave him no more than 40 coins, he complained . . . swearing to God that they would need him again soon, as later happened.

For, having treated her with aromatic smoke and ointments which he had left the said woman, she worsened, in such a way that the demons returned to possess her. She became sick of the head, her mouth twisted and her head fell onto her shoulder. She went for three days without eating or drinking. These were all obvious results of the threat the accused had made on underpayment.[27]

The prosecutor, then, accepts these notions of pacts, invocations and demonic possession quite seriously. What is noticeable is that having had a scholastic–rational education the Inquisitors did not apply their book-learning to everyday life. Instead they developed a gloomy belief system in order to deal with the practical, popular and ingenuous world view of the moriscos. Neither did the Inquisitors realize that it was quite different from their own. Three levels can be identified in the inquisitorial trials in relation to beliefs in devils.[28]

(1) The rational attitude of the Supreme Council of the Inquisition.
(2) The attitude of the provincial Inquisitors: they internalized and transformed the European belief about devils by integrating it

into a rational system based on medieval scholastic formulae. With this transformation they created a superstructure, of which they were completely convinced, and which they tried to impose on the people. They were thus upholding the *status quo* by using a belief system loosely based on the rational attitude of the Supreme Council.

(3) The morisco world of belief, in which demons were a reality, but a different reality from that described in the second level. This world of belief was shown through simple everyday practices by the humble peasants, some of whom were charlatans. In spite of this the Inquisitors took them seriously. Together with this was the religious problem and the rôle of the Inquisition as a destroyer of morisco social structures. We must not forget that medicine and medical practice were part of this social structure.

In the trial quoted above the accused doctor, Román Ramírez, gives a quite different version from the prosecutors. We shall see how he finally explained his experiences with devils. He only did so after three months in prison and under pressure from the Inquisitors. His first declaration made to the Christians was about popular methods of healing, and it is a mixture of folk beliefs and academic science. In the two declarations the dilemma of his existence comes through strongly: the pretences and repressions of a newly converted Moor in a life full of social and personal tensions. In the first declaration he says that he was called to Tajaguerce by the girl's family and on arriving found the girl:

her neck was twisted, her chin thrust into her shoulder. The first thing he did to cure her was tell the parish priest to read the gospels to her . . . then, he asked the apothecary to send him certain herbs, mineral powders (sulphur) and juniper oil. He mixed them and made an ointment which he applied to the patient. He told the family that the illness was serious and that if the symptoms returned they should apply the ointment again, recite the Gospels and invoke the Virgin Mary . . . the family said that when the sick girl was better they would pay him well.[29]

Later I will deal at length with the interesting problems posed by this empirical use of pharmaceutical herbs and in particular that of the sources of his knowledge in this field. Usually these empirical doctors knew of these herbs through the oral tradition and personal experience. (We should not forget that they were mostly country people.) In Román Ramírez, however, a series of interesting features coincide: his ignorance of the Moslem tradition (he could not speak Arabic), a tradition of medicine in his family (his grandfather and mother both practised medicine) and his contact with the medical materials used by Christian doctors. He would have used Andrés Laguna's translation into Castilian of the work of Dioscorides.

Let us return again to the devilish world of our doctor Ramírez. His second declaration reveals the whole Islamic belief in the devil myth. This second statement was only made under great pressure. In it we can see the oral tradition operating – a tradition which preserved the mixture of practice and belief:

I was taught by Juan de Luna, my grandfather, who was a great doctor. When I was ten or twelve years old my grandfather, who was going to die, told me that if I needed anything, between eleven and twelve at night I should call out *Liarde*. He said he had ordered *Liarde* to come and help me. I understood that *Liarde* was a demon with whom my father had a pact. Later I heard my grandfather talking to him a few times from his bed at night. After a year I asked my grandfather who he was talking to. He said again that after he died the person he was talking to would come and help me whenever I called. Since my grandfather died I have called the demon *Liarde* many times between eleven and twelve at night, just as my grandfather told me. The demon has answered many times, although at other times he has not . . .[30]

The family nature of the medical profession (with its roots in the Judaic–Arabic medical tradition) was obviously influential when it came to decide on a future career. In spite of Ramirez's initial lack of enthusiasm for medicine he considered himself obliged to continue the tradition of his grandfather and his mother in medicine.

As we see, Ramírez attributes his own and his grandfather's medical knowledge to the demon *Liarde*. Jerónimo Pachet, the famous morisco doctor from Valencia, did the same. At his trial he said:

When I first worked with the demon, I often cured people with his help (since I did not have much experience). But after fourteen or fifteen years I stopped using him because I knew enough about the properties of herbs and medicines. I have occasionally called him, but only when the case was very serious and I did not understand it by natural means, and when university doctors had given up.[31]

This is a clear attempt to bring medical knowledge together with the Beyond, or the devil. A doctor who could boast of this connection in his practice was thus guaranteeing his knowledge in the eyes of the people. The sacred origins of his science put him above criticism. The morisco doctor thus embodies the rich and complex beliefs held by moriscos and even Old Christians, because the whole population, both Old and New Christians, had lived together for centuries. There was also the possibility of doctors dishonestly exploiting people's beliefs.

Apparently morisco healers were not always called to treat the higher reaches of society. Only when there was no alternative, that is when the (Christian) doctor left the patient 'in the hands of God,' were they consulted. 'Those morisco doctors only treated those whom the Christian doctors had said would die'.[32]

Chronic and incurable diseases were the usual reasons for the high classes and intellectuals calling for healers. As Malinowski has pointed out, magical and religious explanations usually replace natural or scientific ones when we move into the world of unpredictable events, where the human will sees its own inability to control events.[33]

As I have stated, the morisco believed in many kinds of demons. There were the medical specialists who advised certain healers and many others who were evil, who could cause illnesses. To get rid of the evil demons, people did not have to call in a specialist, for it was enough to carry around a piece of paper with a spell and a verse of the Koran written on it. A morisco document advises:

If anyone wants to stop spirits entering the house and upsetting their peace and health, they only have to put the paper into a tube, seal the tube with fish and put it in the main door-way of the cowshed. Also it is good to put it in the roof and in the corners, always inside the walls, so that the spirits cannot find a way in through cracks in the walls.[34]

Now, in the 1980s, these charms can sometimes be found when old houses are demolished in Aragon or Granada or Castile. They can also be identified in Inquisition cases against the moriscos, for example, the young merchant's servant from Alcoy (Alicante) who was found to have a bag which 'was smooth and coloured, containing some rings and a little musk and a small piece of paper with writing on it . . . .'.[35] This writing, which was Arabic, was translated by order of the Inquisition. It read:

It is proven that the man carrying this about his person and writing four of the following will be protected and defended from everything. The words are, *Alguaco, Alguaca, Sogel, Sagel, Mosaguin, Johuage, Jahuage, Guaquimisi a la raig.*[36]

The Jesuit translator added: 'All these names are those of demons and especially *guaquimisi a la raig* which means "lame devil"'. The Inquisition accused the young servant of 'carrying demon's names in Arabic'. The trial was in 1620. Ten years previously, when his mother had to leave the young boy, she gave him the bag and entreated him to keep it to protect himself from all evil and sickness.[37]

A morisco reader of Arabic texts, made a comment in the margin of one text:

The good Muslim should never be without charms for the person who goes without them is like a house which cannot be shut because it has no door. Without a door anyone can enter. Anyone who goes without charms can be entered anywhere by demons.[38]

Morisco doctors often used spells, charms, phrases from the Koran and similar things in their practices. An example comes from 1596 in the trial of the morisco Francisco de Córdoba in Toledo. One witness, an academic, told the story like this:

Don Alonxo Mexía de Tovar, student of the University of Alcalá, after swearing in, said that the previous Lent, in the year 1595, in Villacastin (Segovia) his brother

Antonio Mexía de Tovar was ill. Some said that he had been bewitched. Don Alonso heard of a Morisco called Francisco de Córdoba who lived in Toledo . . . and heard that the said morisco could cure his brother's illness, so the doctor was brought. When he came the witness saw that the said morisco was administering some powders and was telling the family to scatter the powders in the patient's room and also to scatter powder in the room of the woman suspected of sorcery, and also in the eggs the patient was to eat. Each time he made certain signs with a feather and saliva. He also gave them some small written documents and ordered them to be soaked in the patient's wine or water.[39]

Later, when they had been translated by the Arabic professor in Alcalá, they were seen to be fragments of the Koran.

Leaving aside the empirical part of the morisco's medical practice, which was basically pharmacological, it is clear that his medicine was mixed very much with religious belief. Short prayers were common amongst the people. For example those which the abbot of the monastery of Valldigna (Valencia) found on a morisco and which he quickly sent to the Inquisition. Apart from being written in Arabic, 'they seemed to contain something against the Faith'.[40]

The documents which the diligent monk took show quite clearly the duality of empiricism and belief which I have previously indicated. One of them, for example, is a recipe against scabies, which could easily have been written by a medical faculty professor. It says:

Burn two ounces of sulphur and two ounces of alum together. Grind the residue and mix the powder with orange juice and olive oil. Make an ointment and rub it into the parts affected by scabies. Afterwards bathe with boiling water and rosebay and flax-leaved daphne.[41]

I do not think it is a coincidence that we owe the first descriptions of scabies to Arab doctors and that they possessed a richer pharmacological tradition. The above prescription was found with some short prayers for the sick. For example: 'To Our Lord, Healer of those who call him, listener to the dead, grant me what I ask'.[42]

Soon after the expulsion of the majority of moriscos from Granada in 1572, archbishop Pedro Guerrero condemned 'sorcerers' and anyone who used:

Any type of riddle, such as omens, birds, sneezes, so-called proverbs, lucky charms, spells and those who use water, glass, swords or anything which shines, or those who cast spells with metal or anything else, those who perform magic with the heads of corpses or animals or with children's or virgin's palms or bewitch with wedding rings, or who cut the mountain rose because it cures the sickness which they say comes from the mountains, and anything similar to gain health or worldly goods . . .[43]

This text, which was part of the conclusions of the Synod of Granada, sums up the richness and complexity of the baroque world of morisco belief.

Third, after the conquest of the Muslim Kingdom of Granada in 1492 the Spanish kings were left with a large number of people on their hands whose culture was Islamic. Even though their leaders, intellectuals and the better-off emigrated to North Africa in the following decades, there still remained a 'learned' morisco minority in Granada. This minority, which was linked to the royal bureaucracy, formed the centre of the morisco social structure, the members of which came ultimately to live on what were almost reservations. This minority, which hispanicized its names, tried to bridge the gap between itself and the dominant Christian power. The crown and the church began a carefully planned scheme to rob the moriscos of their culture. The intention behind the scheme was to try to turn morisco children into model Christian scholars, and in implementing it schools and later the University of Granada were founded. The scheme was to prove very useful to the Castilian crown during the conquest of the non-European cultures of the New World.[44]

For a number of reasons this scheme failed. The moriscos in Granada rebelled and were only put down after a bloody war (the 'war of the Alpujarras'). Philip II then had the idea of dispersing the moriscos of Granada throughout Castile. This was done between June 1569 and December 1571, but rather than providing solutions, it created new social and political problems in Castile.[45]

It is in this context that we should consider Pedro de Vesga's words when he asked the king in the Castilian Parliament to prevent 'the moriscos who recently revolted in the Kingdom of Granada'[46] and the old moriscos from entering medical faculties and also from practising medicine. Parliament stated that

many moriscos study and practise in the universities of Alcalá and Toledo and others; we implore the king to find a solution because it is very likely that before long all or at least most of our doctors will be moriscos.[47]

The political and religious tensions between Old and New Christians and their old controversies played a vital part in the social alienation of the morisco doctor:

After their rebellions and many other signs we can only conclude that morisco doctors hate the Old Christians, so who wants to be treated by his enemy? We must also say that judging by their confessions to the Inquisition that many doctors treated their own race properly whilst deliberately killing Old Christians and supplying medicines which induced abortion.[48]

The figure of the morisco doctor became a symbol of all the degradation and corruption of which medicine could be capable. Moreover, under the Inquisition's methods of persuasion, morisco doctors admitted to all kinds of professional misconduct. Thus the morisco doctor became something to be eliminated from a society made up of Old Christians. Only Old

Christians should have the right to enjoy the status of a doctor and surgeon, and the traditionally virtuous reputation of the good doctor.

If the moriscos are doctors they will have the status owing to a doctor, they will wear luxurious clothes, and travel by coach. The laws of the kingdom forbid the moriscos the use of these things and to hold honourable professions, and if the medical profession is the most honourable, why must they practise it?

Going into convents to cure nuns, and knowing how imaginative and curious they are, the moriscos could show them things harmful to their faith. There are few positions which require more virtue than that of a doctor, but instead the moriscos have bad tendencies. They do not confess, or if they do confess it is out of a sense of duty. They do not give alms. A doctor must send his patient to confession and heal the poor freely and with charity. How can those who do not call a priest when they are ill or never do good works fulfil the above conditions? With many medicines it is possible to kill secretly and subtly, without being asked, and we can be sure that we are correct when we presume that they use these medicines, and between them kill more people in this kingdom than the Turks, the English and others.[49]

The wickedness of the morisco doctor's practice is clearly shown in the confession forced out of a morisco surgeon by the Valencian Inquisition, 'the said man confessed to having malevolently left Old Christians with only one arm so that they could not carry weapons'.[50] The Old Christians would not allow the morisco doctor out of the social alienation in which he had been put. They blocked all his paths for rising socially, within both the Faith and the University. Their conversion was considered as insincere. We should remember here the important social rôle played by the Christian Faith. '[Morisco doctors] do not confess, or if they do confess it is out of a sense of duty'.[51]

The morisco's great biological vitality could be dangerously capable of shaking social equilibrium in his favour, an equilibrium which was unlawfully held by the Old Christians.

For some years now the moriscos who were expelled from Granada have enrolled their sons in the medical faculty, but then they were not admitted as apothecaries, clerks nor any position of confidence, and this caused many problems because the Old Christians and honourable people did not want to enroll at the faculty of medicine for this reason, since the moriscos who practised medicine could have got revenge on the Old Christians . . . and that before long the majority of doctors will be moriscos.[52]

It was necessary also to close the door to social elevation which the university presented.

For these problems and others which will be omitted for the sake of brevity, it seems advisable that His Majesty make a decree in which he orders the universities not to give degrees to those who cannot prove that they are not moriscos, and to punish the clerk, witnesses and examiners, those who give the degree and the doctors who have a part in it. All this should apply to doctors' diplomas as well as to graduates and bachelors.[53]

But it was possible to be a romanist doctor or surgeon, that is, to obtain a diploma to practise, without going to university; only being examined by the Royal Tribunal of *Protomedicato* on practical knowledge and capabilities.[54] This they also tried to stop.

Item: when they go to be examined at the Tribunal that included in the practical information should be the fact that they are not moriscos, neither old nor modern.[55]

This requirement was introduced into the rules and regulations of the University of Alcalá in 1565–6.[56]

This still leaves a loophole through which the morisco can gain medical knowledge – he can still practise in illicit competition in certain ways, because even though he does not graduate he can still listen to university lectures.

And because they can still practise in secret, even without graduating, we must instruct the university bedels and secretaries, under pain of punishment, not to allow moriscos to enrol, practise nor attend lectures . . .[57]

Fourth, the Kingdom of Granada was seriously affected by the 'war of the Alpujarras' and its major consequence, the deportation of moriscos to other parts of Spain. The university of Granada, and especially its weak medical faculty, collapsed. For example medical publishing in Granada was interrupted in 1580, not to begin again until 1640! As Bernard Vincent[58] has observed, there are hardly any investigations on the subject of moriscos in Granada and Castile between 1570 and 1619, when the moriscos were all finally exiled from Spain. What information there is still lies in general and municipal archives. The long year after the decision to expel them was a crucial one. We should not forget that already in 1569 moriscos from some parts of the kingdom and from Albayzin (a quarter in the city of Granada) had been expelled. The latter was depopulated when twenty thousand inhabitants left.[59] At this time the attitude of the population of Castile was vital to the chances of the integration of the morisco community.

Under what conditions did the move from Granada to Castile take place? How were the moriscos accepted in the different places? What ideas directed the different phases of expulsion? In short what solutions did the Spanish have in mind for the old conflict . . . which, whatever the policy, could disappear or break out again?[60]

We still cannot answer these questions properly and we hardly have any data to judge the repercussions on medicine of such a serious measure. For this reason I shall confine myself to an important piece of evidence which throws up a new problem in the relationship of morisco and academic medicine in Castile.

The dispersion of the moriscos was not only a punitive measure or one of internal security. It was also the only apparently feasible way of trying to integrate them into society . . . deep down the problem was not theological, but social.[61]

They had to be integrated in all respects 'into the society in which until then they had been a foreign body'.[62]

This was the aim of the intellectual Pedro de Valencia in his *Treatise on the Moriscos*.[63] It was written in 1605 and 1606 when the idea of exiling all moriscos from Spain was taking shape amongst the king's closest advisors. This terrible decision was taken in 1609. Ironically, the king who took the decision, Philip III, had been cured as a child of a very serious illness by a morisco doctor.[64]

In the way it was done the dispersion of moriscos through Castile was one of the most atrocious deportations in history. Lapeyre[65] established that 20.7 per cent of the 54 366 moriscos on the census died during the journey. Vincent,[66] however, from archive evidence, has put the figure higher, at 33.5 per cent, at least for six years in Estremadura. We can get an idea of the risk to life when we realize that it was during the exodus that one of the most serious epidemics of louse-borne typhus in the sixteenth century broke out. It is the illness typical of underdevelopment and poverty.

It is precisely this fact which brings out a new aspect of the relationship between moriscos and academic medical men. The latter saw the moriscos as the cause of a hitherto untraced illness: louse-borne typhus, called in Old Castilian *tabardillo*. With this a new problem is thrown up, not to be grasped until the beginning of the twentieth century, by social pathology: the social aetiology of illnesses. Let us look at it a little closer.

During the sixteenth century a number of 'new illnesses' were described. For example, 'English sweats', which flourished between 1485 and 1551, the *nuwe krenckte* of Dusseldorf, the *morbus gallicus*, a new diphtheria. Along with these there was a new form of fever. Although Girolamo Fracastoro in 1546 was the first to describe with any kind of clinical precision an epidemic of this fever and so permit its later identification as louse-borne typhus, the most conscientious study of the disease was by Luis de Toro who was a doctor from Estremadura (Castile).[67] We will leave to one side whether these diseases were all 'new' or if they were only the nosographic consequence of better observation. Luis de Toro's description of what now we know as louse-borne typhus is very correct and direct. His study was part of the contemporary renaissance scientific reach towards reality, which along with a great care to describe the patients he had, led him to distinguish new illnesses and to extricate them from the jumble of 'fevers'. His clinical description hardly differs from that which appears in any of today's medical manuals.

There are four things which I wish to emphasize here: first the rôle of illness in a consciousness of the morisco problem, second the dramatic nature of the illness, third contemporary doctors' own explanation of the social factors for example (cold, or poverty following war) which cause and aid the development of illness, and lastly the causal relationship between illness and the presence or absence of a social group in this case, the moriscos.

Like the majority of Spanish intellectuals and scientists in the second half of the sixteenth century, Luis de Toro saw himself as being involved in the morisco problem. His involvement was a consequence of the deportation of moriscos after the 'war of Alpujarras', which suddenly brought a problem straight under his nose. By carefully reading Luis de Toro's work we can make out an anti-morisco climate; a protest against these people on whose arrival a louse-borne typhus epidemic flared up again, straight on the heels of the previous one.

They caused the disease to return and spread through large parts of Spain, being particularly cruel throughout Extremadura. The saracens were the source of the infection. All those who led and directed the dispersion, those who dealt with them or received them in villages and towns became infected and either died or came very close to it. At the same time those parts through which they did not go remained free of the disease. The disease was quite special amongst the moriscos, owing to the intense cold and poverty after the war in which they had to live.[68]

In all, in two years (1569–71) between seventy thousand and eighty thousand moriscos were dispersed in Castile, not counting those who were sent as slaves to the kingdom of Valencia. In the dedication of his book (1574) Luis de Toro talks of the cause of the disease as something insidious which has infiltrated and spread through Castile. He always refers to the moriscos pejoratively, as saracens (*sarraceni*) or moors (*mauris*).

Fifth, of all the morisco healers that we have found, very few could read or write, except those who were also teachers (*alfaquí*) or those who were trained as physicians outside the faculties of medicine. They were almost all farmers. Therefore, the training these healers received was limited to the oral tradition, usually taking place within the family itself. The lack of institutions through which this knowledge and wider culture could be passed and the repression which the moriscos suffered both contributed to the importance of oral transmission of information. The case of the morisco Román Ramírez, is typical of this situation. He was the grandson of Juan de Luna, 'who was a great doctor' and with whom he was brought up. Juan de Luna taught his daughter (Ramírez's mother) 'medical things' who then, says Ramírez, 'taught him everything he knew about herbs and curing illness'.[69]

Here we have, very clearly, the way in which medical knowledge was passed on. We could apply the same outline to the scientific teaching of surgeons. All this knowledge was based on a concise outline of traditional Galenic medicine which was still taught in the *madrasa* sixty or seventy years before. The *madrasa*, or Islamic university, was maintained by the Moslem community of Saragossa.[70] Alongside this system (or in fact mixed up with it) there existed a rich and complex belief world which had grown up in the absence of institutional control. The institutions had either disappeared with the conquest or led an increasingly difficult life. Their effect on the moriscos diminished or disappeared altogether, as they settled into lifelessness within a larger social structure. Along with this mixture of medical–scientific and belief systems, there existed a rich world of therapeutic knowledge. This knowledge largely centred on medical herbs. In all morisco doctors this is the most striking aspect of their medicine. What are more noticeable are not only the range of herbs they used, but also the complexity and extravagance of their prescriptions. Many ingredients were acquired at pharmacies.[71]

A new and interesting element is brought out in the interrogation of a morisco doctor. It is the use of Dioscorides translated into Castilian by Andrés Laguna. When talking about his mother's medical knowledge Román Ramírez says:

I never had medical books, neither did she write down the medicines she prescribed nor have I had them written down. I only had Dioscorides' book, which I bought thirty years ago in Madrid.[72]

In spite of never going to school 'little by little I learned to read. Everything I read . . . I memorised'.[73] Moreover, we should remember that Ramírez did not know any Arabic.

These facts are clear evidence of how far the Islamic culture of the moriscos, in Castile and Aragon, had disintegrated. They also show the strong attraction of Christian culture; the extent to which science had been spread by printing and the use of romance languages; and also the great popularity of Laguna's *Dioscorides* which our morisco bought in Madrid in about 1560, that is to say, five years after the first edition was published in Amberes (1555). The use of Laguna's *Dioscorides* as the only teaching book and the fact that the tribunal made Ramírez read a medical book written by the doctor Huarte de San Juan (1529–88),[74] as proof of his ability to read Castilian, show an important step in the programme of morisco integration into Christian society, at least in the scientific field. The integration naturally took place at the expense of morisco cultural models. All this existed alongside circulating works written in Spanish with Arab characters (*aljamiado*), such as medical astrology and spells applied to medicine, deeply rooted in Judaic–Arabic tradition.

Even though in the kingdom of Valencia and in other Spanish communities, Arabic remained as a written and oral medium (in its dialect, *algaravia*), we can still ask whether books of Arab medicine circulated amongst the 'professional' practitioners. We will leave to one side the academically-trained morisco doctors' contact with Arab sources and the relative abundance of Arab scientific and medical manuscripts in Spain in the first half of the sixteenth century.[75] What interests us is seeing whether the morisco healer, who had not fitted into Christian society and its science, had any connection with his written scientific tradition. This is to say, how did information pass on outside the university?

While the available documentation makes it difficult to get near the reality of my subject (the morisco healer and the Christian society in which he lived), here we find even greater problems. The Inquisition was very careful to watch for circulation or mere possession of papers written in Arabic. In the second half of the sixteenth century it was enough to be caught with a brief note (even if it were a legal contract) to be charged by the Inquisition under suspicion of being part of 'the abject sect of Mahomet'.[76] Obviously, this has not helped to conserve such literature. Also we should not forget that almost all the moriscos were illiterate. This, despite a clandestine network of teachers (*alfaquies*) who taught people to read and write Arabic and who were thus centres of upkeep of Islamic tradition. In spite of the difficulties, I think we can be sure of the existence and circulation of a medical literature written in Arabic (even though fragmentary) among the morisco communities in Castile, Aragon and Valencia.[77] Obviously it was a literature which was practically reduced to prescriptions. For example, the papers which were intercepted by the abbot of Valldigna included prescriptions. One of them, a treatment for scabies, has been quoted above. During the trial of Jerónimo Jover, who we know could read, write and speak Arabic, and who lived in Valencia in the 1580s and 1590s it was said that

when he left Valencia, (with the intention of enrolling at the Medical Faculty at Lérida, Catalonia) he took with him some books in Arabic. He left a different Arabic book at home, which the witness gave to the Holy Inquisition.[78]

Unfortunately, records do not speak of the contents of this book, nor has it been kept along with the court records. Were they medical books? It is very possible, since Jover was good enough for it to be worth his while going to the Faculty at Lérida to get a medical degree. His status was also high enough for him to marry the widow of the notary Pedro Fuster, an Old Christian. From the testimony of an apothecary friend of his we have been able to find out the names of some of the Christian books in his library. These books show the point to which these learned moriscos had become integrated, and the complex nature of the co-existence of the Islamic and scholastic Christian cultures. The apothecary said:

The said doctor (the morisco Jover) auctioned all the Christian books he had; including a book by St Thomas Aquinas and a book by Friar Luis of Granada and a book called *Memorable Things of Spain*.[79]

In a farm of Ciudad Real, in Castile, about 1600, the Inquisition found a library owned by a morisco with fourteen books. One of them was a medical book in Arabic. The title was *Medical Prescriptions*. Unfortunately it was burned by the Inquisition.[80]

A recently discovered document permits us to trace with precision another channel for the circulation of medical knowledge among the morisco community and to establish, with documentary evidence, the existence of a form of medical training for the morisco doctor other than the empirical that we have seen Román Ramírez take. Ramírez belonged to the world of that medical sub-profession which is covered by the imprecise concept of 'quack', which is specially applied to a healer in sixteenth-century Spain. The morisco doctor we are going to deal with, however, stands within a medical tradition of medical education that still existed in the sixteenth century in which, we should once more emphasize, both medical professional models characteristic of the late middle ages coexist. The doctor in question, Gaspar Capdal, must have practised in the Kingdom of Valencia (Buñol, Requena and Valencia city). His testimony was recorded by the inquisitorial clerks as follows:

He was born in Buñol; as soon as he could talk he became interested in learning how to read and write the language of the *algemía* [foreign language] which he was taught by a son of Martin Hernández, Old Christian, and the parson of Buñol . . . At the age of ten he moved to Requena and Valencia to study medicine . . . He knows how to read and write *algemía*, and not to read and write Arabic and he studied medicine with a doctor named Catalá at Requena and he studied through a book named Metiolosenes [Pietro Andrea Mattioli] and another named compendium of human health which is said to be written by the saints Cosmas and Damian and through another book named a practical manual (*practica*) by Pascual (Miguel Juan Pascual) and through the book by Fragoso (Juan Fragoso) on trees and *The Thesaurus of the Poor* (Spanish translation of *Thesaurus Pauperum* by Petrus Hispanus) and that he has not studied in any other place and has no books but only papers that he, from the cited books, has copied. After studying with Catalá he had conversations for two years with Master Damian, New Christian, resident in Valencia, at the apothecary Ynca's home.[31]

This text clearly shows how his own tradition had been forgotten (he could not read or write Arabic); if the interrogator had suspected him of doing so matters would not have been at all favourable for him. He was a morisco totally integrated in a society consisting of Old and New Christians in which the everyday act of living together with them was more normal and less tense than it appears through the narrow window of the inquisitorial processes. The fascination exerted by academic medicine and its obvious scientific and social prestige is something that shows itself throughout Capdal's testimony. He is proud of his knowledge of the new scientific languages (Spanish, Italian) which allowed him to acquire an adequate scientific training. This training proceeds according to the medieval model of open professional learning, away from the closed, institutional learning of the university. This model, still extant in the sixteenth century, and which was an important tradition in the Arabic and

Christian medicine of the late middle ages, is based upon a learning process, both theoretical and practical, that is carried out under one or several doctors. The learning period usually lasted several years. Through that time, the medical apprentice read medical texts, explained and annotated by his master, who gave him selected books. This period was completed with one or two years of practical medical training under the tuition and vigilance of an experienced doctor who had a licence issued by the authorities. In the case of Valencia this was a jury of doctors appointed by the Town Hall. After this training, whoever wanted to practise legally, obtained the necessary certificate from his masters and appeared before the jury who examined him on theoretical as well as practical aspects of medicine. The jury's judgements varied from rejection to admission, through to licences for a longer or shorter period of practice under an experienced doctor, or ones which did not allow their holders to treat certain diseases which required complicated therapeutics.[82]

Gaspar Capdal followed this model of professional training step by step. First of all, he learned Spanish (*algemía*), a relatively new tool for learning academic medicine; the term *algemia*, in its etymological sense, means 'foreign language'. As the Valencian moriscos remained very islamized they spoke, as their mother tongue, the *algaravía* or dialect Arabic language (which was very corrupt). For them, any other language, Spanish, Latin, Italian, was *algemia*.[83] From the medical literature handled by Capdal, we conclude that it was Spanish that he learned with 'Martín Hernández, an Old Christian, and with the parson of Buñol'. His knowledge of Spanish enabled him to read an Italian medical text. He studied under doctor Catalá, who practised in Requena (Valencia).

According to the cited works, the learning of Capdal had two sources: treatises of practical medicine (which we could call handbooks of internal and external medicine) and writings on medicinal therapeutics, basically on medical herbs. The first consists mainly of Vigo's *Short Practical Manual in Surgery* (1517) translated into Spanish by Miguel Juan Pascual (*c.* 1505–61), professor at the school of medicine in Valencia from 1542. The second, medical therapeutics, is represented by the work of Pietro Andrea Mattioli (1501–77) and Juan Fragoso (*c.* 1530–97).

Miguel Juan Pascual[84] did not, however, merely translate Vigo's handbook into Spanish; he added to it his marginal notes (*addiciones marginales*). To give an idea of the variety – and at the same time the complexity and subtlety – of the contents of this kind of work, it suffices to say that it deals in a more or less systematic way with anatomy, wounds, abscesses, ulcers, syphilis, fractures, simple medicines, mineral remedies, diseases of the different parts of the body, and so on. There are two elements in Pascual's translation that we should stress: one is the arabicized Galenism, whose main source of inspiration is the *Canon* of Avicenna; the other was the growing demand to convert direct contact with reality into a source of knowledge. This reflects a current of thought which originated and had its clearest development in Italian medical circles. Outstanding in this current was Berengario da Carpi (*c.* 1460–*c.* 1530), author, among other writings, of the book which brought up to date the *Anathomia* by Mondino de Luzzi (*c.* 1275–1326), a compendium of Galenist anatomy written in Bologna at the beginning of the fourteenth century (1316). The modern authors were frequently mentioned by Miguel Juan Pascual in his marginal notes. The traditional component is represented, above all, by Vigo's own work, which is more or less a simple compilation of that arabicized Galenism we mentioned above; on the other hand, many of Pascual's additions are intended to criticize or correct Avicenna's opinions. Where this aspect can be most clearly seen is in the sections on anatomy where Pascual gives priority to his own personal experience over the authority of Avicenna. His argument is quite simple: 'I have seen it myself'.[85]

If we have dwelt at some length on all these details, it is because we want to draw attention to the rich and complex world of medical thought and subject matter in which Gaspar Capdal (born *c.* 1579) was involved during his medical training in the Valencia of the 1590s.

The second of the sources around which our morisco doctor's learning evolved, was that of therapeutics. This was represented, as we have said, in his medical education and practice by the works of the Italian Pietro Andrea Mattioli (1501–77) and the Spaniard Juan Fragoso (*c.* 1530–97). The former became doctor to the Austrian Court (Ferdinand I and Maximilian II) in Prague. Right from the very start of his medical studies in Padua he showed a special interest in natural history and particularly in herbal medicine. This interest led him to publish in Venice (1544) the work which was to make him famous: his annotated translation into Italian of the classical treatise on therapeutics written by Dioscorides. The first Italian edition has as its title: *The five books by Pedanius Dioscorides of Anazarbus on Natural History and Therapeutics translated into the Italian language by M. Pietro Andrea Mattioli of Siena with extensive commentaries, notes and learned annotations and criticism by the translator himself.*[86] The Italian edition was the one the morisco Gaspar Capdal studied and later used in his pharmaceutical and medical practice. Indeed, when he tells the Inquisitors of the medical books that he handled, he refers to Mattioli's work in its Italian edition: 'And (I) studied through a book called Matiolosanes (=*Mathiolo Sanese*)'.[87] Ten years later (Venice, 1554) Mattioli was to publish the Latin edition of Dioscorides' work aimed at an academic and more-demanding public. The aim of the Italian translation was more modest but no less useful: he wanted to provide doctors and apothecaries with a practical manual which would enable them to identify, pick, store and supply medicinal herbs. The success of the Italian edition was so great that it was published in a fuller revised and illustrated edition in 1548, 1550 and 1552.[88]

Juan Fragoso (*c.* 1530–97) – the second of the authors mentioned from whose works the morisco doctor acquired knowledge of therapeutics – was surgeon to the Court of Philip II from 1570 onwards and he, too, was preoccupied by herbal medicine, which he summarized in a series of works written in Latin. In 1572 he did, however, publish a book in Spanish on simple medicines entitled *A Description of Aromatic Herbs, Trees, Fruit Trees, and many other simple medicines brought from the East Indies, which are of use in medicine*, which is based on the contributions of the naturalists García d'Orta and Nicolás Monardes.[89] This was the work used by Caspar Capdal.

To these sources we have to add a handbook, probably about hygiene, a sort of compendium that was a part of the artisan learning supported by the guild of barbers and surgeons under the protection of saints Cosmas and Damien,[90] and a *Thesaurus of the Poor*, supposedly written by Petrus Hispanus (*c.* 1277), a very popular handbook on therapy. He did not, probably, have sufficient money to acquire a necessary minimum of books, and this was why he resorted to the medieval procedure, which was completely normal by then among physicians and surgeons, of making a copy of medical writings, or the parts he was most interested in, for his medical practice. His training on patients and his expertise in the preparation of drugs he received from a morisco doctor, 'Master Damien, a New Christian', and the apothecary Ynca from Valencia.

As we have seen, this medical 'knowledge' which fed morisco healers outside universities circulated through identifiable channels: the oral tradition; empirical practice; training in which the medical doctor is seen as a craftsman and medicine as a craft; and the contact, however weak, with a double written tradition which, despite its academic origins, was popular. This tradition was linked, on the one hand, to the most interesting aspects of Arab therapeutics (like the treatment for scabies) and, on the other, to the therapy of the Christian academic world of 'medical humanism', such as the translation of the book of therapeutic pharmacology of Dioscorides into Italian and Spanish by Mattioli and Laguna respectively, or the current medical literature produced in the Christian faculties of medicine and written in non-Latin languages.

Notes

Notes to Chapter 1, C. B. Schmitt

* I should like to thank my fellow participants for a number of comments which were very valuable in revising for publication the first draft of this paper. In addition I am grateful to Katharine Park Dyer and Jill Kraye for many useful suggestions.

1 This is, on the whole, true only for those scholars who treat the Italian universities as a subject of study in its own right. Far too much of the general literature on medieval universities takes the northern universities as generalizable models and fails to recognize (1) the absence of theological faculties and (2) the presence of combined arts and medical faculties in Italian universities. On the general relationship between philosophy and medicine during the renaissance, specifically in relation to theories of generation see L. A. Deer, 'Academic Theories of Generation in the Renaissance: The Contemporaries and Successors of Jean Fernel (1497–1558)' (Ph.D. thesis, University of London [Warburg Institute], 1980), esp. pp. 127–464. Some useful information and a general orientation is contained in the entry 'Medizin' (by H. Diller, H. Schipperges, R. Toellner and H. Probst) in *Historisches Wörterbuch der Philosophie* (Basel-Stuttgart, 1971f.) V, pp. 967–1002, though the Renaissance is given unduly short shrift.

2 C. Malagola, *Statuti delle Università e delle Collegi dello Studio Bolognese* (Bologna, 1888; reprint Turin, 1966), pp. 274–7.

3 There is a large literature on this. See esp. the following: A. Crescini, *Le Origini del Metodo Analitico: il Cinquecento* (Udine, 1965); *idem, Il Problema Metodologico alle Origini della Scienza Moderna* (Rome, 1972); N. W. Gilbert, *Renaissance Concepts of Method* (New York, 1960); N. Jardine, 'Galileo's Road to Truth and Demonstrative Regress', *Studies in the History and Philosophy of Science*, VII (1976), 277–318; D. P. Lockwood, *Ugo Benzi, Medieval Philosopher and Physician* (Chicago, 1951), pp. 222–7; D. Mugnai Carrara, 'Profilo di Nicolò Leoniceno', *Interpres*, II (1979), 169–212; *idem*, 'Una Polemica umanistico-scolastica circa l'Interpretazione delle tre Dottrine Ordinate di Galeno', *Annali dell'Istituto e Museo di Storia della Scienza di Firenze*, VIII (1983), 31–57; G. Papuli, *Girolamo Balduino: Ricerche sulla Logica della Scuola di Padova nel*

Rinascimento (Manduria, 1967); J. H. Randall, *The Development of Scientific Method in the School of Padua* (Padua, 1961); P. Rossi, 'Aristotelici e "Moderni": le Ipotesi e la Natura', in *Aristotelismo veneto e Scienza Moderna*, ed. L. Olivieri (Padua, 1983), pp. 125–54; C. Vasoli, *Studi sulla Cultura del Rinascimento* (Manduria, 1968), pp. 257–344; *idem*, 'La logica', in *Storia della Cultura Veneta*, vol. IV (Vicenza, 1981), pp. 35–73; and W. P. D. Wightman, 'Quid sit methodus? "Method" in Sixteenth-Century Medical Teaching and "Discovery"', *Journal of the History of Medicine*, XIX (1964), 360–76.

4 This is one of the themes traced in W. Pagel, *William Harvey's Biological Ideas* (Basel–New York, 1967).

5 *Decorum* V in *Hippocrates with an English Translation*, ed. W. H. S. Jones (London, 1923–31), II, 286–9.

6 To the best of my knowledge there is not a coherent and comprehensive study of Galen's philosophy. For some information see O. Temkin, *Galenism: Rise and Decline of a Medical Philosophy* (Ithaca–London, 1973), esp. ch. 2.

7 This work is found in Galen, *Opera Omnia*, ed. G. C. Kühn (Leipzig, 1821–30; reprint Hildesheim, 1964) I, pp. 53–63. For critical literature on the work and its ideas see the bibliography collected in V. Nutton, *Karl Gottlob Kühn and His Edition of the Works of Galen* (Oxford, 1976). The Erasmus translation first appeared in *Galeni . . . exhortatio ad bonas Arteis, praesertim Medicinam . . .* (Basel and Paris, 1526). For further details see R. J. Durling, 'A Chronological Census of Renaissance Editions and Translations of Galen', *Journal of the Warburg and Courtauld Institutes*, XXIV (1961), 230–305, at pp. 254, 295 (§143) and *passim*.

8 This work went through many editions beginning with that of Venice, 1607. Undergoing periodic revisions it remained a standard reference work until the eighteenth century. The work and its author have not been studied very thoroughly, but see *Dizionario Biografico degli Italiani*, XXI (1978), 685–6 (by A. De Ferrari).

9 Several times Aristotle refers to a work of his entitled *Dissections* ('Ανατομαι), e.g. *Hist. An.* 497a32, 509b23. For further references see H. Bonitz, *Index Aristotelicus* (Berlin, 1870; reprint Graz, 1955), p. 104. Diogenes Laertius (V, 25) lists two separate works by Aristotle on anatomy. On the question in general see P. Moraux, *Les Listes Anciennes des Ouvrages d'Aristote* (Louvain, 1951), pp. 108, 265–6, 318; E. Heitz, *Die verlorenen Schriften des Aristoteles* (Leipzig, 1865), pp. 70–6; and V. Rose, *Aristoteles Pseudepigraphus* (Leipzig, 1863; reprint Hildesheim, 1971), pp. 276–326. It has been argued that a Roman painting made between 320 and 350 AD depicts Aristotle carrying out an anatomy lesson. This interpretation has not, however, been universally accepted. See P. Boyancé, 'Aristote sur une Peinture de la Via Latina', in *Mélanges Eugène Tisserant* (Vatican City, 1964) IV, pp. 107–24.

10 480b22–30. For a discussion of this text and its place in the Aristotelian *corpus* see my 'Aristotelian Textual Studies at Padua: the Case of Francesco Cavalli', in A. Poppi (ed.), *Scienza e filosofia all'Università di Padova nel Quattrocento* (Trieste, 1983), pp. 287–314, esp. 302–5, 314.

11 See esp. A. Z. Iskandar, 'An Attempted Reconstruction of the Late
    Alexandrian Medical Curriculum', *Medical History*, XX (1976), 235–58.
    The close relation between medicine and philosophy also comes out
    clearly in two recently-published late ancient Latin commentaries on
    Galen. See Agnellus of Raverna, *Lectures on Galen's De sectis* (Buffalo,
    1981) and Johannes Alexandrinus, *Commentaria in librum de sectis Galeni*,
    ed. C. D. Pritchet (Leiden, 1982).
12 Still fundamental is M. Meyerhof, 'Von Alexandrien nach Bagdad. Ein
    Beitrag zur Geschichte des philosophischen und medizinischen
    Unterrichts bei den Arabern', *Sitzungsberichte der preussische Akademie der
    Wissenschaften*, Philos.-hist. Kl. (1930), 389–429.
13 For Averroës see E. Torre, *Averroës y la Ciencia Médica* (Madrid, 1974)
    and for the later influence, D. Gracia, 'En Torno al Averroísmo Médico
    Latino', *Asclepio* XXX–XXXI (1978–9), 233–64. There is widely
    scattered literature on Avicenna, but for a general orientation see the
    article (by G. C. Anawati and A. Z. Iskandar) in *Dictionary of Scientific
    Biography*, XV (1978), pp. 494–501.
14 There is a large literature on the subject, but see esp. S. de Renzi, *Storia
    documentata della Scuola Medica di Salerno*, second edn (Naples, 1857;
    reprint Milan, 1967); P. O. Kristeller, 'The School of Salerno. Its
    Development and Contribution to the History of Learning', *Bull. Hist.
    Med.*, XVII (1945), 138–94 [reprinted in his *Studies in Renaissance Thought
    and Letters* (Rome, 1956), pp. 495–551]; *idem*, 'Bartholomaeus
    Musandinus and Maurus of Salerno and Other Commentators of the
    Articella with a Tentative List of Manuscripts', *Italia Medioevale e
    Umanistica*, XIX (1976), 57–87 [with recent bibliography]; and B. Lawn,
    The Salernitan Questions (Oxford, 1983), among others.
15 Note 14 (1956 edn), 511f. The distinction between 'theoretical' and
    'practical' medicine which was to play so central a role in Italian medical
    education is already apparent in the opening word's of the *Isagoge* of
    Johannitius [Hunayn ibn Isḥāq] (808–73), which was one of the key texts
    of the Salernitan school and which retained a position of eminence into
    the sixteenth century. The work begins: 'Medicina dividitur in duas
    partes idest theoricam et practicam . . .', as cited in L. Thorndike and
    P. Kibre, *Catalogue of Incipits*, rev. edn (Cambridge, Mass., 1963),
    p. 856. On Johannitius see the article by A. Z. Iskandar in *Dictionary of
    Scientific Biography*, XV (1979), 230–49.
16 'La rôle joué par les médecins et les naturalistes dans la réception
    d'Aristote au XIIe et XIIIe siècles' (Warsaw, 1930) [cited from the reprint
    in Birkenmajer's *Études d'histoire des Sciences et de la Philosophie du moyen
    âge* (Wrocław, etc., 1970), p. 73–87]. See also P. O. Kristeller,
    'Philosophy and Medicine in Medieval and Renaissance Italy', in
    S. F. Spicker (ed.), *Organism, Medicine and Metaphysics* (Dordrecht, 1978),
    pp. 29–40; N. G. Siraisi, *Taddeo Alderotti and His Pupils* (Princeton, 1981);
    P. G. Ottosson, *Scholastic Medicine and Philosophy: A Study of
    Commentaries on Galen's Tegni* (*c. 1300–1450*) (Uppsala, 1982); and
    J. Agrimi and C. Crisciani, '*Doctus et expertus*: la formazione del medico
    tra Due e Trecento', *Quaderni* XXIII (1983), 149–71, among recent
    publications.

17　See Siraisi (note 16), esp. ch. 3.

18　For the importance of this work see S. Ferrari, *I Tempi, la Vita, le Dottrine di Pietro d'Abano* (Genoa, 1900); *idem, Per la Biografiae per gli Scritti di Pietro d'Abano* (Rome, 1918); L. Thorndike, *History of Magic and Experimental Science*, 8 vols. (New York, 1923–58) II, 874–947; L. Norpoth, 'Zur Bio-bibliographie und Wissenschaftslehre des Pietro d'Abano', *Kyklos*, III (1930), 292–353; and N. G. Siraisi, *Arts and Sciences at Padua. The Studium before 1350* (Toronto, 1973). The *Conciliator* was printed at least eighteen times before 1600.

19　*Conciliator* (Venice, 1526), fos. 3r–4r.

20　See, for example, the material found in M. Fournier (ed.), *Les Statuts et Privilèges des Universités Françaises depuis leur fondation jusqu'en 1789* (Paris, 1891) I, pp. 1–300. There is a large literature on the subject, but see esp. L. Dulieu, *La Médecine à Montpellier* (Paris, 1975–9); R. G. Lewis, Guillaume Rondelet and His Circle (Oxford D. Phil. Thesis, 1967); and R. Antonioli, *Rabelais et la Médecine* (Geneva, 1976).

21　See R. J. Durling, 'An Early Manual for the Medical Student and the Newly-fledged Practitioner: Martin Stainpeis' *Liber de Modo Studendi seu Legendi in Medicina* ([Vienna] 1520)', *Clio Medica*, V (1970), 7–33.

22　The statutes are printed in A. Gherardi, *Statuti dell'Università e studio Fiorentino dell'anno* MCCCLXXXVII (Florence, 1881; reprint Bologna, 1973). K. Park Dyer is preparing a study of medicine in Florence during the period.

23　See above note 2.

24　*Statuta dominorum artistarum Achademiae Patavinae* (Venice, c. 1496). There is a microfilm of the imperfect Marciana copy of this rare edition (shelfmark 12.c.141) at the Wellcome Library (microfilm 89) which I have used. The same statutes were printed with little change several times in the sixteenth century, including at Venice in 1551 and 1589.

25　They are printed in F. Buonamici, 'Sull'antico statuto della Università di Pisa: alcuni preliminari notizie storiche', *Annali delle Università Toscane*, XXX (1911), iii–xvii, 1–80. For some other examples and a discussion of the question see Deer (note 1).

26　This can be determined by consulting the *rotuli* for any Italian university of the sixteenth century. The highest-paid professor of philosophy seldom made as much as even junior professors of medicine. Moreover, professors of theoretical medicine were systematically better rewarded than those of practical medicine.

27　This pattern can be traced in the careers of many of the most eminent medical figures of the sixteenth century. For example, Ulisse Aldrovandi (1522–1605) taught logic (1554–5) and philosophy (1555–6) before botany and other medical subjects. See *Dizionario Biografico degli Italiani*, II (1960), 118–24 (by G. Montalenti).

28　Though much of Pico's effort was devoted to demolishing philosophy and showing that the subject is positively harmful to the Christian, he was forced to admit at one point: 'Medicus enim a philosopho principia et fundamenta haurit medicinae, multaque mutuatur, quibus ad conciliandam sanitatem utatur.' *De studio Divinae et Humanae*

Philosophiae, I, 5 (first edn, 1496), cited from G. F. Pico, *Opera quae extant Omnia* . . . (Basel, 1601), p. 13.

29 . . . non autem in inani philosophia plus temporis terere [*scil.* medici], quam medicinae usus requirat.' F. Patrizi, *Discussionum Peripateticarum tomi IV* . . . (Basel, 1581), p. 173. I am indebted to Dr. Michael Wilmott for drawing this text to my attention.

30 However, Vives, here as elsewhere, rejected the scholastic accretions to classical learning (for example, the doctrine of intension and remission of forms). He says nothing about philosophy in general being harmful to medical studies. See J. L. Vives, *Opera Omnia*, ed. G. Majans (Valencia, 1782–90; reprint London, 1964), VI, pp. 198–203.

31 See esp. the well known letter 'contra senes dyaleticos' to Tommaso da Messina, dated *c*. 1350. The text is printed in his *Le Familiari*, ed. V. Rossi (Florence, 1933–42), I, 35–8. On this letter and the problems of interpreting it see N. W. Gilbert, 'The Early Italian Humanists and Disputation', in *Renaissance Essays in Honor of Hans Baron*, ed. A. Molho & J. A. Tedeschi (Florence, 1971), pp. 201–26.

32 *Taddeo Alderotti* (note 17), 150. It is also worth noting that Coluccio Salutati emphasized that medicine and philosophy are clearly linked, and that medicine is regulated by 'speculative reason', i.e. philosophy. See Coluccio Salutati, *De Nobilitate Legum et Medicinae*, ed. E. Garin (Florence, 1947), pp. 28–30.

33 There is now a substantial literature on the subject. For a basic orientation see M. Clagett, *The Science of Mechanics in the Middle Ages* (Madison, 1959), ch. 11. For more specific studies see, *inter alia*, D. P. Lockwood, *Ugo Benzi. Medieval Philosopher and Physician (1376–1439)* (Chicago, 1951); G. Federici Vescovini, *Astrologia e Scienza. La Crisi dell'Aristotelismo sul cadere del Trecento e Biagio Pelicani da Parma* (Florence, 1979); and F. Bottin, *La Scienza degli Occamisti* (Rimini, 1982).

34 The first question, as with many later treatises, is 'Utrum medicinalis habitus sit ars vel scientia, et an theoreticus vel practicus', *Summa Thome de Garbo* (Lyon, 1529), fo. aiir. There is relatively little literature on the author (d. 1370), but see M. A. Mannelli, 'Tommaso del Garbo ed Ugo Benzi da Siena, lettori di medicina nello *Studium generale* di Firenze', *Rivista di Storia della Medicina*, VIII (1964), 183–90; A. Oberti, 'L'insegnamento medico dei Del Garbo nell'autunno del medioevo' and F. Guido, 'Cenni biografici su Dino e Tommaso del Garbo', *Atti del XXI Congresso internazionale di Storia della Medicina* (Rome, 1970), 40–5, 156–63.

35 For Peter of Mantua see T. E. James (ed.), *Petrus Alboinus, De primo et ultimo Instanti* (Columbia University Ph.D. thesis, 1968). For a guide to the scattered literature on Paul of Venice see C. H. Lohr in *Traditio*, XXVIII (1972), 314–20 and F. Bottin, 'Logica e Filosofia Naturale nelle opere di Paolo Veneto', in A. Poppi (ed.), *Scienza e Filosofia* (note 10), pp. 85–134. For Blasius see Federici Vescovini (note 33) and A. Harrison, 'Blasius of Parma's Critique of Bradwardine's *Tractatus de Proportionibus*' in Poppi, *op. cit.*, pp. 19–69.

36 This generalization is based upon consulting a fairly wide range of Nifo's

commentaries on Aristotle. Undoubtedly, some more dedicated student of Nifo's voluminous writings will be able to hit upon a passage or two relevant to the point at issue. The best guide to Nifo's work on Aristotle is C. H. Lohr, 'Renaissance Latin Aristotle Commentaries: Authors N-Ph', *Renaissance Quarterly*, XXXII (1979), 529–88, at 532–9. Nifo's medical works have been little studied, but see F. Garfano-Venosta, 'Il *De Ratione Medendi* di Agostino Nifo', *Pagine di Storia della Medicina*, XV (1971), 59–74.

37 I have consulted Agostino Nifo, *Expositio super octo Aristotelis libris de physico auditu* (Venice, 1569); Lodovico Boccadiferro, *Explanatio libri I physicorum Aristotelis* . . . (Venice, 1558); and Giampaolo Pernumia, *Philosophia Naturalis ordine definitivo tradita* (Padua, 1570).

38 I have used the edition M. A. Zimara, *Tabula dilucidationum in dictis Aristotelis et Averrois* (Venice, 1562), as part of the edition of Aristoteles-Averroës, *Opera* (Venice, 1562–74; reprint Frankfurt, 1962). There are a number of references to *medicus* and *medicina* (fos. 236r–237v), though the majority refer to Averroës' *Colliget*.

39 '. . . quod eodem modo utitur Aristoteles in invenienda intentione libri physicorum, quo utitur medicus in inveniendis mediis et causis ad sanitatem introducendam. Nam medicus tria facit antequam introducat sanitatem, primo praecognoscit ipsam sanitatem tanquam finem. Secundo resoluit ipsum finem, id est sanitatem in omnia illa media per quae acquiri possit, quae media isthaec sunt scilicet adaequatio humorum, inductio caloris, et exhibitio medelae calidae, et tertio ipse medicus incipit procedere ab ipsis mediis et causis inventis ad sanitatem introducendam et acquirendam. Sic etiam facit Aristoteles in venanda intentione libri physicorum.' Girolamo Balduino, *Primi libri physicorum Aristotelis prooemii Expositio* . . . (Naples, 1559), fo. 2v.

40 Cesare Cremonini, *Explanatio prooemii librorum Aristotelis de physico auditu* . . . (Padua, 1596).

41 Sic igitur ostendimus utilitatem scientiae de anima ad scientias omnes communiter, et ad quasdam particulariter, nempe et ad moralem, et ad divinam. Possemus etiam de multis effectricibus artibus id ostendere, ut de arte medica, quae multa sumit a libris de anima, ut hic considerat Paulus Venetus, sed hoc aliis considerandum relinquimus. Restat considerandum, quomodo scientia de anima sit utilis ad scientiam naturalem, sed hoc videtur clarum cum ab ipso Aristotele declaretur dum ait, "Est enim tanquam principium animalium."' Jacopo Zabarella, *In tres Aristotelis libros de Anima Commentarii* . . . (Venice, 1605), fo. 6v [to *De Anima* I, text 2]. Further on (fo. 7r) there is an interesting discussion of the importance of the subject matter of the *De Anima* for understanding nature, but nothing specific on medicine.

42 This is argued especially in ch. 33 of the work.

43 'Quamobrem sicut bonus medicus esse non potest, qui non sit philosophus naturalis, ita nec bonus legislator, qui non calleat moralem philosophiam. Inter eas tamen illud interest, quid medicina solam effectionem respicit, philosophia naturalis non effectionem, sed solam scientiam . . .' Jacopo Zabarella, *De Rebus Naturalibus libri XXX* (Frankfurt, 1607), 102 [*De Naturalis Scientiae Constitutione*, ch. 33].

44 'Ex hac potissimum naturalis philosophiae parte sumit ars medica partem illam, quae physiologia dicitur, in qua de humano corpore, ac de eius partibus sermo fit, quum medico illas curaturo necessaria penitus sit earum cognitio.' *Ibid.*, 93 [ch. 32].

45 '. . . ob id medici, qui artificiosam ac fructuosam facere volunt humani corporis anatomen, imitari Aristotelem debent, non in libris de historia, sed in libris de partibus methodice de ipsis partibus agentem . . .' *Ibid.*

46 See his *Opera Logica* (Cologne, 1603). For a discussion of his application of logic to a wide range of disciplines see W. F. Edwards, 'Jacopo Zabarella: a Renaissance Aristotelian's view of Rhetoric and Poetry, and Their Relation to Philosophy', in *Arts libéraux et Philosophie au Moyen Âge* (Montréal-Paris, 1969), pp. 843–54.

47 'Philosophus naturalis nil a medico sumit, sed medicus multus a naturali.' *Opera Logica*, 61 [*De Natura Logicae* II, 4].

48 Especially in *De Natura Logicae* II, 4.

49 See esp. *De Methodis* II, 11–14 (edn. *cit.*, 193–212).

50 For Zabarella in Germany see P. Petersen, *Geschichte der Aristotelischen Philosophie in Protestantischen Deutschland* (Leipzig, 1921; reprint Stuttgart-Bad Cannstatt, 1964), pp. 196–9. For Britain see my *John Case and Aristotelianism in Renaissance England* (Kingston-Montréal, 1983), pp. 35–7.

51 From the point of view of the present enquiry possibly the most interesting work is his *De Differentiis* (Padua, 1562). It is also available in an expanded form as *De Differentiis Doctrinarum sive de Methodis liber*, printed in Girolamo Capivacci, *Opera Omnia*, ed. Johannes Hartmann Beyer (Frankfurt, 1603), pp. 1004–51. He begins by discussing whether this subject is the task of the logician alone or also that of the philosopher and physician (1004). In chapter VI (1014–19) he treats 'De ordine resolutivo', 'De ordine compositivo', and 'De ordine definitivo'. In each case, after the subject has been explained from a logical point of view, he illustrates the results by both an *exemplum philosophicum* and an *exemplum medicum*.

52 Particularly relevant is Joannes Baptista Montanus, *In Artem Parvam Galeni Explanationes a Valentino Lublino Polono editae* (Venice, 1554). On this work see the studies of Crescini and Wightman cited in note 3.

53 *De Sensu 436a18–b2*. The translation is taken from Aristotle, *On the Soul, Parva Naturalia, On Breath*, transl. W. S. Hett (London-Cambridge, Mass., 1936), pp. 215–17.

54 The *Aristoteles Latinus* lists over 250 manuscripts of the medieval versions. During the sixteenth century the work was printed in Greek at least fifteen times and in Latin more than a hundred times. See F. E. Cranz-C. B. Schmitt, *A Bibliography of Aristotle Editions, 1501–1600*, 2nd edn (Baden-Baden, 1984), pp. 201–2. There appear to be relatively few medieval commentaries on the work, at least not very many easily available in printed form. I have consulted the following two: Thomas Aquinas, *In Aristotelis libros de Sensu et Sensato, de Memoria et Reminiscentia commentarium*, ed. R. M. Spiazza, 3rd edn (Turin-Rome, 1949), and John of Jandun, *Quaestiones super Parvis Naturalibus* (Venice, 1570). Thomas comments upon the text in question, emphasizing that the problem of

health and sickness are concerns both of the natural philosopher and the physician (p. 6), but in not nearly so much detail as the sixteenth-century commentaries discussed below. John of Jandun does not take up the point in question.

55 e.g. *Post. An.* I. 27 (87a30f.).

56 Among others see Domingo Gundisalvo, *De Scientiis*, ed. M. Alonso Alonso (Madrid-Granada, 1954); Hugh of St Victor's *Didiscalia* in *Patrologia Latina* 176, cols. 738–838; and Robert Kilwardby, *De Ortu Scientiarum*, ed. A. G. Judy (London-Toronto, 1976). There is a large literature on the subject, but see the various contributions in *Arts libéraux et Philosophie au moyen âge* (Montréal-Paris, 1969).

57 Simone Simoni, *In librum Aristotelis . . . de Sensuum Instrumentis et de his quae sub sensum cadunt Commentarius unus . . .* (Geneva, 1566), pp. 22–6; Mainetto Mainetti, *Commentarius mire perspicuus nec minus utilis in librum Aristotelis . . . de Sensu et Sensilibus . . .* (Florence, 1555), pp. 10–12.

58 'Dicamus in summa, corpus vivum qua sanum a physico consideratur.' Simoni (note 57), p. 23.

59 'Subiectum enim in physiologia est res naturae, medicinae vero artis.' *Ibid.*, p. 25.

60 'At res artis et res naturae essentialiter distinguuntur'. *Ibid.*

61 'Rectius igitur, qui dixerunt medicinam ex pluribus fere scientiis coalescere, atque a physico universalia principia sanitatis et aegritudinis, elementa, humores, plantarumque cognitionem accipere.' *Ibid.*, p. 26.

62 See, for example, Isidore of Seville, *Etymologiarum sive Originum libri XX*, W. M. Lindsay (Oxford, 1911), book IV, ch. 13.

63 'Ex pluribus fere medicina coalescit scientiis, cum a physiologo quidem ipsam sumpserit anatomiam, elementa, humores ac plantarum cognitionem et vires.' Mainetti (note 57), 11.

64 *Ibid.*

65 Simoni (note 57), p. 24. Even if the pithy formulation is not quite present, the sentiment is in Salutati's *De Nobilitate Legum et Medicinae*, where he says: '. . . hoc non crediderim te neque medicorum aliquem contendere vel negare, quoniam verissimum est, ubi speculatio desinat philosophi principium sumere medicinam, que quidem ars est, sicuti tui diffiniunt, operativa.' edn. cit. (note 32), pp. 28–30.

66 M. A. Zimara, *Quaestio est, an Medicina nobilior atque praestantior sit Iure Civili*, in E. Garin (ed.), *La Disputa delle arti nel Quattrocento* (Florence, 1947), pp. 111–23, esp. 113, 117–18 (where the passage is quoted), and 123. The *Quaestio* is dated 1482.

67 Jacopo Zabarella, *De Doctrinae Ordine Apologia* (Cologne, 1602), pp. 77–9.

68 Cremonini (note 40), fo. 33v. The passage is noted by Deer (note 1), p. 230.

69 'Unde dico quod medicina subalternatur philosophiae naturali per additamentum, eo quia additur corpori humano ipsa sanitas a medico; quod corpus ut corpus humanum tantum erat substantia in philosophia, sed medicus habet considerare corpus humanum sanabile, quatenus sanabile est. Quare patet etiam quomodo medicina sit scientia, quomodo theorica et practica simul . . .' Montanus (note 52), fo. 6r.

70 '. . . quod idem assignat Aristoteles in libro de sensu et sensato inquirens, ubi desinit philosphus, qui desinit a speciebus animalibus, incipit medicus determinans a forma etiam rationem'. *Ibid.*, fo. 5v.

71 Oddo degli Oddi, *In primam totam fen libri Canonis Avicennae dilucidissima et expectatissima Expositio* . . . (Venice, 1575), p. 80.

72 'Physica vero et mathesis tam sunt in rem medici, quam ethica iurisconsulti. Ubi enim desinit physicus, ibi incipit medicus.' This is published with Herman Conring, *In universam artem Medicam singulas partes eius Introductio* . . ., ed. G. C. Schelhammer (Speyer, 1687). The text quoted is at vol. II, p. 10.

73 *De Respiratione* 480b22–30. The translation is taken from Aristotle (note 53), 480.

74 I give the evidence in my article cited in note 10, pp. 302–5.

75 See the discussion in Simoni (note 57), pp. 22–6.

76 Among recent studies see C. Vasoli, *L'Enciclopedismo del '600* (Naples, 1978) and W. Schmidt-Biggemann, *Topica Universalis* (Hamburg, 1983).

77 The text is printed (II, 17–68) in the same volume containing similar works of Conring and Bartholin cited in note 72.

78 *Ibid.*, 30–1.

79 *Ibid.*, 31.

80 'Metaphysica enim nullum pene usum medico praestat . . .', *op. cit.* (note 72), p. 10.

81 The work was printed at least seventeen times between 1608 and 1676. For further information see C. H. Lohr in *Studies in the Renaissance*, XXI (1974), 261–2.

82 *Op. cit.* (note 77), p. 28.

83 *Op. cit.* (note 72), p. 9.

84 Various significant points are made regarding the relationship of Aristotle's zoological works to medical studies during the renaissance by Deer (note 1). Her analysis of the *Interpretatio obscuriorum locorum et sententiarum omnium operum Aristotelis* (Rome, 1590) of Felice Accoromboni (fl. 1590–1604) deserves particular attention with regard to the problems discussed in this paper (pp. 135–8). It should also be pointed out that the article on *philosophia* in Bartolomeo Castelli's *Lexicon Medicum* is favourable to the subject and sees philosophy as a positive aid to medical studies. See above note 8. Castelli followed the normal pattern of being interested in both philosophy and medicine, publishing, *inter alia*, a *Brevis et dilucida ad Logicam Aristotelis Introductio* (Messina, 1596).

Notes to Chapter 2, N. G. Siraisi

1 This chapter is part of a broader study of the place of Avicenna in renaissance and early modern Italian medicine which will focus upon the content of commentaries written after 1500. Grants from the National Endowment for the Humanities and the Research Foundation of the City University of New York in 1981 and from the John Simon Guggenheim Memorial Foundation in 1982–3 enabled me to pursue this research. The

discussion at the 1983 Cambridge Conference on Sixteenth-Century Medicine was extremely useful both for this chapter and regarding the larger project of which it is a part, and I should like to thank all those who took part.

2 The count of editions may well be incomplete, especially as regards the seventeenth century. For the sixteenth century I have for the most part followed the *Index Aureliensis*, part 1, vol. II, pp. 448–54, s.v. Avicenna. However, the list there provided does not include excerpts from the *Canon* contained in anthologies such as the *Articella*; these I have added to the extent that they are known to me. Furthermore, in the numerous cases where text and commentary are found in the same volume, I have simply followed the lead of the title pages provided by the sixteenth-century editors and of the *Index Aureliensis* in determining whether to count the book as an edition of the text or as an edition of a commentary. As a result, a good many editions of commentaries, including some of those written in the sixteenth century, which do in fact contain portions of the text are not discussed in the present chapter. Of the various library catalogues consulted, special mention must be made of Richard Durling, *A Catalogue of Sixteenth-Century Printed Books in the National Library of Medicine* (Bethesda, Md., 1967) and *A Catalogue of Printed Books in the Wellcome Historical Medical Library*, I, *Books Printed Before 1641* (London, 1962) and II and III, *Books Printed from 1641 to 1850* (London, 1966, 1976), A-L. In the notes that follow, I indicate only the libraries where I consulted the works, locations being abbreviated as follows:

BL   British Library
NLM   National Library of Medicine, History of Medicine Division, Bethesda, Md, USA.
NYAM   New York Academy of Medicine, Rare Book Room.
WL   Wellcome Historical Medical Library.

I am grateful to all those who helped me at these libraries.
The editions in Arabic referred to are those of the whole work, Rome, 1593, IA 110.626; *Liber Secundus de Canone Canonis a filio Sina studio sumptibus ac typis Arabicis Petri Kirsteni . . .* (Breslau, 1609), NLM; and *Georgii Hieronymi Velschii Exercitatio de Vena Medinensi ad Mentem Ebnsinae, sive De dracunculis veterum. Specimen exhibens novae versionis ex Arabico . . . [Canon 4:3:2:21–2]* (Augsburg, 1674), NLM. In the notes that follow, punctuation has been modernized and Latin abbreviations silently expanded.

3 Francesca Lucchetta, *Il Medico e Filosofo Bellunese Andrea Alpago (1522) traduttore di Avicenna* (Padua, 1964); M. T. d'Alverny, 'Avicenne et les Médecins de Venise', in *Medioevo e Rinascimento. Studi in onore di Bruno Nardi*, 2 vols. (Florence, 1955), I, pp. 175–98; *idem*, 'Les Traductions d'Avicenne (Moyen Age et Renaissance), in *Avicenna nella Storia della Cultura Medioevale (Problemi attuali di scienza e di cultura dell'Accademia Nazionale de' Lincei)*, Quaderno no. 40 (Rome, 1955, pp. 71–87, at pp. 84–7; and *idem*, 'Andrea Alpago Interprète et Commentateur d'Avicenne,' in *Atti del XII Congresso Internazionale di Filosofia*, IX

(Florence, 1960), 1–6. We look forward to the appearance of the studies of the Gerard of Cremona translation currently being undertaken by Danielle Jacquart and Ilona Opelt, respectively.

4 For preliminary discussion of some of these commentaries and a list of published commentaries, see Siraisi, 'Renaissance Commentaries on Avicenna's *Canon*, book I, part 1, and the Teaching of Medical *Theoria* in the Italian Universities,' forthcoming *History of Universities*, IV. 'Part' is here and in this chapter used to render the Arabo–Latin term 'fen' for the subdivisions of the *Canon*.

5 At Padua, *Canon* 1:1 was retained until 1767; see Bartolo Bertolaso, 'Richerche d'Archivio su alcuni Aspetti dell'Insegnamento Medico presso l'Università di Padova nel Sette e Ottocento,' *Acta Medicae Historiae Patavina*, V (1958–9), p. 8. At Bologna, the use of *Canon* 1:1 as a text was abandoned in 1721, reintroduced in 1737, and retained until 1800; see Umberto Dallari, ed., *I Rotuli dei Lettori Legisti e Artisti dello Studio Bolognese*, 3 vols. (Bologna, 1888–9), III, 1, pp. 260 and 282, and III, 2, pp. 5 and 326. I am grateful to Dr Herbert Matsen for drawing my attention to the latter point.

6 So long as students were actually examined on the texts, no matter how cursorily, the texts were presumably read, even if only rapidly and reluctantly; and such examinations were still administered when Morgagni first came to teach at Padua in 1711. See G. Battista Morgagni, *Opera Postuma. IV. Lezioni di Medicina Teorica: Commento ad Avicenna*, ed. Adalberto Pazzini (Rome, 1969), p. 6. However, Morgagni also noted that very few students were involved. Morgagni's own lectures on *Canon* 1:1 remained unpublished until the twentieth century.

7 A. C. Klebs, *Incunabula Scientifica et Medica* (Bruges, 1938), nos. 131.1–14.

8 The *Canon* was extensively used by the author of the *Anatomia Vivorum*, with a probable date of around 1225; see Georg Corner, *Anatomical Texts of the Earlier Middle Ages* (Washington, 1927), pp. 38–44. It was probably known to Albertus Magnus in the 1240s, and certainly in the late 1250s and early 1260s when he was working on his *De Animalibus*; see Siraisi, 'The Medical Learning of Albertus Magnus', in *Albertus Magnus and the Sciences*, ed. James A. Weisheipl, O. P. (Toronto, 1980), pp. 392–3.

9 Commentaries on short sections were written by Johannes de Sancto Amando, *c.* 1280 (see Lynn Thorndike and Pearl Kibre, *A Catalogue of Incipits of Mediaeval Scientific Writings in Latin*, 2nd edn (Cambridge, Mass., 1963), cols. 361, 492), and by Taddeo Alderotti (d. 1295 – see Siraisi, *Taddeo Alderotti and His Pupils* (Princeton, 1981), pp. 416–17).

10 For example, Luis Garcia Ballester has shown that the *Canon* was introduced at Montpellier in the middle years of the thirteenth century; see his 'Arnau de Vilanova (*c.* 1240–1311) y la Reforma de los Estudios Médicos en Montpellier (1309): El Hipócrates Latino y la Introduccion del Nuevo Galeno', *Dynamis*, II (1982), 103–4. Avicenna is among the authors listed in the papal bull of 1309 specifying the Montpellier curriculum; see *Cartulaire de l'Université de Montpellier*, 2 vols. (Montpellier, 1890), I, pp. 219–21, no. 25.

11 Carlo Malagola, ed., *Statuti delle Universitá e dei Collegi dello Studio Bolognese* (Bologna, 1888), pp. 276–7.

12 For examples, see Thorndike and Kibre, *A Catalogue*, cols. 227, 695, 860, 1307; one may also note the set of *Flores Avicennae* contained in a fifteenth-century Latin manuscript (7047) in the Bibliothèque Nationale. I have seen only the last of these manuscripts at the time of writing. Tiziana Pesenti Marangon, '"Professores Chirurgie," "Medici Ciroici" e "Barbitonsores" a Padova nell'età di Leonardo Buffi da Bertipaglia († dopo il 1448)', *Quaderni per la Storia dell'Università di Padova*, XI (1978), 1–38, contains some interesting information about the use of medical authorities by practitioners and their connections with the world of university medicine.

13 On Gentile's career, see Fausto Bonora and George Kern, 'Does anyone really know the life of Gentile da Foligno,' *Medicina nei Secoli*, IX (1972), 29–53.

14 On Giacomo's biography, see Paolo Sambin, 'Su Giacomo della Torre (†1414)', *Quaderni par la storia dell'Università di Padova*, I (1968), 15–47.

15 On Ugo, see D. P. Lockwood, *Ugo Benzi: Medieval Philosopher and Physician 1376–1439* (Chicago, 1951). On the reputation of these figures, see Siraisi, 'The Physician's Task: Medical Reputations in Humanist Collective Biographies,' forthcoming in a volume in the series *Smith College Studies in History*.

16 *Liber Canonis Avicenne revisus et ab omni errore mendaque purgatus summaque cum diligentia impressus* (Venice, 1505), IA 110.581, NLM, and *Liber Canonis Avicenne revisus et ab omni errore mendaque purgatus summaque cum diligentia impressus* (Venice, 1507, facsimile Hildesheim, 1964), IA 110.582. A number of the incunabular editions are also of this type.

17 The surviving manuscripts of Gentile's exposition of book three appear all to be on subsections of that part of the *Canon*, and were presumably put together by the early sixteenth-century editors; some sections are missing in the editions. See Thorndike and Kibre, *A Catalogue*, cols. 265, 543, 735, 1009, 1506, 1701, and, for example, *Tertius Canonis Avicenne cum dilucidissimis Expositionibus Gentile Fulginate . . .*, 3 vols. (Venice, *c.* 1505), IA 110.580, WL. The impression that Gentile's commentaries were printed more frequently than those of other authors *c.* 1500–25, is based on volumes classified on the basis of the principles indicated in note 2, above, as editions of the text, accompanied by commentary. Gentile's works would not necessarily predominate if editions of commentaries were also taken into account.

18 On Jacques Despars, see Danielle Jacquart, 'Le Regard d'un Médecin sur son Temps: Jacques Despars (1380?–1458),' *Bibliothèque de l'Ecole des Chartes*, CXXXVIII (1980), 35–86.

19 For a summary of Dino del Garbo's career, see Siraisi, *Taddeo Alderotti*, pp. 55–64.

20 On Ferrari da Grado, see H. M. Ferrari da Grado, *Une Chaire de Médecine au XVᵉ Siècle: un professeur a l'Université de Pavie de 1432 à 1472* (Paris, 1899).

21 See note 17, above. Despite its title, this work includes book four.

22 *Praesens Maximus Codex est totius Scientiae Medicinae Principis Aboali Abinsene cum expositionibus omnium . . . interpretum ejus . . .* 5 vols. (Venice, 1523), IA 110.595, NLM.

23 On his career and writings, see Siraisi, *Taddeo Alderotti*.

24 To take the single, but not uncharacteristic example of Ugo Benzi, chosen because the printing history of his works has already been the subject of scholarly investigation: between 1478 and 1524, Ugo's commentary on *Canon* 1:1–2 appeared in five editions; his commentary on *Canon* 1:4 was printed eleven, perhaps twelve, times; and his commentary on *Canon* 4:1 five times. No further editions of any of these commentaries appeared after 1524. These data are taken from Lockwood, *Ugo Benzi*, pp. 382–98. However, some early commentaries were occasionally reprinted thereafter; for example, that of Giovanni Arcolano (d. 1458) on *Canon* 4:1 was reissued at Padua in 1685 as *De Febribus Ioannis Arculani in Avicennae IV Canonis Fen primam dilucida atque optima expositio . . .*, BL.

25 *Flores Avicenne* (Lyons, 1508), IA 110.583, NLM. The preface is by Michael de Capella, *artium et medicine magister*. I have not investigated what relationship, if any, this work has to that mentioned in note 12, above.

26 *Flores Avicenne collecti super quinque Canonibus quos edidit in Medicina: nec non super decem et novem libris de Animalibus cum Canticis eiusdem ad longum positis* (Lyons, 1514, 1528), IA 110.588, 599, NLM, WL.

27 *Soli Deo. Memoriale Medicorum Canonice Practicantium a Rustico medicine cultore ordinatum . . .* (Pavia, 1517), NYAM.

28 *Textus Principis Avicenne par ordinem alphabeti in sententia reportatus cum quibusdam Additionibus et Concordantiis Galieni et quorundam aliorum doctorum . . .* This is the third of five separately foliated booklets in a work entitled *Habes humane lector Gabrielis de Tarrega Burgdalensis civitatis medici Regentis et Ordinarii Opera brevissima Theoricam et Prathicam (sic) medicinalis scientie. . . .* The second item in the collection has a colophon on fol. 63r giving the date 1520; the fourth item is dated 1524 on fol. 90v; the title page of the fifth item indicates that the place of printing was Bordeaux. The compendium of, or index to, Avicenna is 59 fols. in length. IA 110.589, BL. Another handbook popular later in the century was *Methodus Generalis et Compendaria ex Hippocratis, Galeni, et Avicennae Placitis deprompta ac in ordinem redacta . . . Alfonsi Bertotii Fanensis opera hinc inde collecta . . .* (Venice, 1556), IA 118.063, BL. It was reprinted at Lyons in 1558, and at Geneva in 1588, IA 118.064–65, both NYAM.

29 On the formation of the *Articella* see Paul Oskar Kristeller, 'Bartholomaeus, Musandinus, and Maurus of Salerno and other Early Commentators on the "Articella," with a Tentative List of Texts and Manuscripts', *Italia Medioevale e Umanistica*, XIX (1976), 57–87. The *Canon* excerpts were not part of the *Articella* as it existed in the twelfth or thirteenth century. Their inclusion in early sixteenth-century editions may have been an innovation of that period, since they are not found in the incunabular editions of the *Articella* (Klebs 116.1–6).

30 [*Articella.*] *In hoc Volumine parvo in quantitate, maximo in virtute, continentur infrascripti Codices . . . Textus duarum primarum fen primi Avicenne in theorica. Textus fen quarte primi, et prime quarti in practica* (Pavia, 1506), WL; '*nova impressio*' of same (Venice, 1507), IA 109.132, NLM.

31 *Articella nuperrime impressa cum quamplurimis Tractatibus pristine impressioni*

superadditis . . . (Lyons, 1515), IA 109.135, NYAM, and *Articella nuperrime impressa cum quamplurimis Tractatibus pristine impressioni superadditis* . . . (Lyons, 1534), IA 109.140, WL. This collection was also reissued Lyons, 1519 and 1525, IA 109. 136, 138, both NLM.

32 The anatomical chapters of *Canon* 1:1:5 , *De membris*, are omitted from the commentary on *Canon* 1:1 by Antonio da Parma (fl. 1310), who probably taught medicine at Bologna; see MS Vat.lat.4452, fos. 1r–47v. Gentile da Foligno commented unfavourably on the practice of commenting only on the introductory chapter of this section but nonetheless followed it; see *Primus Avicenne Canonis cum argutissima Gentilis Expositione* (Pavia, 1510, at NYAM), fo. 54v. The Bologna statutes of 1405 endorsed the practice (Malagola, *Statute*, p. 274).

33 Much current work on renaissance Galenism and medical humanism in general is summarized in Richard J. Durling, 'Linacre and Medical Humanism', in *Linacre Studies: Essays on the Life and Work of Thomas Linacre, ca. 1460–1524*, ed. Francis Maddison, Margaret Pelling, and Charles Webster (Oxford, 1977), 77–106; Vivian Nutton, 'John Caius and the Linacre Tradition', *Medical History*, XXXIII (1979), 373–89; and Andrew Wear, 'Galen in the Renaissance', in *Galen: Problems and Prospects*, ed. Vivian Nutton (London, 1981), pp. 229–62; see also Owsei Temkin, *Galenism* (Ithaca, 1973), pp. 125–74.

34 Leoniceno's *De Plinii et plurium aliorum Medicorum in Medicina Erroribus* contains numerous attacks on Avicenna as well as on Pliny. I have consulted this in *Nicolai Leoniceni . . . Opuscula . . .* (Basel, 1532, at NYAM), but the work was first published in 1492. On Leoniceno's work and the fairly widespread debate over it in humanist, medical, and botanical circles, see Charles G. Nauert, Jr, 'Humanists, Scientists, and Pliny: Changing Approaches to a Classical Author', *The American Historical Review*, LXXXIV (1979), 72–85; on Leoniceno's intellectual position in general, Daniela Mugnai Carrara, 'Profilo di Nicolo Leoniceno', *Interpres*, II (1978), 169–212. In the first letter of his *Epistolae Medicinales*, a general justification of the whole work, Manardi referred to the *Canon* as containing 'densam caliginem, infinitum ambagum chaos', *Epistolae Medicinales in quibus multa recentiorum errata et antiquorum decreta reserantur . . .* (Ferrara, 1521, NYAM). Manardi's *Epistolae* were reprinted at Paris in 1528, Basel in 1535 and 1540, and Venice in 1542, the later editions being greatly expanded (all those mentioned are at NYAM).

35 On the opposition to the Arabs, see Felix Klein-Franke, *Die klassische Antike in der Tradition des Islam* (Darmstadt, 1980), pp. 17–66; E. Wickersheimer, 'Laurent Fries et la Querelle de l'Arabisme en Médecine (1530),' *Les Cahiers de Tunisie*, IX (1955), 56–103; Gerhard Baader, 'Medizinisches Reformdenken und Arabismus im Deutschland des 16 Jahrhunderts', *Sudhoffs Archiv: Zeitschrift für Wissenschaftgeschichte*, XLIII (1979), 261–96; for Montpellier, Roland Antonioli, *Rabelais et la Médecine* (*Etudes Rabelaisiennes XII, Travaux d'Humanisme et de Renaissance 143*) (Geneva, 1976), ch. 3.

36 The complaints of Avicenna's critics were well summarized by Girolamo Cardano, who emphatically did not agree with them:

adduci autem solent quatuor rationes, quibus Avicennae scripta
refelluntur. Prima quod ipse falsas habuit interpretationes Graecorum
Authorum . . . Secunda, quod corruptus ad nos pervenit, inditio est
varietas codicum emendatio, inconstans, barbara elocutio. Tertia
quod cum habeamus omnes libros a quibus sumpsit, nunc optime
conversos, stultum est quaerere in stagno, quod inveniri potest in
flumine . . . Quarta quod in simplicibus erravit insignis confudit. In
curatione ut quamcumque artem exercuerit fide dignus non habetur.
*Commentaria in quatuor primas principis primae sectionis Doctrinas, seu
Floridorum libri duo in Hieronymi Cardani . . . Operum tomus nonus qui est
Medicinalium quartus* (Lyons, 1663), p. 456. The passage comes from the
preface to lectures on *Canon* 1:1 delivered by Cardano at Pavia in 1561.

37 Leoniceno's complaints about Avicenna fell mostly into this, Cardano's
fourth category: for example 'Error Avicennae, multas herbas figura et
natura diversas uno capite confundentis', *Opuscula*, 1532, fos. 9r–v.

38 On the Arabic studies and translations of the physicians Girolamo
Ramusio (d. 1486) and Andrea Alpago (d. 1522) see the works of
Lucchetta and d'Alverny cited in note 3 above; as these authors have
pointed out, much of Alpago's interest was in Avicenna's philosophical
works. Ramusio was a Latin poet with connections with the circle of Pico
della Mirandola; see Francesco Flamini, 'Girolamo Ramusio (1450–1486)
e i suoi Versi latini e volgari', *Accademia di Scienze, Lettere, ed Arti in
Padova, Atti e memorie,* new ser. XVI (1899–1900), 11–41.

39 On the use of *Canon* 4:1, on fevers, in the sixteenth century, see Iain M.
Lonie, 'Fever Pathology in the Sixteenth Century: Tradition and
Innovation', in *Theories of Fever from Antiquity to the Enlightenment,* ed.
W. F. Bynum and V. Nutton, *Medical History*, Supplement No. 1 (1981),
pp. 19–44. *Canon* 1:1 contains a survey of the so-called things natural,
namely elements, *complexiones*, humours, members, and faculties or
virtues, that is almost entirely Galenic.

40 *Liber Canonis totius Medicine ab Avicenna arabum doctissimo excussus, a
Gerardo Cremonensi ab arabica lingua in latinam reductus. Et a Petro Antonio
Rustico Placentino in philosophia non mediocriter erudito ad limam ex omni parte
ab erroribus et omni barbarie castigatus; Necnon a domino Symphoriano
Camperio lugdunensi fecundis annotationibus terminisque arabicis et eorum
expositionibus nuper illustratus . . .* (Lyons, 1522), IA 110.592, NYAM.

41 On Champier, see Brian P. Copenhaver, *Symphorien Champier and the
Reception of the Occultist Tradition in Renaissance France* (The Hague, Paris,
New York, 1978), especially, for his role as a critic of the Arabs,
pp. 67–9, also, on the same topic, Antonioli, *Rabelais,* pp. 46–7.
Copenhaver points out that Champier's repudiation of Avicenna was far
from complete.

42 *Principis Avicennae Libri Canonis, necnon de Medicinis Cordialibus et Cantica
ab Andrea Bellunensi ex antiquis arabum originalibus ingenti labore summaque
diligentia correcti atque in integrum restituti . . .* (Venice, 1527), IA 110.598,
WL. One or both of the two short medical works had also been printed
with the *Canon* in a number of earlier editions; see Klebs, p. 69.

43 Lucchetta, *Il Medico,* pp. 33–56.

44 The privileges are printed at the beginning of the 1527 edition.

45 *Avicenna liber Canonis, De Medicinis Cordialibus, et Cantica. Cum castigationibus Andreae Alpagi Bellunensis, una cum eiusdem nominum arabicorum interpretatione. Quibus recens quamplurimae accesserunt ab eodem ex multis Arabum excerptae huiusmodi asterico notatae* (Venice, 1544), IA 110.606, NLM. For Massa's career and writings, see Richard Palmer, 'Nicolo Massa, His Family and His Fortune', *Medical History*, XXXV (1981), 385–410. Regarding biographies of Avicenna included in editions of the *Canon*, see further below.

46 *Avicennae Quarta fen primi libri de Universali Ratione Medendi: nunc primum M. Jacobi Mantini medici hebrei opera latinitate donata* (Venice, 1530), IA 110.600, NLM. For the career of Mantino (d. 1549), at one time a papal physician, who also translated works of Averroës and became involved in the controversy over Henry VIII's divorce, see D. Kaufman, 'Jacob Mantino. Un Page d'Histoire de la Renaissance', *Revue des Etudes Juives*, XXVII (1893), 30–60, 207–38; see also regarding both Mantino and the role of Jewish physicians in the Veneto in general P. C. Ioly Zorattini, 'Gli Ebrei a Venezia, Padova e Verona', *Storia della Cultura Veneta*, 3, I (Vicenza, 1980), pp. 560–7.

47 Klebs 132.1. For the translators and manuscripts of the various Hebrew versions of parts of the *Canon* made in the thirteenth to fifteenth centuries and regarding the edition, see Moritz Steinschneider, *Die hebraeischen Übersetzungen des Mittelalters und die Juden als Dolmetscher* (Berlin, 1893, facsimile Graz, 1956), pp. 678–85, and Benjamin Richler, 'Manuscripts of Avicenna's Kanon in Hebrew Translation; a revised and up-to-date list', *Koroth*, VIII (1982), 145–68.

48 One enthusiast for Mantino's versions was Amatus Lusitanus, who praised their superiority to those of earlier interpreters (presumably including Alpago) and expressed his regret that Mantino had not lived to complete the work; see *Curationum Medicinalium Amati Lusitani medici physici praestantissimi . . .*, I (Venice, 1566), scholium to *Cent.* I. 1, pp. 37–8. Amatus suggested Bartolomeo Eustachio should take up the task. The first *Centuria* was composed in 1551.

49 *Avicennae Arabis medicorum ob succinctam brevitatis copiam facile principis Quarta fen primi de Universale Ratione Medendi nunc primum M. Jacobi Mantini medici hebraei latinitate donata . . .* (Ettlingen, 1531), IA 110.601, consulted at Biblioteca Nazionale, Rome; *Avicennae . . . Quarta fen primi de Universali Ratione Medendi. Interprete Iacob Mantino medico hebreo* (Paris, 1532), IA 110.602, NLM; *Quarta fen primi: de Universali Ratione Medendi. Interprete Iacob Mantino medico hebreo* (Paris, 1555), IA 110.611 (I have not seen this edition, and take the title from the Wellcome Library's *Catalogue of Printed Books*, I, p. 31, no. 585); *Avicennae . . . Quarta fen primi de Universali Ratione Medendi per M. Iacob Mantinum medicum hebreum latinitate donata . . .* (The Hague, 1532), IA 110.603, NLM. Mantino also translated a chapter on headache from book three (3:1:1:29), which is printed in *Methodus Universae Artis Medicae formulis expressa . . . Cornelio a Baersdorp . . . autore* (n.p., 1538) at sig. Viir–Vvv, BL.

50 *Avicennae primi libri fen prima nunc primum per Magistrum Iacobum*

Mantimam (sic) medicum hebreum ex hebraico in latinum translatum [Venice, *c.* 1540], IA 110.604, WL; *Primi libri fen prima nunc primum per Iacobum Mantinum ex hebraico in latinam translata et diligentius nuper emendata* (Padua, 1547), IA 110.608 (I have not seen this edition).

51 *Oddi de Oddis patavini physici ac medici celeberrimi . . . In primam totam fen primi libri Canonis Avicennae dilucidissima et expectatissima Expositio . . .* (Venice, 1575), NYAM. The author died in 1558.

52 *Avicennae . . . libri tertii fen secunda . . . ad fidem codicis hebraici latinus factus. Interprete Iohanne Quinquarboreo Aurilacensi . . .* (Paris, 1570), IA 110.620, NLM; *Avicennae . . . libri tertii fen primae tractatus quartus . . . in linguam latinam conversus . . . interprete J. Quinquarboreo* (Paris, 1572), BL: *Libri tertii fen primae tractatus quintus . . . ad fidem hebraici exemplaris, latinus factus ac emendatus. Interprete Iohanne Quinquarboreo* (Paris, 1586), IA 110.625 (I have not seen this edition).

53 *Avicennae Liber Canonis, De Medicinis Cordialibus, et Cantica . . . Nunc autem demum a Benedicto Rinio Veneto, philosopho et medico eminentissimo, eruditissimis accuratissimis lucubrationibus illustrata. Qui et Castigationes ab Alpago factas suis quasque locis aptissime inseruit . . .* (Venice, 1555), IA 110.612, BL. Rinio was a collateral descendant of an earlier Benedetto Rinio, author of an illuminated manuscript book of simples now preserved in the Biblioteca Marciana, which was at one time in the younger Rinio's possession. See Ettore de Toni, 'Il libro dei Semplici di Benedetto Rinio', *Memorie della Pontificia Accademia Romana dei Nuovi Lincei*, 2nd ser., V (1919), 171–279; VII (1924), 275–398; VIII (1925), 124–264; and V (1919), 173, 181. The Benedetto Rinio with whom we are here concerned apparently died before 1566, when his son Fabrizio prepared his father's brief *Tractatus de Morbo Gallico* for publication; see *De Morbo Gallico omnia quae extant . . .* 2 vols. in 1 (Venice, 1566), II, p. 14. That Rinio was a practising physician is indicated not only by this treatise, which is in fact a *consilium* for a priest, and also by his ownership of a collection of treatises on empirical medicine, namely *Benedicti Victorii Faventini . . . Opera* (Venice, 1550). The copy of the latter work at the New York Academy of Medicine contains Rinio's ownership signature and recipes in his hand on front and back flyleaves.

54 *De Removendis Nocumentis, quae accidunt in regimine sanitatis* and *De Syrupo Acetoso*; Alpago's translation of these two works was first published, along with his translation of two Arabic commentaries on parts of the *Canon*, Venice, 1547.

55 *Avicennae medicorum Arabum principis, Liber Canonis, De Medicinis Cordialibus, et Cantica . . .* (Basel, 1556), IA 110.613, NYAM.

56 *Avicennae Liber Canonis, De medicinis cordialibus, Cantica, De removendis nocumentis in regimine sanitatis, De syrupo acetoso. Quorum priores tres primo quidem Andreas Alpagus Bellunensis . . . Arabicaeque linguae peritissimis (qui duos etiam ultimos tractatus ex Arabico in Latinum transtulit) infinitis pene ex codicum Arabicorum collatione emendationibus . . . ornaverat. Postea vero Benedictus Rinius Venetus . . . eruditissimis lucubrationibus decoraverat: castigationes Alpagi suis locis inserens, plurimasque alias in margine addens, locosque etiam quam plurimos in margina indicans, in quibus Avicenna, aut*

eandem oppositamve sententiam scribit, aut aliquid ab aliis auctoribus . . .
Novissime autem idem Rinius in hac editione toto volumine summa iterum
diligentia perlecto, adhibitis etiam exemplaribus manu Alpagis scriptis (quorum
copiam nuper nobis fecerunt eius haeredes) innumeris pene aliis tum
castigationibus, tum locorum citationibus . . . illustravit (Venice, 1562), IA
110.616, NYAM.

57 *Avicennae . . . Libri in Re Medica Omnes, qui hactenus ad nos pervenere . . .*
omnia novissime post aliorum omnium operam a Ioanne Paulo Mongio
Hydruntino , et Ioanne Costaeo Laudensi recognita . . . (Venice, 1564), IA
110.618, WL.

58 According to *Biographisches Lexikon der hervorragenden Ärzte alle Zeiten*
und Völker, II, 2nd edn (Berlin and Vienna), 1930, pp. 122–3. However,
his name can be found in the Bologna *rotuli* only for the years 1581–98,
when he held an extraordinary or supraordinary lectureship first in
practical and later in theoretical medicine; see Dallari, *I Rotuli*, II, under
the years indicated.

59 *Disquisitionum Physiologicarum Ioannis Costaei Laudensis, In primam primi*
Canonis Avicennae sectionem Libri sex. . . (Bologna, 1589), NLM.

60 C. G. Jöcher, *Allgemeines Gelehrten Lexicon . . .* (Leipzig, 1751), III,
p. 615.

61 On Paterno's career at Padua, see Bartolo Bertolaso, 'Ricerche
d'Archivio su alcuni Aspetti dell'Insegnamento Medico presso la
Università di Padova nel Cinque- e Seicento', *Acta Medicae Historiae*
Patavina, VI (1959–60), 23, and I. P. Tomasini, *Patavini Illustrium Virorum*
Elogia iconibus exornata (Padua, 1630), pp. 151-3. Paterno's commentary,
Bernardini Paterni Salodiensis philosophi, et medici clarissimi, . . .
Explanationes in primam fen primi Canonis . . ., was printed at Venice, 1596
(NYAM). The others are Nicolo Sanmichele and Francesco Modegnano,
identified as professors of theory at Padua and Pavia respectively
(although Sanmichele is not listed as a professor by Bertolaso
[1959–60]). On Cortuso (1513–1603), from 1590 the third head of the
Paduan botanic garden, see G. B. de Toni, 'Spigolature Aldrovandiane
XIX: Il Botanico Giacomo Antonio Cortuso nelle sue Relazione con
Ulisse Aldrovandi', in *Monografie Storiche sullo Studio di Padova:*
Contributo del R. Istituto Veneto di Scienze, Lettere ed Arti alla VII Centenario
della Università (Venice, 1922), pp. 217–51.

62 *Canon* (Venice, 1595), I, pp. 101–2, referring to Paterno's time as a
professor at Pisa, which, acording to Angelo Fabroni, *Historia Academiae*
pisanae, II (Pisa, 1792), p. 468, occupied the years 1555–8.

63 'Institutum autem in primis tuum sequuti, Paterne clarissime, antiquam
versionem delegimus, puriorem certe et plerunque meliorem nisi paulo
esset obscurior. Sed iam illustravimus varia lectione adhibita, quam in
libri margine . . . apposuimus.' *Canon* (Venice, 1564), I, dedication to
Paterno preceding book one.

64 *Principis Avicennae Liber primus. De Universalibus Medicae Scientiae*
Praeceptis. Andrea Gratiolo Salodiano interprete . . . (Venice, 1580), IA
110.622, NYAM. Graziolo referred to Oddo as his preceptor in his
preface to the reader. At the time of writing, I have not yet secured access

to Lino Agrifoglio, 'Argomentazione sulla Peste in un libro di Andrea Graziolo Medico del XVI secolo', *Rev. Ital. Igiene*, XX (1961), 492–9.

65 These and other statements in Graziolo's preface are discussed in d'Alverny, 'Avicenne et les Médecins de Venise', pp. 182–4.

66 See note 61 above.

67 Similar ties bound some of those involved in the Alpago and Rinio editions. Lucchetta, *Il Medico*, pp. 61–2, draws attention to the personal links between Paolo Alpago and Nicolo Massa; and we have seen that Rinio had the confidence of Alpago's heirs.

68 Lucchetta, *Il Medico*, p. 90.

69 *Avicennae Liber Canonis, De Medicinis Cordialibus, Cantica, De Removendis Nocumentis in Regimine Sanitatis, De Syropo Acetoso . . .* (Venice, 1582), IA 110.623, NLM.

70 *Avicennae Arabum medicorum principis. Ex Gerardi Cremonensis versione, et Andreae Alpagi Bellunensis castigatione, a Ioanne Costaeo, et Ioanne Paolo Mongio annotationibus iampridem illustratus. Nunc vero ab eodem Costaeo recognitus . . .* (Venice, 1595), IA 110.627, NLM, and *Avicennae . . . ex Gerardi Cremonensis versione, et Andreas Alpagi Bellunensis castigatione. A Joanne Costaeo et Joanne Paulo Mongio annotationibus jampridem illustratus. Nunc vero ab eodem Costaeo recognitus . . .*, 2 vols. (Venice, 1608), NYAM, WL.

71 D. P. Walker, *Spiritual and Demonic Magic From Ficino to Campanella* (reprint, Notre Dame, 1975), p. 126. On Paolino and the Uranici in general, see *ibid.*, pp. 126–42. Walker also throws light on a possible reason for the interest of Paolino in the *Canon*, when he notes, p. 162, 'Erastus' most violent attack on Ficino is as a follower of Avicenna.' On Paolino's career, see G. G. Liruti, *Notizie della Vite ed Opere Scritte da Letterati di Friuli*, (Venice, 1760), III, pp. 352–72, and Pietro Someda da Marco, *Medici Forojuliensi dal sec. XIII al sec. XVIII* (Udine, 1963), pp. 70–1. However, the date of Paolino's death is established as 16 September, 1604, by Archivio di Stato di Venezia, Provveditori alla Santà, Reg. 832, *Necrologio*, anno 1604. I have not seen this document myself and owe the reference, as also the information that the dates of Paolino's lectureship in Venice (1588–1604) are established by documentary evidence, to the kindness of Dr Richard Palmer.

72 Liruti states that Paolino learned Arabic; however in Paolino's own epistle to 'medicinae studiosis' prefaced to the *Canon* (Venice, 1595), he remarked of the work's critics: 'in quo melius fortasse, et gratius fecissent, si vicem tanti scriptoris, et optime de se meriti dolentes, Arabum percepta lingua, in qua aureum illius esse dicendi genus tradunt, latine eum loqui explosa barbarie fecissent.' The use of 'tradunt' seems not to imply evaluation from personal judgement. Perhaps Paolino's Arabic studies were at an early stage, since he added he had reason to think such a translation would soon be made.

73 Lorenzo Massa was a nephew of Nicolo and a successful Venetian official; see Palmer, 'Nicolo Massa'.

74 See J. R. Jones, 'The Arabic and Persian Studies of Giovan Battista Raimondi, *c.* 1536–1614' (Warburg Institute M.Phil. thesis, 1981), and

G. E. Saltini 'Della Stamperia Orientale Medicea e di Giovan Battista Raimondi', *Giornale Storico degli Archivi Toscani*, IV (1860), 257–308. I am grateful to Dr Charles B. Schmitt for drawing my attention to the work of Mr Jones, and to Mr Jones for corresponding with me on the subject. I hope to provide more extended consideration of Raimondi's medical contacts and possible access to his edition by some European physicians in my forthcoming study. Meanwhile, it may be noted that conceivably Paolino's remark, referred to in the previous note, about the likelihood of a forthcoming translation of the *Canon* from the Arabic may be an allusion to the existence of the Rome edition, which would facilitate such a project.

75 *Canon*, 2, Kirsten (Breslau, 1609), p. 7. On Kirsten (1577–1640), who became rector of the university of Breslau, see Jöcher, II (1750), 2105–7.

76 Paolo Camerini, *Annali dei Giunti*. I. *Venezia*, part 1 (Florence, 1962), p. 23, characterizes the publication policy of the Venetian branch as 'fondata su libri di facile smercio.'

77 See note 16, above.

78 *Avicennae summi inter medicos nominis Fen I, Lib. I Canonis . . .* (Vicenza, 1611), BL.

79 *Avicennae summi inter Arabes medici Fen I, Lib. I Canonis in usum Gymnasii Patavini editio correctior . . .* (Padua, 1636), BL.

80 *Avicennae Arabum medicorum summi Fen I, Lib. I Canonis. Gerardo Cremonense interprete. In usum Gymnasii Patavini. Nova editio castigatior* (Padua, 1648), NLM.

81 *Schola Medica in qua Hippocratis, Galeni, Avicennaeque, medicinae facile principum, pro tyronibus habentur Fundamenta . . .* (Venice, 1647), BL.

82 *Avicennae quarti libri Canonis Fen prima de Febribus. Nova editio ceteris accuratior . . .* (Padua, 1659), BL. Books such as this and those mentioned in the last few notes presumably supplied the need served in the previous century by the *Articella*, the abbreviations and compendia, and perhaps also the translations of Jacob Mantino which circulated in small and doubtless inexpensive volumes.

83 Preface to edition of Vicenza, 1611, reprinted before *Canon* 1:1 in *Schola Medica* (Venice, 1547) (the sections of the *Canon* included in *Schola Medica* are separately paginated from the other parts of the collection).

84 'Prudenti majorum instituto usque ad nostram memoriam Avicennae dogmata Italiae Gymnasia retinuerent.' *Canon* 1:1 (Padua, 1636), p. 3.

85 *Schola Medica* (Venice, 1647), p. 143. The *puncta* from the two sections of the *Canon* occupy pp. 143–5.

86 Kirsten (Breslau, 1609), Plemp (Louvain, 1658), and Welsch (Augsburg, 1674) all review a number of the editions already discussed. In addition, Plemp and Welsch provide some tantalizing hints in their introductions about a number of other more or less contemporary comments on the desirability of a new translation of the *Canon* and projects to undertake one that seem to have come to nothing. I hope to discuss some of these aspects of interest in the *Canon* more fully in my larger study.

87 On the development of Arabic studies, see Johann Fück, *Die Arabischen Studien in Europa bis in den Anfang des 20 Jahrhunderts* (Leipzig, 1955), and,

for the rise of Leyden to prominence, J. Brugman and F. Schröder, *Arabic Studies in the Netherlands* (Leyden, 1979), pp. 3–49.

88 *Petri Kirsteni Wratisl. Phil. et Med. D. Grammatices Arabi Liber I. Sive Orthographia et Prosodia Arabicc* (Breslau, 1608), p. 3. See also notes 2 and 75, above.

89 '"verus medicus, potius linguam latinam carere posset, quam vel Arabicam, vel Graecam"', *ibid.*, p. 7.

90 *Petri Kirsteni . . . Notae in Evangelium S. Matthaei ex collatione textuum Arabicorum, Hebraeorum, Syriacorum, Graecorum, Latinorum . . .* (Breslau [1611]), and *Petri Kirsteni . . . Vitae Evangelistarum Quatuor nunc primum ex antiquissimo codice manuscripto Arabico Caesario erutae . . .* (Breslau [1608]), New York Public Library.

91 *Clarissimi et praecellentissimi doctoris Abualj Ibn-Tsina qui hactenus perperam dictus est Avicenna Canon Medicinae interprete et scholiaste Vopisco Fortunato Plempio. I. Librum primum et secundum Canonis exhibens, atque ex libro quarto tractatum de Febribus* (Louvain, 1658), fo. 2v. On Plemp (1601–71), who was a professor at Louvain from 1633 until his death, see *Biogr. Lexikon*, IV (1885), p. 589.

92 *Abugali filii Sinae sive, ut vulgc dicitur, Avicennae . . . De Morbis Mentis tractatus, Editus in specimen normae medicorum universae ex Arabico in Latinum . . . interprete Petro Vatterio . . .* (Paris, 1659). Consulted on microfilm NYAM. On Vattier, see Moritz Steinschneider, *Die europäischen Übersetzungen aus dem Arabischen bis Mitte des 17 Jahrhunderts* (*Sitzungsberichten der Kais. Akademie der Wissenschaften in Wien, Phil.-Hist. Klasse*, 149) (Vienna, 1904), 79, no. 117.

93 novam hanc versionem a me non ex vetere interpolatam, sed vere ac plane novam factam esse. Hoc ideo dico, quod ex eiusmodi interpolatione magni viri non parvam nec sane immeritam laudem consecuti sint, Iacobus Sylvius ex Mesue librorum trium, Vesalius ex nono Rhasis ad Almansorem; vanitatis tamen in hoc cujusdam non absolvendi, qui ex Arabico horum autorum sermone Latinum suum expressisse videri quasi voluerint, qui neque aspexerant unquam, neque si aspexissent, ullam eius literam legere potuissent, homines alias quidem doctissimi, sed in Arabum idiomate prorsus hospites, magis ingenue facturi. *Canon* 3:1 (excerpts), transl. Vattier (Paris, 1659), dedicatory letter.

94 See note 2 above. On Welsch, see C. F. von Schnurrer, *Bibliotheca Arabica* (Halle, 1811), pp. 452–4.

95 'Quem librum Vopiscus Fortunatus Plempius, ante hos quinque et quinquaginta annos, ex arabico, non indiserte latinum fecit; nostra, tamen, haec celeberrima academia venustissimo, atque adeo primo omnium interprete utitur Gerardo Carmonense . . .,' Morgagni, comm. *Canon* 1:1, *Opera postuma*, IV, p. 16.

96 See note 3, above. As regards the translating techniques of Gerard of Cremona in rendering an Arabic version of a Greek original, see Ilona Opelt, 'Zur Übersetzungstechnik des Gerhard von Cremona', *Glotta*, XXXVIII (1960), 135 ff. I owe this reference to Dr Charles Burnett.

97 *Biblia Iatrica, sive Bibliotheca Medica . . . auctore Ioanne Georgio Schenkio* (Frankfurt, 1609), pp. 80–2.

98 Nunc autem demum a Benedicto Rinio Veneto . . . lucubrationibus
    illustrata. Qui et castigationes ab Alpago factas suis quasque locis
    aptissime inseruit: Et quam plurimas alias depravatas lectiones in
    margine ingeniosissime emendavit. . . . . Plurimis etiam arabicis
    vocibus nunque antea expositis, latinum nomen invenit: Indicemque
    latinum medicamentorum simplicium in secundum librum
    composuit.

Title page, *Canon* (Venice, 1555):

> Sed eam illustravimus varia lectione adhibita, quam in libri margine
> tum ex Bellunensis correctione, et Mantini versione; tum ex variis
> vetustis codicibus; tum ex nostra et aliorum coniectura apposuimus.
> Difficiliores interdum Arabicas in contextu voces latinas reddidimus,
> ut facilior et expeditior legendi esset cursus; sequuti hac in re et
> doctiorum interpretum, et Bellunensis iudicium; ita tamen, ut antiqua
> vocabula in margina integra adhuc sint conservata, et asterisco
> indicata.

Costeo, dedicatory letter to Paterno, prefaced to book one, *Canon* (1564).

99 See previous note. Amatus Lusitanus believed himself to have
    demonstrated that not only Rinio, but even Alpago himself emended
    from sources other than the Arabic:

> unde satis conscius sum quod Belunensis, et Rinus ipse, ac iis alii
> similes viri, suas in Avicenna restitutiones, ab Hebraico contexto, vel
> saltem ad eius enarratoribus, emendicarunt, non vero a puro fonte
> Arabico eas contraxerunt, quem si recte callerent Avicennam de novo
> interpretarentur, et tam ingentem errorem non praetermitterent, ut
> alios infinitos sileam: non deerit tamen aliquis qui brevi Avicennam ex
> integro nobis latinissimum et sincerum ac purum pro veritate
> Arabica, reddat; sed mea sententia pro hac conficiundo opere, non
> unius viri, sed duorum et trium labor emergat, decet.

Curationum Medicinalium (Venice, 1566), II, pp. 94–5, *Cent.* 7.54.

100 Of course, use of Gerard of Cremona and Alpago is not necessarily *ipso
    facto* unsatisfactory. When G. B. Raimondi, the Arabic scholar
    responsible for the publication of the *Canon* in the original language
    (Rome, 1593), tried his hand at translating a passage of book one, part
    one, into Latin, he too used their work as a basis; see Jones, 'Raimondi',
    Appendix VI, pp. 205 ff., where Raimondi's translation is shown side by
    side with Gerard's as revised by Alpago.

101 See Fück, *Arabischen Studien*, pp. 35–55; Karl H. Dannenfeldt, 'The
    Renaissance Humanists and the Knowledge of Arabic', *Studies in the
    Renaissance*, II (1955), 96–117.

102 Lucchetta, *Il Medico*, p. 39, basing the conclusion on the assertion in
    Nicolo Massa's life of Avicenna that the Arabic manuscript of the life had
    been supplied for the 1544 edition by Paolo, having previously belonged
    to Andrea, but that no one could be found who was able to translate it; see

Vita, transl. Massa (1544), fo. 24r (the life is placed at the end of this edition of the *Canon* in a separately foliated section). See also in the same sense, d'Alverny, 'Avicenne et les Médecines de Venise', p. 189.

103 Massa commissioned a translation of the life into Italian from an interpreter for the Venetian merchant community in Damascus and himself translated the Italian into Latin; see *Vita* (1544), p. 24.

104 'nescio litteras Arabes', and 'sive modo ita stet littera Arabica sive non, ego id nescio quoniam ignarus sum', G. B. Da Monte, . . . *In secundam Fen primi Canonis Avicennae* (Venice, 1557), pp. 93, 247, NLM.

105 'ut enim nihil de Avicennae eloquentia, qui Arabice scripsit, decernere possimus, credendum tamen est, virum sublimi ingenio, politissimisque disciplinis ornatum, hac etiam in parte, quantum ferat idioma illud, non fuisse infelicem.' *Canon* 1:1, Graziolo (Venice, 1580), preface to the reader [b3r].

106 *Ibid.* [b3v–4r]; D'Alverny, 'Avicenne et les Médecins de Venise', pp. 183–4.

107 On Arabic biographical material concerning Avicenna, see William E. Gohlman, *The Life of Ibn Sina: A Critical Edition and Annotated Translation* (1974), Albany, NY, USA.

108 *Avicenne cordube principis Vita a Francisco Calphurnio vindocinensi declarata* . . . *Canon* (Lyons, 1522), fo. 1v. The supposed letter of Avicenna to Augustine survives in manuscript; see M. T. d'Alverny, 'Avicenna latinus, III', *Archives d'Histoire Doctrinale et Littéraire du Moyen Age*, 1963 (1964), pp. 269–71, describing ms. Vat.lat. 5108, where the letter occupies fos. 107–8 and has the incipit 'Apparuisti compatriota noster . . .'

109 This note, headed *De arabicorum nominum significatu*, appears in various positions in most of the subsequent major editions.

110 See note 102, above. The life in question is edited and translated by Gohlman.

111 For example *Tertius Canonis Avicenne cum amplissima Gentilis Fulginatis Expositione* . . . (Venice, 1522; WL) opens with a *Tabula Dubiorum prime partis Gentilis super III Avicerna*. Some separate editions of older commentaries on the *Canon* contain subject indices to the commentaries; for example *Iacobi Foroliviensis in primum Avicenne Canonem Expositio* . . . (Venice, 1518; BL), and *Iacobi Foroliviensis* . . . *Expositio et Quaestiones in primum Canonem Avicennae* . . . (Venice, 1547; NYAM).

112 *Index in Avicennae libros nuper Venetiis editos* . . . *Julio Palamede Adriensi medico auctore* (Venice, 1557), BL, where it is bound with *Canon*, Rinio (Venice, 1555).

113 In *Canon*, Rinio (Venice, 1562), Palamede's index is found with its own title page and separately foliated; the shorter index found in *Canon*, Rinio (Basel, 1556) after *De Syrupo Acetoso* and before Alpago's glossary has been dropped. Palamede's index was again reissued by Junta in 1584, presumably to accompany the reissue of Rinio's edition of the *Canon* in 1582, with which the copy owned by NLM is bound.

114 See note 98 above. It would be interesting to explore the possibility of a

relationship between this list and the alphabetical index in the book of simples of the elder Rinio, printed E. de Toni (1925), pp. 206–64, and owned by the younger Rinio (see note 53 above).

115 On Alpago's glossary, see Lucchetta, *Il Medico*, pp. 39–47.

116 *Canon*, Champier and Rustico (Lyons, 1522), ff. 2r–10r.

117 Rustico's 'castigations' may be incorporated in some of these *dubia*, as some of them seem to parallel the subject matter of one of his other works; in particular, nos. 7, 8, 9 and 10 deal with *bubones, ignis persicus*, and *pruna*, conditions on which Rustico had discussed Avicenna's views in *Qui Venenosa Formidas Apostemata et pestiferos Paves Bubones ecce dicta Avicene Arabis de Igne Persico Pruna vel Carbone . . . ordinata, exposita, discussa Rustico medicine cultore . . .*, printed with Baviero Baviera, *Consilia* (Pavia, 1521; NYAM).

118 Letter of dedication to Giorgio Cornelio; *Paulus Alpago ad lectorem* (*Canon*, 1527).

119 Benedictus Rinius Fabricio, Scipioni, Alberto, et Claudio, filiis iucundissimis, *Canon*, Rinio (Venice, 1555), ff. iiir–ivv. Aspects of this preface are discussed in d'Alverny, 'Avicenne et les Médecines de Venise', pp. 196–7.

120 Preface to book one, Costeo to Paterno; to book two, Mongio and Costeo to Cortuso, *Canon* (Venice, 1564).

121 Eget Avicennae, eget Arabum doctrina acri, solerti, et accurata plerunque lectione: quam ii, qui ad medicinam nullo vel dialectices, vel philosophiae studio initiati se se contulere, non satis assequi possunt; proptereaque huic hominum generi soli placent Graeci medici, displicent modis omnibus Arabes; Graeci quidem verborum suavitate, et effusa dicendi copia intellectu non difficiles; Arabes vero sententiarum gravitate, et recondita quadam brevitate non faciles.
Preface to book three, Mongio and Costeo to Sammichele, *Canon* (Venice, 1564)

122 verum quia Galenus id non scripserit, non audere aliquid proferre confiteantur, quasi piaculum sit ad Galeni scripta quidquam adijcere; aut nihil scire fas fit quod is non norit. . . . At vero non ita Galenus. . . . Non ita quicunque in omni scientiarum genere illustres
ibid., preface to book four, Costeo to Modegnano.

123 *Andreas Gratiolus lectori*, *Canon* 1, Graziolo (Venice, 1580), br–cv.

124 See note 105, above. Compare:

Avicenna est elegantissimus in sua lingua, ut nullus Arabum, est eloquentissimus et utitur maxima proprietate loquendi, sicut mihi retulit D. Diegus Orator illius Imperatoris, quod in publicis scholis Avicenna propter linguem ornatum, sicut apud nos Cicero et Boccaccius apud nostros vulgares praelegit,

and

ego nihil scio, sed ita puto, quia nescio litteras Arabes, tamen unum scio, quod Avicenna est multum elegans in suo sermone

Da Monte, comm. *Canon* 1:2 (Venice, 1557), pp. 35, 93.

125 Fabius Paulinus medicus medicinae studiosis, *Canon* (Venice, 1595), a6r–v.

126 Costeo to Paterno, preface to book one, *Canon* (Venice, 1564).

127 These topics are discussed in Costeo and Mongio's annotations to *Canon* 1:1 (Venice, 1595), pp. 33, 34, 13–14. For discussions of the same topics by late thirteenth- and early fourteenth-century Italian physicians, see Siraisi, *Taddeo Alderotti*, pp. 342, 338–9, 321.

128 . . . *In primam Fen libri primi Canonis Avicennae Explanatio* (Venice, 1554); a second edition, with some additions, was published at Venice, 1557. On the content of this commentary see Siraisi, *History of Universities* IV (in press). On innovation during this period in commentaries on the *Canon* written in Spain, see L. Garcia Ballester, 'The Circulation and Use of Medical Manuscripts in Arabic in sixteenth-century Spain', *Journal for the History of Arabic Science*, III (1979), 183–99 at p. 189.

129 See note 51, above.

130 See note 61, above.

131 See note 59, above.

132 *Canon* 1, Graziolo (Venice, 1580), fos. 13v–14r.

133 *Io. Fernelii Ambiani Medicina . . .* (Paris, 1554; NYAM), p. 85. The *Physiologiae Libri*, in which the passage is found, were first published under the title *De Naturali Parte Medicinae* in 1542.

134 F. E. Cranz, 'Alexander Aphrodisiensis', *Catalogus Translationum et Commentariorum*, I (Washington, DC, 1960), pp. 81, 113–14. The scope of renaissance interest in Alexander is well illustrated in idem, 'The Prefaces to the Greek Editions and Latin Translations of Alexander of Aphrodisias', *Proceedings of the American Philosophical Society*, CII (1958), 510–46.

135 Da Monte, comm. *Canon* 1:1 (Venice, 1557; NYAM), pp. 114–27.

136 *Canon*, Costeo and Mongio (Venice, 1595), pp. 259–60.

137 Doctissimus Ioannes Costaeus, in sumtuosa sua hujus Canonis editione praestiterit, qui mea opinione, melius fecisset, se ex fontibus Arabicis hunc authorem restituere voluisset, quam quod sibi proposuerat eum ex Galeno restituere

Canon 2, Kirsten (Breslau, 1609), p. 131; and

ille [Costaeus] vero leviculis quibusdam totus occupetur, et linguarum orientalium omnium ignarissimus,

Welsch (1674), fol. b1ᵛ; and

Andreas Gratiolus Salodianus librum primum integrum nobis latiniorem dedit, adjectis scholiis Hippocratis et Galeni praecipue loca commonstrantibus. Vocat et interpretem nihil minus quam interpres existens: Arabicae quippe linguae prorsus nesciens fuit; nec sequitur authoris verba aut contextum, set ex commentatoribus sensus hausit, saepe male. Aliquando Galeni integras periodos inseruit. Ea non sunt interpretis.

Plemp (1658), fo. 3r.

Plemp and Welsch were also somewhat critical of Kirsten's grasp of Arabic, although in milder terms; see Plemp (1658), 3r, and Welsch (1674), c2v.

138 On the strength of the adherence to Galen among the Paduan faculty in the 1570s, see Richard J. Palmer, 'The Control of Plague in Northern Italy, 1348–1600' (University of Kent Ph.D. thesis, 1978), pp. 254–66.

139 On the innovatory and reformist nature of humanist medicine up until about the 1550s, see W. Pagel, 'Medical Humanism – a Historical Necessity in the Era of the Renaissance', in *Linacre Studies*, pp. 375–6, and Vivian Nutton, 'Medicine in the Age of Montaigne', in *Montaigne and His Age*, ed. K. Cameron (Exeter, 1981), p. 17.

Notes to Chapter 3, R. K. French

1 L. R. Lind, *Studies in Pre-Vesalian Anatomy. Biography, Translations, Documents* (Philadelphia, 1975): Lind, *Studies*. Lind has also translated Berengario's brief introductory work, the *Isagoge Breves*, but this gives us only an inkling of what is in the commentary. See Jacopo Berengario da Carpi, *A Short Introduction to Anatomy* (*Isagoge Breves*), transl. L. R. Lind (University of Chicago Press, 1959).

2 C. D. O'Malley presents a brief account in C. C. Gillispie (ed.), *Dictionary of Scientific Biography*, 15 vols. (New York, 1970–80). One of the few modern historians to study the text seriously is V. Putti, *Berengario da Carpi Saggio Biografico e Bibliografico* (Bologna, 1937): Putti, *Berengario*. See also Thorndike, *History* (note 4).

3 Jacopo Berengario da Carpi, *Commentaria cum amplissimus additionibus super Anatomia Mundini* (Bologna, 1521): Berengario, *Commentary*. It consists of approximately one thousand pages, in which Berengario quotes about eighty authors on substantial points (a further sixty are quoted once only).

4 We can agree with Thorndike's impression that Berengario seems 'to show a command of pretty much the entire literature of medieval Latin and Arabic medicine'. L. Thorndike, *A History of Magic and Experimental Science*, 8 vols. (New York (Columbia University Press, 1923–58)), vol. V (1941), p. 502.

5 Thorndike, *History*, p. 503.

6 The nature of a humanist commentary will be set out by I. Lonie and A. Cunningham in a forthcoming book on renaissance Hippocratism.

7 G. W. Corner, *Anatomical Texts of the Earlier Middle Ages* (Washington, 1927).

8 Jacopo Berengario da Carpi, *Tractatus de Fractura Calvae sive Cranei* (Bologna, 1518), p. 61r. Most of the biographical details that follow in this paper are taken from Putti, *Berengario*.

9 Berengario, *Commentary*, p. 225r.

10 See M. Lowry, *The World of Aldus Manutius* (Oxford (Blackwell) 1979), p. 56.

11 Lowry, *Aldus*, p. 57.

12 Berengario, *Isagoge*, dedication.

13 Jacopo Berengario da Carpi, *Galeni Pergameni Libri Anatomici* (Bologna, 1529), dedication.

14 It was not printed but parts of it have been published by C. Singer, 'A Study in Early Renaissance Anatomy, with a new Text: The Anothomia of Hieronymo Manfredi', in Singer, C., ed., *Studies in the History and Method of Science* (Oxford, 1917), pp. 79–164.

15 G. de Zerbi, *Liber Anathomie Corporis Humani et singulorum Membrorum illius* (Venice, 1502).

16 A. Benedetti, *Historia Corporis Humani; sive Anatomice* (Venice, 1502). The dedication is dated 1497, but there is confusion in the bibliographies over the existence of editions earlier than 1502.

17 For the *accessus* see R. K. French, 'A note on the anatomical accessus of the middle ages', *Medical History*, XXIII (1979), 461–8. Brief biographical details of Zerbi are given in Lind, *Studies*.

18 Lowry, *Aldus*, p. 117.

19 Berengario often addresses his commentary to the *iuniores* and his *scholares*, for example 360v, 398r, 492v.

20 Taddeo Alderotti (Thaddeus Florentinus), *Expositiones in arduum Aphorismum Ipocratis volumen. In divinum Pronosticorum Ipocratis librum. In praeclarum Regiminis Acutorum Ipocratis opus. In subtilissimum Joannitius Isagogarum libellum* (Venice, Junta, 1527); for example in the *Isagoge*, 343r. See also N. Siraisi, *Taddeo Alderotti and His Pupils* (Princeton University Press, 1981).

21 Gentile da Foligno, *Expositio et Quaestiones subtilissimae super primo libro Microtechni Galeni*; and his printed commentary on book three of the *Canon* (Venice, 1505). Gentile also applies his causality analysis in his bibliographical exercise on the works of Galen, which was sometimes printed with the *Articella*, for example that of Venice, 1483, p. 210r–v.

22 Gentile's commentary in the edition of 1505 stops at fen 22 and its place is supplied by that of Matthaeus de Gradibus, which has the same structure.

23 In his commentary on the *Aphorisms* (note 20).

24 Thus Taddeo in expounding *Regimen in Acute Diseases* (note 20). The difference is marked: for in the late thirteenth century, it was *Galen* who was the commentator (upon Hippocrates) not the contemporary expositors.

25 Thus Taddeo in expounding the first aphorism (note 20: p. 2r) distinguishes 'experience' from 'reason' (in relation to 'experience is fallacious and judgement difficult' etc.) and enlarges on the sensory nature of experience. See also his remarks on what is visible in medicine, in his commentary on the *Isagoge*, 351r.

26 In the proemium to his first commentary (see note 20).

27 See N. Siraisi, *Arts and Sciences at Padua. The Studium of Padua before 1350* (Toronto, 1973): Siraisi, *Arts and Sciences*.

28 In the proemium (note 20).

29 The stories of ancient giants (*Commentary*, 14r) that were to enable Sylvius to 'save' Galen by historicizing the *body* (and not the texts, as the

other humanists were doing) did not convince Berengario that the body had changed.

30 John of Alexandria's commentary on Galen's *De Sectis* was a germinal work for medieval anatomy. Galen is here discussing the attitude of the different sects towards anatomy, and the rival advantages of dissection and vivisection, and John's remarks on the status of anatomy, the *accessus* or *occasiones* of observables in dissection and other things were of great interest to anatomists up to the renaissance. The commentary has been printed in the *Primum Galeni Volumen. Quarta Impressio ornatissima* (Pavia, 1515).

31 Putti, *Berengario*, p. 219: in 1511 Berengario and 16 others, illegally armed, pursued one Johannes Baptista into the house of a neighbour, uttering threats against his life and those of his parents. Berengario's servant, on his orders, inflicted a wound on the mother.

32 Lind's translation of the *Isagoge*, p. 160.

33 Siraisi (1973) gives a useful picture of the early years of Padua. Illumination from a different direction is supplied by Q. Skinner, *The Foundations of Modern Political Thought*, 2 vols. (Cambridge, 1978), I: Skinner, *Foundations*.

34 See B. Lawn, *The Salernitan Questions* (Oxford, 1963).

35 Skinner, *Foundations*, I, pp. 205, 208.

36 Putti, *Berengario*, p. 64.

37 Skinner, *Foundations*, I, p. 206.

38 The most important work missing from the contemporary Galenic canon was the *Anatomical Procedures*, of which Berengario published an edition in 1529.

39 For example in the *De Fractura Calvae*, 103v, and several times in the *Commentary*: see note 19.

40 See for example D. J. Geanakoplos, *Byzantium and the Renaissance* (Connecticut, 1973).

41 N. Leoniceno, *Opuscula* (Basel, 1532); p. 126v is 'Contra suarum translationum obtrectatores apologia.'

42 See R. K. French, 'De Juvamentis Membrorum and the reception of Galenic physiological anatomy', *Isis* LXX (1979), 96–109.

43 Galen, *On the Usefulness of the Parts of the Body*, transl. M. T. May, 2 vols. (Cornell University Press, 1968), I, p. 269; and Galen, *De Juvamentis Membrorum* in the *Opera* (Pavia, 1515–16) (unpaginated: book 6, chapter 3).

44 As claimed by Lind, *Studies*, p. 147.

45 In the dedication to the works of Galen (1529).

Notes to Chapter 4, V. Nutton

1 The old survey by J. F. Malgaigne, *Paré; Oeuvres Complètes* (Paris, London, 1840); Eng. transl., *Surgery and Ambroise Paré* (Norman, 1965), conveys some of the complexities of sixteenth-century surgery better than, e.g., W. J. Bishop, *The Early History of Surgery* (London, 1961), pp. 76–94, or O. H. and S. D. Wangensteen, *The Rise of Surgery*

(Folkestone, 1978). As a collection of raw data, E. J. Gurlt, *Geschichte der Chirurgie*, 3 vols. (Berlin, 1898), remains essential. On the availability of the surgeon, see M. Pelling, C. Webster, 'Medical practitioners', in C. Webster (ed.), *Health, Medicine and Mortality in the Sixteenth Century* (Cambridge, 1979), pp. 164–234; M. Pelling, 'Occupational diversity: barbersurgeons and the trades of Norwich, 1550–1640', *Bull. Hist. Med.*, LVI (1982), 484–511.

2 Montaigne, *Essais*, II.37.

3 C. Wickersheimer, *La Médecine et les Médecins en France* (Paris, 1906), p. 176.

4 P. Kibre, 'Hippocrates Latinus', *Traditio*, XXXIV (1978), 194, 208; no. 38 (1982), 176.

5 J. E. Pétrequin, *La Chirurgie d'Hippocrate* (Paris, 1877), I. p. 137.

6 E. T. Nauck, 'Der Ingolstädter medizinische Lehrplan aus der Mitte des 16 Jahrhunderts', *Sudhoffs Archiv*, XL (1956), 1–15.

7 The earliest published commentary on this text, by Falloppia, 1566, represents his lectures of 1559. In the fifty years that separate his edition from that of Paaw in 1616, eight further authors published commentaries.

8 Aëtius, *Libri Medicinales, (C(orpus) M(edicorum) G(raecorum) VIII.1)* (Leipzig, Berlin, 1935), p. XIV.

9 Oribasius, *Collectiones (CMG VI.1.1)* (Leipzig, Berlin, 1928), p. VII.

10 See below p. 87 f.·

11 Paulus, *De Re Medica* (Paris, 1532), sig. A ii.

12 N. Leoniceno, *De Morbo Gallico* (Venice, 1497), *passim*.

13 On the editions of Paul, see E. F. Rice, Jr, 'Paulus Aegineta', *Catalogus Translationum et Commentariorum*, no. 4 (1980), 145–91.

14 By Albanus Thorinus in March 1532 but lacking book 6 which was supplied by G. B. Feliciano in August 1532; by Guenther of Andernacht in 1532; also by Janus Cornarius who probably translated part of book 7 in 1532 and hearing of the other translations, left the project. He came back to it later in life and published his version in 1556.

15 R. J. Durling, 'A Chronological Census of Renaissance Editions and Translations of Galen', *Journ. Warburg and Courtauld Inst.*, XXIV (1961), 293, 295.

16 E. Legrand, *Bibliographie Hellénique* (Paris, 1885), I, p. 75.

17 R. J. Durling, 'Linacre and Medical Humanism', in F. Maddison, M. Pelling, C. Webster (eds.), *Linacre Studies* (Oxford, 1977), pp. 84–9.

18 Rice, 'Paulus', pp. 157–61.

19 Durling, 'Census', p. 295.

20 A. Toledo-Pereyra, 'Galen's Contribution to Surgery', *Journ. Hist. Med.*, xxviii (1973), 357–75; all his references from p. 367 onwards are, in fact, to the pseudo-Galenic *Introduction*.

21 A. Grafton, *Joseph Scaliger* (Oxford, 1983), I, pp. 180–4.

22 At Montpellier the demands of the medical students in 1550 caused the courses for surgical apprentices and medical students to be amalgamated again after a three year separation, see L. Dulieu, *La Médecine à Montpellier* (Avignon, 1979), II, p. 261.

23 G. Maloney, R. Savoie, *Cinq cent ans de Bibliographie Hippocratique* (St

Jean Chrysostome, 1982), nos. 540, 581, 730, 836, 998, 1124, but their data should be treated with caution.

24 M. Curtius, *Quaestio de Phlobotomia in Pleuresi* (Venice, 1534); J. Veyras, *Traicté de Chirurgie . . . avec l'avis de M. Laur. Joubert* (Lyons, 1581).

25 L. Gryllus, *Oratio de Peregrinatione Studii Medicinalis ergo Suscepta* (Prague, 1566), fo. 6v. For the unusual participation in surgical lectures by the leading members of the medical faculty at Montpellier, cf. Dulieu, *Montpellier*, p. 262.

26 G. Ferrabino, 'La Tradizione e la Gloria dell'Insegnamento della Chirurgia nell'Università di Pisa', *Boll. Ist. Stor. It. d. Arte Sanitaria*, no. 8 (1928), 82.

27 See the chapter on Berengario in this volume.

28 On de Leonibus, J. Lange, *Epistulae Medicinales* (Frankfurt, 1589), p. 231. The claim for Berengario goes back to Gurlt, *Allgemeine Deutsche Biographie* (Leipzig, 1883), XVII, p. 637, and is repeated by V. Fossel, 'Aus dem medizinischen Briefen des pfalzgräflichen Leibarztes Johannes Lange', *Sudhoffs Archiv*, vii (1914), 238.

29 T. Pesenti Marengon, 'Professores chirurgie, medici ciroici e barbitonsores a Padova nell'età di Leonardo Buffo da Bertipaglia (†dopo il 1448)', *Quaderni per la Storia dell. Univ. di Padova*, xi (1978), 1–38.

30 H. Stone, 'The French Language in Renaissance Medicine', *Bibl. d'Humanisme et Renaissance*, xv (1953), 315–46.

31 J. Canappe, *Opuscules de Divers Auteurs Médecins* (Lyons, 1552), pp. 386–92. The whole preface by Isaac Joubert to *Annotations de M. Laurent Joubert sur Toute la Chirurgie de M. Guy de Chauliac* (Thournon, 1598), pp. 3–20, is of interest in this regard, especially in its suggestion of a deep division between the humanist (or Latin) surgeons, whose complaints mirror those of the physicians, and the other surgeons.

32 Durling, 'Census', p. 241.

33 Rice, 'Paulus', p. 186.

34 J. Canappe, *Opuscules*, pp. 386–7.

35 J. Daléchamps, *Chirurgie Françoise* (Lyons, 1569), title. cf. also M. Dusseau, *Enchirid ou Manipul des Miropoles* (Lyons, 1561), p. 40.

36 *Le second livre de Claude Galien à Glaucon* (Paris, n.d.), sig. a 2v., quoted by Durling, 'Census', p. 240.

37 J. Canappe, *Opuscules*, p. 389.

38 Brief biographies of Canappe and Tolet are given by H. Joly, J. Lacassagne, 'Médecins et Imprimeurs Lyonnais', *Rev. Lyon. de Médecine*, 1958, 91, 113.

39 J. Canappe, *Opuscules*, sig. 2r., pp. 38, 40, 115–19, 144.

40 Archagathus, whose career was described by Pliny, *Nat. Hist.* XXIX.6, was the standard example of the incompetent classical surgeon, see, e.g., Ravisius Textor, *Officina* (Venice, 1617), p. 332 (the first edition appeared at Paris in 1520 and was frequently reprinted). He was mentioned by almost every writer on surgery, even if, like F. le Fevre, *Les trois premiers livres de la Chirurgie d'Hippocrate*, (Paris, 1555), sig. c.1, he had no idea how to spell the Greek name.

41 J. Canappe, *Opuscules*, pp. 115–29.

42 *Traicté familier des Noms Grecz, Latins et Arabicques ou Vulgaires . . . extr.*
    du septiesme livre des Epistres de Maistre Jehan Manard (Paris, 1555).

43 On Daléchamps, see, in particular, C. B. Schmitt, 'The correspondence
    of Jacques Daléchamps', *Viator*, viii (1977), 399–434; Rice, 'Paulus',
    pp. 186–7.

44 Hence the curious entry in Maloney and Savoie, *Bibliographie*
    Hippocratique, no. 433, who, like Rice, 'Paulus', p. 148, did not know of
    the 1569 edition, of which a copy exists in the Wellcome Institute Library.

45 J. Daléchamps, *Chirurgie*, pp. 4v–7r.

46 W. Brockbank, 'The man who was Vidius', *Ann. R. Coll. Surgeons*,
    no. xix (1956), 269–95; C. E. Kellett, 'The school of Salviati', *Med. Hist.*,
    xi (1958), 164–8; id., *Santorinos of Rhodes and the illustrations to the Chirurgia*
    of Vidus Vidius (Newcastle, 1959); M. D. Grmek, 'Vidius et les
    Illustrations Anatomiques et Chirurgicales de la Renaissance', *Actes VIIIe*
    Congr. Int. de Tours, 1973, 175–85; id., 'Contribution à la Biographie de
    Vidius', *Rev. hist. des sciences*, xxxi (1978), 289–99.

47 Brockbank, 'Vidius', pp. 286–7.

48 G. C. Aranzi, *In Hippocratis Librum de Vulneribus* (Lyons, 1579); I cite it
    from the edition of Leyden, 1639, p. 11.

49 *Ibid.*, pp. 6, 4.

50 On the increasing tendency to set Hippocrates supreme by himself, see
    A. Foes, *Oeconomia Hippocratis* (Frankfurt, 1588), p. *3v; id., *Hippocratis*
    Opera (Frankfurt, 1594), Sect. VI, pp. 738, 899.

51 Maloney and Savoie, *Bibliographie Hippocratique*, nos. 486 (=494), 487,
    497, 498 (unless these are merely different bibliographical listings of
    486–7), 830.

52 *Ibid.*, no. 810.

53 *Ibid.*, nos. 325, 326.

54 F. Lehoux, *Le Cadre de Vie des Médecins Parisiens* (Paris, 1976), p. 481.
    Brockbank, 'Vidius', p. 279, in ascribing to Botallo the opinion that the
    book was very rare in Vidius' own day, misunderstands the comment of
    the Leyden editors of Botallo's *Opera Omnia* (Leyden, 1660), p. 667 n.,
    and pf., sig. +8r., who were referring to their own time.

55 L. Botalli, *De Curandis Vulneribus Sclopetorum* (Lyons, 1560), pp. 7–8.
    This edition was reprinted unchanged by A. Coninx at Antwerp in 1583.

56 L. Botalli, *Commentarioli Duo* (Lyons, 1565), pp. 448–54. Brockbank, in
    particular, cites this edition and its Leyden reprint without understanding
    that the section of instruments and the long commentary on the last
    chapter of Galen's *Method of Healing*, book six, were not included in the
    first edition.

57 C. Gesner, *De Chirurgia Scriptores optimi quique Veteres et Recentiores,*
    plerique in Germania antehac non editi (Zurich, 1555), sig. *2r–3r. Tagault's
    elegant style found much favourable comment, e.g. G. Falloppia, *Opera*
    Omnia (Frankfurt, 1584), p.. 696.

58 Gesner, *Chirurgia*, sig. +2r.

59 Gurlt, *Geschichte*, I, p. 947. Malgaigne, *Paré*, pp. 191–4, is rather more
    charitable, although he in turn, p. 260, damns Ferri.

60 G. Baader, G. Keil, *Medizin im mittelalterlichen Abendland* (Darmstadt,

1982), pp. 25–37; P. Assion, 'Der Hof Herzog Siegmunds von Tirol als Zentrum spätmittelalterlicher Fachliteratur', in G. Keil (ed.), *Fachprosa-Studien* (Berlin, 1982), pp. 37–75.

61 Gurlt, *Geschichte*, II, pp. 200–34, is still useful.

62 K. Pielmeyer, *Statuten der Deutschen Medizinischen Fakultäten im Mittelalter* (Bonn, 1981), pp. 48, 51–2.

63 H. Decker-Hauff, W. Setzler, *Die Universität Tübingen* (Tübingen, 1977), p. 65.

64 A full study of the relationship between the medicine of Germany and Italy in the renaissance is a desideratum. See, e.g., G. Baader, 'Mittelalter und Neuzeit im Werk von Otto Brunfels', *Med.-hist. Journal*, xiii (1978), 186–203; *id.*, 'Medizinisches Reformdenken und Arabismus im Deutschland des 16 Jahrhunderts', *Sudhoffs Archiv*, lxiii (1979), 261–96.

65 Decker-Hauff, Setzler, *Tübingen*, pp. 68–74; Pielmeyer, *Statuten*, pp. 57–78.

66 Decker-Hauff, Setzler, *Tübingen*, pp. 88–90; Nauck, 'Ingolstadt', *passim*.

67 E. Giese, B. von Hagen, *Geschichte der Medizinischen Fakultät der Universität Jena* (Jena, 1958), pp. 5–80. Three letters of Cornarius to Lange are in the Sammlung Trew at Erlangen, see E. Schmidt-Herrling, *Die Briefsammlung des Nürnberger Arztes Christoph Jacob Trew* (Erlangen, 1940), s.v. Cornarius.

68 On Lange, see Fossel, 'Lange', pp. 238–52, and V. Nutton, 'John Caius und Johannes Lange; medizinischer Humanismus zur Zeit Vesals', *NTM* (forthcoming in 1984), References in the present chapter to Lange's *Epistulae Medicinales* are to the edition of G. Wirth and N. Reusner (Frankfurt, 1589).

69 *Ep. Med.*, p. 356, unless the whole series of letters about Gerard, the Venetians and the drug trade, Epp. I.63–7, is a literary artifice; but cf. p. 418.

70 H. de Vocht, *History of the Foundation and Rise of the Collegium Trilingue Lovaniense, 1517–1550* (Louvain, 1953), II, p. 389. The lady in question stood her ground, 'ceu hinnulus viso elephanto'.

71 Lange, *Ep. Med.*, p. 563, with his earlier comments, p. 39.

72 *Id., Medicum de Re Publica Symposium* (Basel or Augsburg, 1554). Fossel, 'Lange', p. 251, believes in an earlier publication of *c.* 1547.

73 E. Stübler, *Geschichte der medizinischen Fakultät der Universität Heidelberg, 1386–1925* (Heidelberg, 1926), pp. 33–42.

74 This explains the celebrated absence of Erastus at Frankfurt in 1569 recorded by T. Puschmann, *A History of Medical Education* (London, 1891), p. 334.

75 Stübler, *Heidelberg*, pp. 33, 68. cf. the similar complaints of Georg Bartisch, *Ophthalmodouleia* (Dresden, 1583), sig. A 6r–v. and Caspar Stromayr, *Practica Copiosa*, ed. W. F. Kümmel (Munich, 1983), pp. 6–9.

76 Stübler, *Heidelberg*, pp. 37, 59–65; Pielmeyer, *Statuten*, p. 33.

77 Stübler, *Heidelberg*, pp. 37–8; Pielmeyer, *Statuten*, pp. 67–8.

78 P. Monaw, in L. Scholz (ed.), *J. Cratonis . . . Consilia et Epistulae* (Hanover, 1619), V, pp. 431–2, discussed by G. Ongaro, 'La Scoperta della Circolazione Polmonare e la Diffusione della Christianismi

Restitutio di Michele Servetc nel XVI secolo in Italia e nel Veneto',
Episteme, V (1971), 36–7. Ongaro's argument for Pigafetta's use of
Servetus is inconclusive, and he misdates Fabrizio's anatomy of January
1576. He also fails to note that another member of Crato's circle was
moved by the same demonstration by Fabrizio, but this time carried out
three years later, in 1579, to recall similarly the Heidelberg anatomy of
Pigafetta, see Scholz, *Cratonis Epistulae,* VI (Hanover, 1611), p. 95.
79 John Venn, 'John Caius', in E. Roberts (ed.), *The Works of John Caius*
(Cambridge, 1912), is fundamental. See also V. Nutton, 'John Caius and
the Linacre tradition', *Med Hist.,* xxiii (1979), 373–91.
80 W. Langdon-Brown, 'John Caius and the Revival of Learning', *Proc. R.
Soc. Med., Sect. Hist. Med.,* xxxv (1941), 61–9.
81 W. Bullein, *Bulleins Bulwarke of Defence against all Sicknes, Sorenes and
Woundes. (here after insueth a little dialogue . . .)* (London, 1562), *Dial.,* fo.
iiiir.
82 M. Pelling, C. Webster, 'Medical Practitioners', pp. 185, 230.
83 W. Bullein, *Dialogue,* fo. iv v.–v v.
84 W. Clowes, *Selected Writings.* ed. F. N. L. Poynter (London, 1948),
pp. 76–83.
85 On their activities as translators, see Durling, 'Census', pp. 293, 284,
292. They receive little attention from P. Slack, 'Mirrors of Health and
Treasures of Poor men; the Uses of the Vernacular Medical Literature of
Tudor England', in Webster, *Health, Medicine and Mortality,* pp. 237–73.
86 P. Lowe, *The whole Course of Chirurgerie. Whereunto is annexed the Presages
of Hippocrates* (London, 1597), not noted by Maloney and Savoie,
Bibliographie Hippocratique. The book was reprinted in 1612, 1634 and
1654.
87 J. D. Comrie, *A History of Scottish Medicine* (London, 1932), I, pp. 351–3;
D. Hamilton, *The Healers* (Edinburgh, 1981), pp. 64–7.
88 J. T. Lanning, *Pedro della Torre* (Baton Rouge, 1974), p. 7.
89 [Although even sympathizers might have their doubts about the
'prerogative of antiquity']. So A. Dudith, in L. Scholz, *Cratonis Epistulae,*
VI, p. 44.

Notes to Chapter 5, R. Palmer

1 Pietro Andrea Mattioli, *Il Dioscoride . . .* (Venice, 1548), dedication. cf.
Jerry Stannard, 'P. A. Mattioli: sixteenth century Commentator on
Dioscorides', *University of Kansas Libraries Bibliographical Contributions,* I
(1969), 59–81.
2 Charles B. Schmitt, 'Theophrastus', in *Catalogus Translationum et
Commentariorum,* vol. 2, ed. P. O. Kristeller and F. E. Cranz
(Washington, 1971), pp. 239–322. J. M. Riddle, 'Dioscorides', *ibid.,* vol.
4, ed. F. E. Cranz and P. O. Kristeller (Washington, 1980), pp. 1–143.
Theophrastus was virtually unknown in the West in the middle ages.
Dioscorides' *Materia Medica* circulated only in a revised alphabetical
version which exerted little direct influence.

3 P. A. Mattioli, *Commentarii in sex libros Pedacii Dioscoridis . . . de Materia Medica* (Venice, 1565), dedication, dated Prague, January 1565.

4 L. Sabbatini, 'La Cattedra dei Semplici fondata a Bologna da Luca Ghini, *Studi e Memorie per la Storia dell'Università di Bologna*, IX (1926), 13–53.

5 P. A. Mattioli, *I Discorsi nei sei libri di Pedacio Dioscoride* (Venice, 1559), Mattioli's introductory note to his readers.

6 *Dizionario Biografico degli Italiani*, vol. 11 (Rome, 1969), pp. 490–2. cf. Roberto de Visiani, *Della vita e degli scritti di Francesco Bonafede* (Padua, 1845). Bonafede had practised medicine in Venice before teaching at Padua from 1524.

7 Padua, *Archivio Antico dell'Università*, Reg. 677, f. 207r.

8 *Ibid.*, Reg. 675, f. 117r, the Arts University to the *Riformatori* 14 Feb. 1544; Venice, Archivio di Stato (hereafter ASV), *Senato, Terra*, Reg. 34, ff. 57v–58v, 31 July 1545.

9 ASV, *Riformatori dello Studio di Padova*, Filza 63, *Riformatori* to the *Capitanio* of Padua, 12 May 1555.

10 *Ibid.*, Filza 419, Cortusio to the *Riformatori*, 20 May 1602.

11 G. B. de Toni, 'Nuovi documenti intorno Luigi Anguillara', *Atti del R. Istituto Veneto di Scienze, Lettere ed Arti*, LXX (1910–11), 289–96.

12 G. B. de Toni, 'Intorno alle relazioni del botanico Melchiorre Guilandino con Ulisse Aldrovandi', *Atti della I. R. Accademia di Scienze, Lettere, ed Arti degli Agiati in Rovereto,* 3rd ser., XVII (1911), 149–71.

13 Luigi Anguillara, *Semplici* (Venice, 1561), pp. 19, 88, 298. cf. R. Palmer, 'Physicians and Surgeons in sixteenth century Venice', *Medical History*, XXIII (1979), 451–60, and R. Palmer, *The Studio of Venice* (Trieste, 1983), pp. 89, 192.

14 G. Ongaro, 'Contributi alla biografia di Prospero Alpini', *Acta Medicae Historiae Patavina*, VIII–IX (1961–2 and 1962–3), 79–168.

15 Petrus Pena and Mathias de Lobel, *Stirpium Adversaria nova* (London, 1570), p. 54. (Hereafter *Stirpium*.)

16 Prospero Borgarucci, *La Fabrica de gli Spetiali* (Venice, 1567), p. 404. (Hereafter *Fabrica*.)

17 P. A. Mattioli, *Il Dioscoride* (Venice, 1548), p. 333.

18 Pietro Antonio Michiel, *I cinque libri di Piante*, ed. E. de Toni (Venice, 1940). cf. footnote 24 below.

19 Luigi Anguillara, *Semplici* (Venice, 1561), p. 34.

20 Conrad Gesner, *De Hortis Germaniae* (Strasburg, 1561), f. 239v.

21 Quoted in Lynn Thorndike, *A History of Magic and Experimental Science*, 8 vols. (New York, 1923–1958), IV, p. 598. (Hereafter *History*.)

22 M. Cermenati, 'Francesco Calzolari e le sue lettere all'Aldrovandi', *Annali di Botanica*, VII (1908–9), 83–138.

23 C. Raimondi, 'Lettere di P. A. Mattioli ad Ulisse Aldrovandi', *Bullettino Senese di Storia Patria*, XIII (1906), 121–85, especially p. 178, Mattioli to Aldrovandi, 20 March 1572. (Hereafter Raimondi, 'Lettere'.)

24 G. B. de Toni, 'Contributo alla conoscenza delle relazioni del patrizio veneziano Pietro Antonio Michiel con Ulisse Aldrovandi', *Memorie dell'Accademia di Scienze, Lettere ed Arti in Modena*, 3rd ser., IX (1908), 21–70.

25 Ioannes Crato a Kraftheim, *Consiliorum et Epistolarum Medicinalium*, 3 vols. (Frankfurt, 1592–95), III, pp. 376–8, Cordus to Andrea Aurifabrus, from Venice, April 1544.

26 Charles Salzmann, 'Francesco Calzolari . . . und seine Pflanzensendungen an Conrad Gesner in Zürich', *Gesnerus*, XVI (1959), 81–103.

27 C. C. Gillispie (ed.), *Dictionary of Scientific Biography*, 15 vols. (New York, 1970–80), XI, 527–8. (Hereafter DSB).

28 Bologna, Biblioteca Universitaria, *MS Aldrovandi* 38², vol. 1, f. 266r; vol. 3, ff. 9, 175r, 229r. cf. Raimondi, 'Lettere', p. 141.

29 Pena and de Lobel, *Stirpium*, pp. 37, 64.

30 P. A. Mattioli, *Il Dioscoride* (Venice, 1548), pp. 333, 361. Raimondi, 'Lettere', pp. 177–8 on Mattioli's visit to Venice in 1571.

31 Camerarius' visit to Venice in 1562, when Michiel refused to see him, is noted in Bologna, Biblioteca Universitaria, *MS Aldrovandi* 38², vol. 1, f. 267r.

32 Leoniceno justified his criticism of Pliny on this basis. Thorndike, however, thought Leoniceno insincere (Thorndike, *History*, iv, p. 603).

33 See footnote 8.

34 Venice, Museo Civico Correr (hereafter MCV), *Mariegola* 209, vol. 1, f. 70r–v. On pharmacy in general in Venice, see especially Girolamo Dian, *Cenni Storici sulla Farmacia Veneta*, 7 parts (Venice, 1900–8).

35 The original statutes of the College compiled from 1565 are in Venice, Biblioteca Nazionale Marciana (hereafter BMV), *MSS. Italiani* VII 1971 (=9042). These were also published in 1565 and reprinted by Dian in 1891. The minute books of the College are in MCV, *Mariegola* 209.

36 MCV, *Mariegola* 209, vol. 1, f. 115v.

37 *Ibid.*, f. 31r.

38 ASV, *Giustizia Vecchia*, Busta 112, Reg. 152, *Accordi dei garzoni 1582–3*, f. 42r.

39 MCV, *Mariegola* 209, vol. 1, f. 231 *et seq.*

40 Borgarucci, *Fabrica*, p. 2.

41 P. A. Mattioli, *Il Dioscoride* (Venice, 1548), dedication.

42 Bologna, Biblioteca Universitaria, *MS Aldrovandi* 38², vol. 3, ff. 97–183, especially f. 98r. Fulcheri wrote of the *Coral*, 'I am there for experience' (*exercitio*). The *Coral* seems to have been a large pharmacy since it was chosen to supply the Venetian lazarettos with medicines during the plagues of 1527–9 and 1555–6. Galeazzo Corniani's bill for medicines supplied between March 1555 and October 1556 came to nearly 11 000 lire, though the epidemic was a minor one. From October 1556 he lost the contract to Zuan Francesco Corniani at the *Medico* (ASV, *Provveditori alla Sanità*, Reg. 727, f. 144r–v; Reg. 730, ff. 71r, 78v–79v, 87r–v).

43 G. B. de Toni, 'Nuovi documenti intorno a Giacomo Raynaud, farmacista di Marsiglia e alle sue relazioni con Ulisse Aldrovandi', *Atti del R. Istituto Veneto di Scienze, Lettere ed Arti*, LXVIII (1908–9), 117–31.

44 Bologna, Biblioteca Universitaria, *MS Aldrovandi* 38², vol. 3, ff. 229–34.

45 *Ibid.*, ff. 241–3. On the *Medico* pharmacy, cf. above, footnote 42, and W. Schupbach, 'Doctor Parma's medicinal macaronic', *Journal of the Warburg and Courtauld Institutes*, XLI (1978), 147–91, especially p. 172. Francesco

Corniani at the *Medico* supplied drugs worth over 38 000 lire to the
Venetian lazarettos between April and October 1576 during the plague
(ASV, *Provveditori alla Sanità*, Reg. 733, f. 66v).

46 MCV, *Mariegola* 209, vol. 1, f. 33r, the statutes of 1565. An early
manuscript price list, presented to the *Giustizia Vecchia* in 1584 survives
in ASV, *Giustizia Vecchia*, Busta 211. Such lists were printed from at least
1566, and some 40 editions printed between 1636 and 1696 are in the
archive of the *Ospedale di Santa Maria dei Battuti* preserved in the
Seminario Arcivescovile at Udine. A printed Paduan price list for 1579 is
in Padua, Archivio di Stato, *Fraglia degli Speziali*, Busta 17. A unique set
of 16 price lists for Bergamo, 1579–1600, is amongst the printed books in
the Wellcome Institute.

47 Scipione Mercurio, *De gli Errori Popolari d'Italia* (Venice, 1603), f. 151r.

48 Borgarucci, *Fabrica*, pp. 215–16.

49 ASV, *Avogaria di Comun*, Busta 3632/1, 4 June 1543. Bartolomeo
Agolante of Treviso graduated at Bologna in 1516, joined the College of
Physicians of Treviso in 1517, and was *medico condotto* at Serravalle
1527–9.

50 BMV, *MSS Italiani* VII 2356 (=9709), f. 4v; Hvar, Yugoslavia,
Biskupski Musej, Minute book of the Venetian College of Physicians
1534–55 (hereafter Hvar MS), f. 53v.

51 ASV, *Sant'Uffizio*, Busta 35, 8 May 1572.

52 Venice, Istituzioni di Ricovero e di Educazione (hereafter IRE), *Zitelle*,
Commissaria di Maria Massa, the draft will of Nicolò Massa of 1562 refers
to his relations with di Megi in Venice from 1526. These papers also
include notes of medicines from the *Campana* prescribed for his patients
in the nunnery of S. Servolo. On another of Massa's patients supplied
from the *Campana*, cf. ASV, *Sant'Uffizio*, Busta 39, the trial of Lorenzo
de Madiis in 1575.

53 ASV, *Sant'Uffizio*, Busta 39. In his 1553 trial, Donzellini was frequently
described as a doctor practising at the Sarasin pharmacy (*medico solito
praticar alla spiciaria del sarasin*).

54 ASV, *Collegio, Notatorio*, Reg. 24, f. 137r.

55 MCV, *Mariegola*, 209, vol. 1, f. 38. The statutes accordingly laid down
the maximum which the physician could be given in presents each year.

56 IRE, *Ospedale dei Derelitti, Commissaria di Silvestro di Silvestri*. The
pharmacist at the *Cerva*, Zuan Battista Silvestrini, also lent money to
Silvestri.

57 E. A. Cicogna, *Delle Inscrizioni Veneziane*, vol. 2 (Venice, 1827), p. 451.

58 ASV, *Provveditori alla Sanità*, Reg. 727, f. 310r.

59 On Pietro (d. 1563), see R. Palmer, *The Studio of Venice*, p. 105. Andrea
(d. 1570), graduated at Padua in 1547 and was physician at Chioggia. The
relationships are clear from Pietro's will, ASV, *Miscellanea atti di notai
diversi della Cancelleria Inferiore*, Busta 66, cedula 48. Zuan Alberto figures
prominently in MCV, *Mariegola* 209, vol. 1.

60 Giorgio Melichio, *Avertimenti* (Venice, 1575), dedication and ff. 27r,
89v. On Marini, see R. Palmer, *The Studio of Venice*, p. 116. On Mongio,
see Avicenna, *Libri in Re Medica omnes* (Venice, 1564), and the letter to

him from Costa in Mesuë, *Opera* (Venice, 1589 – I have not seen the first edition of 1568). Mongio's service as *medico condotto* at Monselice is mentioned in Scipione Mercurio's *De gli Errori Popolari d'Italia*, f. 160v.

61 Bellebuono died in the Lazaretto Vecchio of Venice, during plague, probably in 1577 (ASV, *Provveditori alla Sanità*, Reg. 734, f. 75r, September 1578). This confirms the date of Fioravanti's *Della Fisica*, published in Venice in 1582 with a letter to Bellebuono deceased, but written earlier, in 1577.

62 ASV, *Sant'Uffizio*, Busta 27. Decio and Galeno Bellebuono were key figures in the trial of Francesco Anovazzo 1568–9.

63 Leonardo Fioravanti, *Dello Specchio di Scientia universale* (Venice, 1572), f. 43r.

64 MCV, *Mariegola* 209, vol. 1, ff. 44r–48v. Di Romani was given a patent for his invention in 1594, but persuaded to share it with his colleagues in the *Collegio degli Spetiali* in 1597. A consultation of the College of Physicians of Padua on the invention is contained in Padua, *Archivio Antico dell'Università*, Reg. 421, ff. 12–31, and further details on di Romani are in the Venice 1605 edition of Melichio's *Avertimenti*.

65 Bologna, Biblioteca Universitaria, *MS Aldrovandi* 38[2], vol. 3, ff. 1–25r.

66 MCV, *Mariegola* 209, vol. 1, ff. 33v–34r.

67 Antonio Musa Brasavola, *Examen Omnium Simplicium* (Rome, 1563), f. 2v. On di Megi, who was certainly at the *Campana* by 1551, cf. note 52 above. He was another of the Venetian correspondents of Aldrovandi (Bologna, Biblioteca Universitaria, *MS Aldrovandi* 38[2], vol. 3, f. 244r, August 1558).

68 P. A. Mattioli, *Il Dioscoride* (Venice, 1548), p. 361.

69 *Ibid.*, p. 395.

70 Borgarucci, *Fabrica*, especially pp. 467, 499.

71 P. A. Mattioli, *Commentarii, op. cit.* (Venice, 1565), dedication. Francesco Calzolari, *Il viaggio di Monte Baldo* (Venice, 1566), p. 15. Borgarucci, *Fabrica*, pp. 499, 506.

72 Pena and de Lobel, *Stirpium*, p. 64.

73 U. Tergolina-Gislanzoni-Brasco, 'Francesco Calzolare speziale veronese', *Bollettino dell'Istituto Storico Italiano dell'Arte Sanitaria*, XIV (1934), 293–310.

74 Giovanni Battista Olivi, *De Reconditis et Praecipuis Collectaneis ab honestissimo et solertissimo Francisco Calceolario veronensi in museo adservantis* (Venice, 1583).

75 M. Cermenati, 'Francesco Calzolari e le sue Lettere all'Aldrovandi', pp. 119, 135.

76 P. A. Mattioli, *I Discorsi . . .* (Venice, 1573), dedication, dated Innsbruck, 1568.

77 On Venetian exports of theriac, see for instance the testimony to the importance of Venetian theriac and mithridatum in their countries given in 1621 by the Ambassadors of Britain and France and the Consuls of the Low Countries and Germany (ASV, *Giustizia Vecchia*, Busta 211). Of Germany, for instance, it was said that, 'throughout Germany, Venetian theriac and mithridatum have always been in customary use as antidotes

precious above all others, and the most excellent and best that are made anywhere.' On theriac in general, see G. Watson, *Theriac and Mithridatium* (London, 1966), and G. Olmi, 'Farmacopea Antica e Medicina Moderna: la Disputa sulla Teriaca nel Cinquecento bolognese', *Physis*, XIX (1977), 197–246.

78 Bartolomeo Maranta, *Della Theriaca et del Mithridato* (Venice, 1572), p. 9. (Hereafter *Theriaca*.)

79 Horatio Guarguanti, *Della Theriaca e sue mirabili Virtù* (Venice, 1596). (Hereafter *Theriaca . . . Virtù*.)

80 Maranta, *Theriaca*, p. 9.

81 As an instance of the quantities of theriac which a single pharmacist might make, Orazio Zattabella, at the *S. Girolamo* in Venice, made 170 pounds weight in 1580, 338 pounds in 1586, 342 pounds in 1589, 444 pounds in 1592, 510 pounds in 1595, 260 pounds in 1598, 352 pounds in 1599 and 433 pounds in 1600 (MCV, *Mariegola* 209, vol. 1, ff. 144v–159v).

82 P. A. Mattioli, *Il Dioscoride* (Venice, 1548), book six, p. 31.

83 *Ibid., I discorsi . . . nei sei libri di Pedacio Dioscoride* (Venice, 1559), dedication.

84 Maranta, *Theriaca*, p. 9.

85 Guarguanti, *Theriaca . . . Virtù*, p. 6.

86 See the translation of Alpino's *De Balsamo Dialogus* in Luciano Cremonini, 'Breve commento al «Prospero Alpini de Balsamo Dialogus»', *Acta Medicae Historiae Patavina*, VIII–IX (1961–62 and 1962–63), 171–203, especially p. 177.

87 On the ingredients of theriac, see the recipe in Maranta, *Theriaca*, pp. 12–14. Recipes for theriacs and mithridata made in Venice between 1580 and 1609 are given in full in MCV, *Mariegola* 209, vol. 1, ff. 144v–164v.

88 P. A. Mattioli, *Il Dioscoride* (Venice, 1548), book six, p. 31.

89 Hvar MS, ff. 122r–124r. A few decades later, manufacture in Venice was far more frequent. Vipers for theriac and mithridatum were killed for instance at the *Anzolo*, the *San Marco* and the *Coral* in May 1572; the *Struzzo* (twice) and the *S. Giovanni* in May 1573; the *Anzolo* (twice), the *S. Giovanni* and the *Coral* in May 1575 (BMV, *MSS Italiani* VII, 2342 (=9695), ff. 121r–135v).

90 P. A. Mattioli, *Commentarii, op. cit.* (Venice, 1565), p. 1405.

91 Verona, *Archivio di Stato, Antico Archivio del Comune*, Reg. 610 (Minutes of the College of Physicians 1469–1569), f. 197v on Calzolari's 1561 theriac; f. 221r–v on his 1566 theriac.

92 Francesco Calzolari, *Lettera . . . intorno ad alcune Menzogne e Calonnie date alla sua Theriaca* (Cremona, 1566).

93 ASV, *Giustizia Vecchia*, Busta 211, 7 October 1568

> . . . in our judgement the said juice is the juice called acacia, since it has the characteristics observed by the ancient doctors who have written about acacia, and especially since we have seen the certificates which testify that this juice comes from the area where the tree called acacia grows.

94 Maranta, *Theriaca*, pp. 82–3
95 *Ibid.*, p. 105.
96 Bologna, Biblioteca Universitaria, *MS Aldrovandi* 38², vol. 3, f. 2r.
97 Borgarucci, *Fabrica*, pp. 499, 506.
98 *Ibid.*, p. 460.
99 Maranta, *Theriaca*, pp. 33–5
100 Calzolari, *Lettera, op. cit.*
101 P. A. Mattioli, *I Discorsi* . . (Venice, 1568), p. 955. Mattioli describes cases successfully treated with Calzolari's theriac by leading Italian physicians.
102 Verona, Archivio di Stato, *Antico Archivio del Comune*, Reg. 611, ff. 151r–152r.
103 To keep this chapter within limits I leave aside other influences on *materia medica*, such as the study of plants from the New World and the Indies, promoted in Italy by Annibale Briganti's Italian translation of works by Garcia da Orta and Nicolò Monardes (Venice, 1576).
104 In the Venetian Republic the earliest official pharmacopoeia was that of the College of Physicians of Bergamo (Bergamo, 1580). A pharmacopoeia was drawn up for the College of Physicians of Verona by Giuseppe Valdagno in 1581, but after various delays the College decided in 1601 to adopt the pharmacopoeia of Bologna (Verona, Archivio di Stato, *Antico Archivio del Comune*, Reg. 611, ff. 79r, 158r, 162v, 167v). The Venetian College approved a pharmacopoeia drawn up by one of its members, Curtio Marinelli, in 1616, published as *Pharmacopoea* (Venice, 1617).
105 See Cortusio's letter to Borgarucci, October 1565, published in the latter's *Fabrica*.
106 P. A. Mattioli, *I Discorsi* . . (Venice, 1573), p. 692.
107 Castore Durante, *Herbario Nuovo* (Rome, 1585), pp. 6, 160.
108 Conrad Gesner, *Epistolarum Medicinalium libri tres* (Zurich, 1577), ff. 11r–12v, 74r–v, 78r. Camerarius took a similar view in commenting on Mattioli, see P. A. Mattioli, *De Plantis Epitome* (Frankfurt, 1586), p. 824.
109 Though in comparing the Florentine pharmacopoeias of 1498 and 1567 a distinct change of emphasis can be observed in favour of ancient Greek and new renaissance drugs – see Alfonso Corradi, *Le Prime Farmacopee Italiane* (Milan, 1887), pp. 45–50 – a glance at any of the late sixteenth century pharmacopoeias shows the continuing fundamental importance in composite remedies of Arabic writers such as Mesuë. Commentaries on Mesuë, like that of Marini published in 1562, could however be well illustrated with drawings of plants, and contain the same sort of critical discussion which Mattioli applied to Dioscorides.
110 Marco Ferrari, 'Alcune vie di diffusione in Italia di idee e di testi di Paracelso', in Istituto Nazionale di Studi sul Rinascimento, *Scienze, Credenze occulte, Livelli di Cultura* (Florence, 1982), pp. 21–9.
111 Claudio Gelli, *Risposta . . . el Flagello contra Medici Rationali* (Venice, 1626), p. 28. I have not seen the first edition published in Venice in 1584.
112 Walter Pagel, *Paracelsus* (Basel, 1958), pp. 12–13.

113 *Idem.*, 'Paracelsus', DSB, x, 304–13 .

114 Aldo Stella, *Dall'Anabattismo al Socinianismo nel Cinquecento veneto*
     (Padua, 1967), p. 140. Paracelsus does not, however, appear in the
     editions of the *Index Librorum Prohibitorum* which I have examined
     (Venice, 1564, 1568, 1570, 1575, 1585).

115 *Ibid.*, p. 179.

116 The statute was published, for instance, in *Privilegia magnificae Civitatis
     Veronae* (Venice, 1588), p. 83. The motivation for the statute was the
     belief that alchemical equipment was used to counterfeit coinage.

117 Gabriele Falloppia, *Opera Genuina Omnia* (Venice, 1606), pp. 330–416.

118 Tommaso Zefiriele Bovio, *Fulmine contro de'Medici putatitii Rationali*
     (Verona, 1592), f. 7v. (Hereafter *Fulmine*.)

119 Orazio Augenio, *Epistolarum et Consultationum Medicinalium libri XXIIII*
     (Frankfurt, 1597), p. 451.

120 Gianfranco Garosi, 'L'opera di Angelo Forte medico del Cinquecento',
     Acta Medicae Historiae Patavina, VI (1959–60), 83–105. Mario Vitti,
     'Βιβλιογραφικα στον 16° αιονα ὁ κερκυραιος γιατρος 'Αγγελος
     Φορτιας', [Bibliography of the sixteenth century: the Corfiote physician
     Angelo Forte], 'Ο 'Ερανιστης, III (1965), 273–6. The following
     information is based on Forte's works and on archival sources which I
     hope to discuss in a future publication.

121 Simon Arborsellus, *Angelo Fortio Naturae Investigatori exquisitissimo* [no
     place or date, *c.* 1543–4].

122 On Fioravanti, see especially Davide Giordano, *Leonardo Fioravanti,
     Bolognese* (Bologna, 1920).

123 On his move to Venice in 1558, Leonardo Fioravanti, *Il Tesoro della Vita
     Humana* (Venice, 1582), f. 80v. He was still in Venice in 1571 when he
     wrote the dedication of his *Reggimento della Peste* (Venice, 1571), but may
     have left for good thereafter. He was in Milan in 1573, in Spain 1576–7,
     and in Naples in 1581.

124 Lynn Thorndike, *History*, V. chapter 29.

125 Fioravanti, *Dello Specchio* (Venice, 1572), f. 14v.

126 *Idem, Il Reggimento della Peste* (Venice, 1571), ff. 8r–9r.

127 *Ibid.*, ff. 7r, 9r, 117v–118v.

128 *Idem, Il Tesoro della Vita Humana*, f. 27v.

129 *Idem, Il Reggimento della Peste*, ff. 43r–52r.

130 *Idem, Dello Specchio; Il tesoro della Vita Humana*, f. 83v.

131 *Idem, Dello Specchio*, f. 220v.

132 N. Latronico, 'Una disavventura milanese di Leonardo Fioravanti',
     L'Ospedale Maggiore, XXIX (1941), 481–2. E. Dall'Osso, 'Due lettere
     inedite di Leonardo Fioravanti', *Rivista di Storia delle Scienze Mediche e
     Naturali*, XLVII (1956), 283–91.

133 G. A. Gentili, 'Leonardo Fioravanti bolognese alla luce di ignorati
     documenti', *Rivista di Storia delle Scienze Mediche e Naturali*, XLII (1951),
     16–41.

134 Fioravanti, *Il Reggimento della Peste*, f. 41r.

135 ASV, *Senato, Mar*, Reg. 35, ff. 36r, 145r; and the original petition of
     Fioravanti to the *Provveditori sopra Beni Inculti* in *Ibid.*, Filza 22.

136 Fioravanti, *Il Reggimento della Peste*, f. 5r–v; *Dello Specchio*, f. 19v.
137 Fioravanti, *Della Fisica*, p. 170.
138 *Ibid.*
139 A. G. Debus, *The English Paracelsians* (London, 1965), p. 67.
140 R. Palmer, *The Studio of Venice*, pp. 24–30.
141 Fioravanti, *Dello Specchio*, introductory matter.
142 Fioravanti, *Il compendio de' Secreti Rationali* (Venice, 1581), prefatory material. This is not in the earlier 1566 edition.
143 Bovio, *Fulmine*, f. 75v.
144 Claudio Gelli, *Risposta . . . ai Flagello contra Medici Rationali*, p. 9.
145 Bovio, *Melampigo*, unpaged.
146 Bovio, *Flagello*, ff. 3v–6r.
147 *Ibid.*, f. 1v, and the *Melampigo*. Bovio's vague references to the Fenari's pharmacy (the *Sarasin*) as the *due Mori* and the *due Sarraceni* may however suggest that he was less familiar with it than he claimed.
148 Marie Boas Hall, 'Humanism in Chemistry', *Chymia*, VIII (1962), 33–9.
149 Melichio, *Avertimenti*, ff. 107v–108r.
150 R. J. Forbes, *Short History of the Art of Distillation* (Leiden, 1948). Robert Multhauf, 'The significance of Distillation in Renaissance Medical Chemistry', *Bull. Hist. Med.*, XXX (1956), 329–45.
151 P. A. Mattioli, *Del modo di Distillare le Acque da tutte le Piante* (Venice, n.d.). This work was first published in Latin to accompany the Valgrisi 1565 edition of the *Commentarii*. The first Italian edition accompanied the *Discorsi* of 1568.
152 Mesuë, *Opera*, edited by Andrea Marini (Venice, 1562), f. 49r–v. Marini, who, as I have noted, practised at the *Struzzo*, commented:

> we therefore owe much to the chemists, who have greatly illuminated the preparation of medicines, especially this separation of the quintessence, as they call it, concerning which they are often consulted by the more elegant doctors.

153 Conrad Gesner, *Tesauro di Evonomo* (Venice: Sessa, 1556), f. 3r–v.
154 Borgarucci, *Fabrica*, p. 806 et seq. on Mesuë's oil of philosophers.
155 Mesuë, *Opera* (Venice, 1562), f. 168v.
156 Borgarucci, *Fabrica*, pp. 398. 733, 810.
157 R. Palmer, *The Studio of Venice*, p. 128. Guttich was in Venice from 1551 to at least 1560.
158 See note 151 above.
159 Borgarucci, *Fabrica*, p. 733.
160 *Ibid.*, introductory matter, Cortusio's letter to Borgarucci 17 October 1565.
161 *L'Horto de i Semplici di Padova* (Venice, 1591), dedication.
162 On Melichio, note 60 above. Calzolari was especially praised in this regard by Mattioli (note 151 above).
163 Fioravanti, *Dello Specchio*, introductory *Raggionamento*.
164 ASV, *Provveditori alla Sanità*, Reg. 735–7, 1580–1607. Coryat, who visited Venice c. 1608, found mountebanks there to be more numerous, eloquent, and more tolerated, than elsewhere in Italy (Thomas Coryat,

Coryat's Crudities (Glasgow, 1905), 2 vols., 1, pp. 409–12). Licences for mountebanks to sell their wares were issued in Venice by the *Provveditori alla Sanità*, who normally took evidence from persons treated with the medicines in question, and consulted the city's College of Physicians, before reaching their decisions.

165 MCV, *Mariegola* 209, vol. 1, ff. 86v–87v, 144r, 173r–175r, 188v.

166 Augenio, *Epistolarum et Consultationum Medicinalium libri XXIII*, pp. 592–7. Contarini, as I have mentioned, was said by Fioravanti to be one of his followers.

167 Dal Pozzo, *Clavis Medica Rationalis, Spagyrica et Chyrurgica*, pp. 41–2, 198.

168 BMV, *MSS Italiani* III, 5 (=4887), *L'idiopedia politica di Galeazzo Cairo, medico*, dated 1628, ff. 137v, 161–162v.

169 See above, note 46.

170 MCV, *Mariegola* 209, vol. 1, f. 144r.

Notes to Chapter 6, A. Wear

1 Jerome Bylebyl has written an important article, 'Teaching *Methodus Medendi* in the Renaissance' which was delivered to the second Galen Conference, Kiel, 1982. The paper gives a good introduction to the *practica* and is concerned with how Galen's *Methodus Medendi* affected the genre. I am grateful to Professor Bylebyl for allowing me to refer to the paper in its preliminary draft stage. The papers of the Kiel conference will be published. On the medieval *practica* there is Luke Demaitre, 'Theory and Practice in Medical Education at the University of Montpellier in the Thirteenth and Fourteenth Centuries', *J. Hist. Med.*, 30 (1975), 103–23 and 'Scholasticism in Compendia of Practical Medicine 1250–1450', *Manuscripta*, 20 (1976), 81–95. Demaitre's, *Doctor Bernard De Gordon: Professor and Practitioner* (Toronto, 1980) also contains rather similar material on the *practica*. C. H. Talbot, *Medicine in Medieval England* (London, 1967) has good accounts of the writers of medieval *practica*. See also N. Siraisi 'Reflections on Italian Medical Writings of the Fourteenth and Fifteenth Centuries' in J. Dauben, V. Dexton (eds.) *History and Philosophy of Science: Selected Papers*, Annals of the N. York Acad. of Sciences Vol. 412 (NY, 1983), pp. 155–68.

2 Often there would be lectures on Rhasis' ninth book *Ad Almansorem* or on the third Book of Avicenna's *Canon*. Both listed affections in a head to toe order.

3 There is confusion as to the exact bibliographical details.

4 P. Bayrus, *De Medendis Humani Corporis Malis ENCHIRIDION. Quod vulgo VENI MECUM vocant* (Basel, 1578), sig. 7r–7v.

5 *Ibid.*, sig. 5v.

6 *Ibid.*, sig. 5v.

7 John of Gaddesden, *Ioannes Angli Praxis Medica 'Rosa Anglica' dicta . . . recens edita opera ac studio . . . Phillip Schoppfii* (Augsburg, 1595), sig. 3v.

8 *Ibid.*, sig. 3v.–4r.

9 *Ibid.*, sig. 3v.

10 *Ibid.*, sig. 3r.

11 L. Fuchs, *De Medendis Singulcrum Humani Corporis Partium A Summo Capite ad Imos Usque Pedes Passionibus ac Febribus* (Basle, 1539), sig. 2r.

12 *Ibid.*, sig. 2r.

13 C. Gesner, *Bibliotheca Universalis* (Zurich, 1545), p. 536v., entry on Paul of Aegina.

14 Paul of Aegina had previously been translated by Albanus Torinus.

15 Paulus Aegineta, *Opera a Ioanne Guinterio . . . conversa et illustrata commentariis* (Lyons, 1551), siз. a 4v.

16 Fuchs, *De Medendis*, sig. 2r.

17 *Ibid.*, sig. 2v.

18 *Ibid.*, sig. 2r.

19 *Ibid.*, sig. 2v.

20 *Ibid.*, sig. 3r.

21 *Ibid.*, sig. 3r. The argument for local remedies can also be found in Timothy Bright's *A Treatise wherein is Declared the Sufficiencie of English Medicines, for cure of all diseases* (London, 1581).

22 D. G. Bates, 'Sydenham and the Medical Meaning of Method', *Bull. Hist. Med.*, 51 (1977), 324–38. For Bylebyl see note 1.

23 I use the terms dogmatic and rationalist interchangeably.

24 J. B. Montanus, *In Nonum Librum Rhasis ad Almansorem Regem Arabum Expositio* (Venice, 1554), p. 6. Jerome Bylebyl in his paper (note 1) has noted Montanus' condemnation of Rhasis for writing empirically.

25 J. Langius, *Epistolarum Medicinalium* (Frankfurt, 1589), p. 999.

26 H. Capivaccius, *Practica Medicina* (Frankfurt, 1594), sig. 2v.

27 *Ibid.*, sig. 2v.

28 *Ibid.*, sig. 2v.

29 *Ibid.*, sig. 4r.

30 P. Forestus, *Observationum et Curationum Medicinalium ac Chirurgicorum Opera Omnia* (Frankfurt, 1634), sig. 1v (to the reader, books 1 and 2, Leyden, 1589).

31 *Ibid.*, sig. 2r (to the reader, books 3; 5, Leyden, 1589).

32 *Ibid.*, sig. 2v (books 1–2).

33 P. Forestus, *De Incerto, Fallaci Urinarum Judicio . . .* (Leyden, 1589).

34 Forestus, *Observationum*, sig. 2r (books 3–5).

35 F. Bacon, *The Advancement of Learning* 1, IV, 5.

36 *Ibid.*, 1, IV, 2.

37 The first use of the head to toe order is given by Demaitre in his *Doctor Bernard De Gordon*, p. 55, n 103 citing C. Talbot *Medicine in Medieval England*, p. 15 who gives Pliny's *Natural History* as an early example (Talbot, despite Demaitre, does not write that the order originates with Pliny) and L. Mackinney, 'Medieval Medical Dictionaries and Glossaries, in J. L. Cate and E. N. Anderson (eds.) *Medieval and Historiographical Essays in Honour of J. W. Thompson* (Chicago, 1938), p. 243, who gives Scribonius Largus as the originator in the *Compositiones Medicamentorum*. Galen used the order in *De Locis Affectis*.

38 See how Manardi discussed whether lycanthropia existed; the fact that the Greeks did write about it was enough to justify its existence for him.

I. Manardus, *Epistolarum Medicinalium, Libri xx* (Venice, 1557), book 4, letter 5, p. 207.

39 *Articella* (Lyons, 1519), p. 363. See text at note 95 for the Galenic significance of the shin.

40 A. Massaria, *Practica Medica* (Venice, 1642), pp. 1–4. In his 'Preaefatio methodica' Massaria wrote that Rhasis 'agit. . . Empirice omnino'. I am grateful to Iain Lonie for drawing my attention to this edition and passage in Massaria's *Practica*.

41 Avicenna, *Liber Canonis* (Venice, 1544), book 3, fen 1, tract. 5, ch. 1, pp. 209v–210v.

42 Constantinus Africanus, *Operum Reliqua* (Basel, 1539), pp. 11–12.

43 Gariopontus, . . . *Ad Totius Corporis Aegritudines Remediorum* ΠΡΑΞΕΩΝ Libri V (Basel, 1531), p. 3r.

44 *Ibid.*, pp. 4r–4v.

45 Arnaldus De Villanova, *Praxis Medicinalis* (Lyons, 1586), p. 35 (second part of book).

46 John of Gaddesden, *Rosa Anglica*, p. 29.

47 *Ibid.*, p. 29.

48 Guy de Chauliac wrote of Gaddesden's work as 'Rosa Fatua'. C. Talbot, *Medicine in Medieval England* thinks better of it. Maybe I am too hard on Gaddesden – he did perceive the relativity of motion.

49 Galen's *De Locis Affectis* was known in the middle ages from a translation by Burgundio of Pisa and one possibly by Peter of Abano. See L. Thorndike and P. Kibre, *A Catalogue of Incipits of Medieval Scientific Writings in Latin* (London, 1963), col. 831.

50 Galen, *De Locis Affectis*, book 3, ch. 12 (Kühn, VIII, pp. 201–4). I have been guided in my rendering by R. Siegel's translation in his *Galen on the Affected Parts* (Basel, 1976), pp. 98–9.

51 *Ibid.*, (Kühn) p. 202.

52 *Ibid.*, p. 202.

53 *Ibid.*, p. 202.

54 *Ibid.*, p. 203.

55 *Ibid.*, pp. 203–4.

56 Aëtius, *Aetii Medici Graeci Contractae ex Veteribus Medicinae Tetrabiblos a I. Cornario . . . Conversa*, 4 vols. (Lyons, 1560), II, p. 204.

57 Paulus Aegineta, *Opera*, p. 127.

58 Aëtius, *Tetrabiblos*, pp. 204–5.

59 Galen, *De Locis Affectis*, (Kühn, VIII) p. 202, Aëtius *Tetrabiblos*, p. 205. The Greek adjectives were also the same: Galen, *De Locis Affectis*, p. 202 and Aëtius, *Librorum Medicinalium Tomus Primus* (Venice, 1534), p. 101.

60 I. Sylvius, *Opera Omnia* (Geneva, 1634), p. 405.

61 *Ibid.*, p. 405.

62 *Ibid.*, p. 405.

63 Bayrus, *Enchiridion*, pp. 45–6.

64 *Ibid.*, p. 45, referring to cutting the arteries behind the ears.

65 Fuchs, *De Medendis*, p. 23.

66 *Ibid.*, pp. 23–4.

67 *Ibid.*, p. 23.

68 *Ibid.*, p. 24; see also note 59.
69 *Ibid.*, p. 23.
70 *Ibid.*, p. 24.
71 *Ibid.*, p. 25.
72 See note 1.
73 Montanus, *Rhasis*, pp. 77r–77v.
74 *Ibid.*, p. 77v.
75 *Ibid.*, pp. 77r–78v.
76 *Ibid.*, pp. 76r–76v.
77 *Ibid.*, p. 89v. In my thesis pp. 219–24 (see note 84) I point out the importance of division for Montanus; J. Bylebyl also does this (note 1).
78 *Ibid.*, p. 89v.
79 *Ibid.*, pp. 89v–90r.
80 *Ibid.*, p. 90r.
81 *Ibid.*, p. 90r.
82 *Ibid.*, p. 90r.
83 *Ibid.*, p. 90v.
84 Montanus wrote that signs formed the bridge between universals and particulars: 'And at this point we begin to show, obscurely, how universals are applied to particulars. And around this order the medical art turns proceeding by means of signs, with which we deal at length afterwards.' The 'universals . . . are to be perceived only by the mind: consequently causes are hidden from the senses'. Causes, therefore, could not be derived from the senses but signs could indicate the cause appropriate to some particular. The causes are already present, the problem is to recognize which is the relevant one: '. . . we ought to proceed to the recognition of causes by way of a sign evident and apparent to the senses. And when that effect is perceived, since it is a particular sign and perceptible to the sense it arouses the sense then is carried back to the intellect and forms a concept in it. Then (the intellect) refers (the sign) to the hidden causes (that is, the universals) and draws an analogy, which is a certain relation (of the nature) of the particular to (that of) the universal'. The three passages come from the *Medicina Universa* (Frankfurt, 1587), p. 26, and *Opuscula Varia* (Basel, 1558), p. 112 and p. 112 respectively. I have cited these passages from my Ph.D. thesis 'Contingency and Logic in Renaissance Anatomy and Physiology' (London University, 1973).
85 Montanus, *Consultationes Medicae* (Basel, 1572), col. 77.
86 See my discussion of this issue in 'Galen in the Renaissance' in V. Nutton (ed.), *Galen: Problems and Prospects* (London, 1981), esp. pp. 239–44.
87 Capivaccio, *Practica*, p. 131.
88 *Ibid.*, p. 132.
89 *Ibid.*, p. 132 'Forma igitur vertiginis, est corrupta imaginatio, cum laesione visus et motus.'
90 A. Massaria, *Practica Medica* (Frankfurt, 1601), pp. 49–50.
91 See Manardus, *Epistolarum*, p. 76.
92 *Ibid.*, p. 77.
93 *Ibid.*, p. 77.
94 The remedies in Lange, *Epistolarum* are concerned to alleviate specific

conditions as well as underlying causes – p. 873, 'Decoctum cephalicum' to be used with appropriate pills for epilepsy, vertigo, dimness of the eyes and floaters; pp. 873–86 decoctions for pain in the teeth, cough and asthma, heat of the liver and choleric fevers, and diseases of black bile; p. 888, infusions for renal stones, for burnt humours and quartan illness; p. 890 'Syrupus Mercurialis' for headache by sympathy from the stomach and the womb; p. 899 syrup in continuous choleric fever. Here one runs through the whole range, from symptoms to internal causes/events to underlying humoural causes.

95 Montanus, *Rhasis*, pp. 89r–89v.
96 Galen went into a little more detail: the condition went from the shin to the thigh and to the ribs and then to the neck and head. Galen, *De Locis Affectis* (Kühn VIII), p. 194 (book 3, ch. 11).
97 Montanus *De Excrementis . . . Tractatus etiam de Morbo Gallico* (Paris, 1555), p. 227r.
98 *Ibid.*, p. 227r.
99 *Ibid.*, p. 227v.
100 *Ibid.*, pp. 227v–28r.
101 Montanus wrote, *ibid.*, p. 230v 'Pariter mirum non debet videri, quod ex parva pustula vel ulcusculo istius morbi venenosi inficiatur totum, si quidem inficiatur hepar, quod est principale membrum toti deserviens: quod cum fuerit ita infectum, necessarium est omnia in deterius labi.'
102 Montanus wrote, *Opuscula* (Basel, 1558), II, p. 34 '. . . quaedam vero tota substantia agere videntur, ut scammonium bilem trahens', and in *De Excrementis*, p. 235v where the reference is to occult qualities: 'Duplex est via, una per ea quae a qualitatibus manifestis operatur, alia quoque a proprietate occulta. Ac quis insurget dicens: tu ergo concedis illam qualitatem occultam sive proprietatem quam tantopere ubique vituperas? Ad hoc dico quod Galenus interdum ad illam confugit, ut exempli gratia quare Scamoneum trahat bilem.' See also a letter by Thomas Erastus: 'Quaeris post haec, an eadem sit putredo, quae ex occultis qualitatibus atque adeo a tota substantia oritur, cum illa, quae e manifesta qualitatibus', in C. Gesner, *Epistolarum Medicinalium* (Zurich, 1577), p. 21.
103 Montanus, *Opuscula*, II, p. 338.
104 *Ibid.*, p. 279.
105 See note 102 the second passage by Montanus.
106 Montanus, *Opuscula*, p. 387.
107 I. Argentarius, *De Morbis* (Florence, 1556), p. 8.
108 *Ibid.*, p. 15.
109 *Ibid.*, p. 15. See Galen, *Methodus Medendi* (Kühn X, p. 895).
110 In C. Gesner, *Epistolarum Medicinalium* (Zurich, 1577), p. 77r. Thomas Erastus wrote at length on *total substantia* in *De Occultis Pharmacorum Potestatis* (Basel, 1574).
111 C. Gesner, *ibid.*, p. 77r.
112 *Ibid.*, p. 77v. On seeds of disease see V. Nutton, 'The Seeds of Disease: An Explanation of Contagion and Infection from the Greeks to the Renaissance', *Medical History*, 27 (1983), 1–34. The wider context of the

issues raised by Erastus' letter are currently being studied by Dr Nutton, and he is also considering the letters of Crato von Krafftheim, Capivaccio and Erastus around these topics.

Notes to Chapter 7, G. Baader

1 See the 'Vita Jacobi Sylvii' in *Jacobi Sylvii Opera Medica*, ed. R. Moreau (Geneva, 1630); also L. Thuasne, 'Rabelaisian: le Sylvius Ocreatus', *Revue des Bibliothèques*, XV (1905), 268–83; M. Salomon, 'Jacques Dubois', in A. Hirsch, W. Haberling, F. Hubotter and H. Vierodt (eds.), *Biographisches Lexikon der hervorragenden Ärzte aller Zeiten und Völker* (Berlin and Vienna, 1929), II, pp. 315 ff.; C. D. O'Malley, 'Jacques Dubois', in C. C. Gillespie (ed.), *Dictionary of Scientific Biography*, 16 vols. (New York, 1971), IV, pp. 98 ff.

2 See C. Elze, 'Jacobus Sylvius, der Lehrer Vesals als Begründer der anatomischen Nomenklatur', *Zeitschrift für Anatomie und Entwicklungsgeschichte*, CIV (1949), 242–50; C. E. Kellet, 'Sylvius and the Reform of Anatomy', *Medical History*, V (1961), 101–16.

3 Sylvius, *Opera Medica*, pp. 1–9.

4 *Ibid.*, pp. 10–22.

5 *Ibid.*, pp. 27–53.

6 *Ibid.*, pp. 54–79.

7 *Ibid.*, p. 495.

8 *Ibid.*, p. 451.

9 *Ibid.*, p. 151.

10 *Ibid.*, pp. 702–864.

11 *Ibid.*, pp. 702–4.

12 *Ibid.*, p. 208.

13 *Ibid.*, p. 312.

14 *Ibid.*, pp. 349–89.

15 *Ibid.*, pp. 389–92.

16 *Ibid.*, pp. 393–9.

17 *Ibid.*, pp. 399–401.

18 *Ibid.*, pp. 401–47.

19 In Marcus Gatinaria, *De Curis Egritudinum Particularium noni Almansoris Practica uberrima. Blasii Astarii de Curis Febrium libellus utilis. Cesaris Landulphi de curis earundem Opusculum. Sebastiani Aquilani Tractatus de Morbo Gallico celeberrimus. Eiusdem Questio de Febre sanguinis* (Vincentius de Portonariis de Tridino de Monteferrato, 1506), fos. AAi–iv, i–lvi.

20 Rhasis, *Opera Parva Abubetri filii Zacharie filii Arasi* (Lyons, 1511), fos. cxliiv–ccxxxiiv.

21 Sylvius, *Opera Medica*, p. 405.

22 *Ibid.*, p. 407.

23 *Ibid.*, p. 408.

24 *Ibid.*, p. 402.

25 cf. for instance H. E. Sigerist, 'Albanus Torinus and the German Edition of the Epitome of Vesalius, *Bull. Hist. Med.*, xiv (1943), 659–66.

26 Avicenna, *Canon*, 3, 1, 3, 3.
27 Gatinaria, *Practica*, fo. IIbr.
28 Sylvius, *Opera Medica*, p. 406.
29 Gatinaria, *Practica*, fo. 1 (II)br.
30 *Ibid.*, fo. IIav.
31 Rhasis, *Ad Almansorem*, 9, 3 (in *Opera Parva*): *oxirodinum*.
32 Gatinaria, *Practica*, fo. Ibv.
33 Sylvius, *Opera Medica*, p. 186.
34 *Ibid.*, pp. 187–91.
35 cf. Salomon, '*Jacques Dubois*', pp. 315 ff.
36 Sylvius, *Opera Medica*, p. 198 ff.
37 *Ibid.*, pp. 196–204.

Notes to Chapter 8, I. M. Lonie

1 Schenck von Grafenberg in the preface to his *Observationes Medicae Rariores*, first published in 1584, speaking of Jacques Houllier's observations, describes their author as 'Hollerii consummatae eruditionis atque Hipprocraticae Medicinae religiosissimi, et post unum Galenum summi interpretis' (cited from the Lyons, 1644 edition). Theodor Zwinger in 1579 wrote of Louis Duret 'De L. Dureto Parisiensis scholae medicae antecessore, summis in arte nostra viris comparando, plerisque praeferendo, in Hippocrate potissimum illustrando (quem ille sibi assiduitate et diligentia familiarissimum reddidisse perhibetur) operam tanto scriptore tantoque commentatore dignam locaturum mihi persuadeo' (*Hippocratis . . . viginti duo Commentarii tabulis illustrati* (Basel, Episcopiorum opera atque impensa, 1579) *Praefatio* to Crato von Krafftheim).
These Parisian scholars will be discussed in a wider context and from a different angle in a study upon which Dr Andrew Cunningham and I are currently engaged.

2 Giorgio Baglivi, *Praxis Medica*, I, x, 11 (quoted from the Lyon 1704 edn, p. 120). He mentions these men together again in a similarly laudatory passage, *ibid.*, II, ii, 3, p. 170. Boerhaave had the same high opinion of Houllier, and called his practical works (to be discussed below) 'nobilis et aureus liber . . . opus absolutum' (H. Boerhaave, *Methodus Studii Medicinae: De Studio Practico*, 2 vols. (Leiden, 1751), II, 867. Haller, in a note in the same edition (II, 605) describes Baillou as 'ex principibus Hippocraticae sectae'.

3 For example, in the chapter 'De pleuritide' in *Praxis Medica*, I, Baglivi refers repeatedly both to Baillou's *Epidemics* and to Duret's commentary upon the Hippocratic work *Coan Prognoses*. This latter text, and Duret's commentary upon it, were especially useful to anyone constructing an account of a particular disease, such as pleuritis, for reasons which will be explained below. Hence Duret earns frequent mention, as well as by Baglivi, in Boerhaave's *Aphorismi* and G. van Swieten's commentary upon them (G. van Swieten, *Commentaria in Hermanni Boerhaave Aphorismos* (Leiden, 1745–72).

4 'Die Wiederherstellung des guten Geschmacks', K. Sprengel, *Versuch einer pragmatischen Geschichte der Arztneikunde*, 3 vols. (Halle, 1792–4), III, p. 4.

5 *Op. cit.* (note 4), III, p. 61. Sprengel's persuasively eloquent reading of history was accepted by historians such as Haeser, Julius Pagel, and Wickersheimer. The last rightly regards Houllier, Duret, Foes, and Baillou as members of a group with common aims, but crudely simplifies history when he says that their close study of Hippocratic texts led them to greater simplicity in treatment, in contrast with Arabic polypharmacy, and to a new emphasis upon observation and the collection of clinical facts. A more cautious version of the same judgement is given by the classical philologist E. Wenkebach in 'John Clement, ein englischer Humanist und Arzt', *Stud. Gesch. Med.* 14 (1925), 14 and note 48.

6 *Op. cit.* (note 4), III, pp. 38–67.

7 For proceedings taken against unqualified practitioners in Paris in the late middle ages see Pearl Kibre, 'The faculty of medicine at Paris, charlatanism, and unlicensed medical practices in the later Middle Ages', *Bull. Hist. Med.* xxvii (1953), 1–20. In the early sixteenth century Wilhelm Kopp in the dedication to his new translation of Hippocrates' *Prognostics* and *Regimen in acute diseases* (Paris: H. Estienne; preface dated April 1511); 'Antonius Albus' in the dedication to an edition of the *Aphorisms* and *Prognostics* (Paris: Chevallon, 1526); Guenther von Andernach in the dedication to his *Institutiones Anatomicae* (Basel, 1536) all eloquently describe the contemporary menace of unlicensed practice, and state that the Hippocratic and Galenic medicine which their texts offer is the only adequate remedy. The same rhetoric reappears later in the introductions and dedications to the works of Houllier and Duret discussed below.

8 The statements were made by the publisher Guillaume Rouillé, who composed a brief biographical note on Houllier for his *Promtuarii Iconum Insigniorum a seculo Hominum, subjectis eorum vitis, per compendium ex probatissimis autoribus desumptis . . . pars secunda*, 2nd edn (Lyons, 1578), p. 266. Marie-Louise Concasty, *Commentaires de la Faculté de Médicine de l'Université de Paris (1516–1560)* (Paris, 1964) (Index under 'Houllier, Jacques').

9 He did however prepare a revised edition of Guenther von Andernach's translation of Galen, *De Remediis Paratu Facilibus* (Paris: J. Gazellus, 1543).

10 Apart from the praise of Houllier by Didier Jacot, Antoine Valet, and Jean Liébault in the dedications which they wrote for their posthumous editions of Houllier's works, Anuce Foes in a passage written in Houllier's lifetime says 'Quo in doctrinae genere palmaris est Jacobi Houllerii praeceptoris doctissimi gloria, qui omnem suam industriam in explicando Hippocrate omnibus semper ita probavit' etc. Foes refers both to Houllier's lectures and to his commentary upon *Coan Prognoses*. This passage was written in 1560, in the preface to Foes' edition of *Epidemics 2 (Hippocratis . . . liber II de Morbis Vulgaribus . . . Commentariis sex et latinitate donatus, Anutio Foesio authore* (Basel: widow of M. Isingrineus, 1560)). It was reprinted as a separate introduction to

Epidemics 2 in Foes' edition of the *Opera Omnia*, Frankfurt, 1595, from which edition the above passage is quoted.

11 Houllier's papers seem to have passed to his son-in-law Andreas Pastoreus, from whom Didier Jacot obtained the manuscript of his lectures on practical medicine, his notes on *Coan Prognoses*, and possibly other notes as well. (This is stated by Jacot in the dedication to *De Morborum Curatione* cited below (note 12)). However, the autograph manuscript of his commentary on *Aphorisms* passed into the keeping of Alexis Gaudin, an ex-pupil of Houllier's who became Royal physician to Henri III. Jean Liébault, who published the commentary on the *Aphorisms*, obtained it from Gaudin.

12 *De Morborum Curatione . . . Desiderii Jacotii Vandoperani et Chrystophori Burgensis Confolentanei Opera . . . in lucem aediti* (Paris, Apud Jacobum Maceum, 1565). The dedication to Andreas Pastoreus by Bourgeois and Jacot is dated March 15, 1565.

13 The circumstances of publication are described by Jacot in the dedication and then again by Bourgeois in a separate prefatory letter. Of Houllier, Jacot says that his 'admirabilis et Hippocratica quaedam doctrina adhuc quasi ob oculos omnium obversatur.' I have been unable to discover anything about Bourgeois. Jacot came from Vandoeuvres, was Town Physician at Arles, and in 1544 wrote a small handbook on the philosophers who were cited by Cicero in his works.

14 *De Morborum Internorum Curatione liber I* (Paris, Apud Jacobum Maceum, 1567). Valet's dedication, dated July 1567, contains the statement that Duret lectured on Houllier's work, which is confirmed by Chartier in his dedication to the 1611 edition (see note 16 below).

15 *Jacobi Hollerii . . . De Morbis Internis libri II. Anto. Valetii Junianensis Opera . . . emendatiores facti* (Paris, Apud Carolum Macaeum, 1571). In this edition Valet removed all trace of Jacot and Bourgeois substituting entirely new introductory material. Jacot complained bitterly about Valet's high-handedness in his dedication to the *Coan Prognoses*, published in 1576 (see note 29 below).

16 The full text of his lecture was not published until the next century, by René Chartier. *De Morbis Internis liber, auctoris scholiis illustratus et L. Dureti scholis (sic) . . . auctus. Has R. Charterius . . . recensuit* (Paris, Ex officina Plantiniana apud A. Perier, 1611).

17 *Op. cit.* (note 15), Dedication. Jacot virtually admitted the truth of this in his reply of 1576, but said that Houllier's notes were so confused that he was obliged to add to them, and in doing so had included material from Jean de Gorris' *Definitiones Medicae* which had not appeared until 1564, after Houllier's death. He asks sarcastically whether Valet had found this also in Houllier's autograph manuscript. The virtues bequeathed by Houllier to his pupils did not include amicability.

18 *Op. cit* (note 4), III, p. 13. Sprengel is here echoing Éloy, *Dictionnaire Historique de la Médicine* (Paris, 1756). Houllier stated his attitude to Arab pharmacology in the preface to his *De Materia Chirurgica*, where he says that it is unjust that Greece alone (Galen and Dioscorides) should be praised for its contribution to pharmacology, and not the Arabs. 'We

should seek remedies from the living sources of the Greeks in the first instance, but without despising the tributaries of the Arabs, nor the genius of posterity.' (*De Materia Chirurgica*, 'Praefatio', in *Joannis Tagaultii . . . de Chirurgica Institutione libri quinque* (Venice: V. Valgrisius, 1549) p. 556.)

19 pp. 382–98 in the edition of 1635.

20 *Ibid.*, pp. 43–51.

21 *Jacobi Hollerii in Aphorismos Hippocratis Commentarii septem. Recens per Joan. Liebautium in lucem editi: eiusdemque scholiis doctissimis illustrati* (Paris, apud Jacobum du Puys, 1582). Liébault's dedication is to Marc Miron, physician to Henri III and an eminent member of the faculty, and is dated July 1582. The edition is adorned by an elegant poem in hendecasyllabics written by Guillaume de Baillou, who had been dean in the preceding year, in which Baillou compliments Hippocrates, Houllier, Duret, and Liébault. It is thus very much a production of the inner establishment. Houllier's commentary was reprinted three more times in the sixteenth century, and in 1613, 1620, 1632, 1646 and 1675.

22 Valet's dedication to the 1567 edition of Houllier's *De Morbis Internis* (*op. cit.*, note 14).

23 Jean Liébault (1534–c. 1596) graduated bachelor in 1557 and received his licence in 1560. He married Nicole, the daughter of Charles Estienne, whose work on agriculture, *Praedium Rusticum*, he translated into the vernacular. He was the author of a work *De Sanitate, Fecunditate et Morbis Mulierum* published in Paris in 1582, the originality of which and of Liébault's own vernacular translation are defended in the article on him in Bayle's Dictionary. He also translated into French the second part of Conrad Gesner's *De Secretis Remediis liber*.

24 *Hieremiae Thriveri Brachelii in primum Aphorismorum Hippocratis librum Commentarius, non minus brevis quam varius* (Antwerp, apud Matthaeum Cromm, 1538); *Antonii Musae Brasavoli . . . in octo libros Aphorismorum Hippocratis et Galeni, Commentaria et Annotationes* (Basel, in officina Frobeniana, 1541); *Aphorismorum sectiones septem, recens e Graeco in Latinum sermonem conversae et luculentissimis, iisdemque brevissimis Commentariis illustratae et expositae . . . per Leonhartium Fuchsium* (Basel, ex officina Joannis Oporini, 1544).

25 Of the scholastic commentators Brasavola writes that although they were perspicacious men, 'bonos authores quos imitari possent non habebant, et tempora incidere, quibus perpulchrum videbatur dialecticam rei medicae et sophisticam artem commiscere' (*op. cit.*, note 24, pp. 5–6). Fuchs in his dedication says of Jacopo and Ugo Benzi 'since they were ignorant of the language of their author, there is no reason why they should have been able to expound him correctly' (sig. A, iiij,r). On *quaestiones* and their value, see Nancy G. Siraisi, *Taddeo Alderotti and his Pupils* (Princeton, 1981), especially chapter 8 and appendix.

26 A discussion of changing attitudes to commentary, with particular reference to Paris, will be a feature of the joint study by Andrew Cunningham and myself, mentioned in note 1.

27 e.g. comments on *Aphorisms*, 3, 5; 3, 8; 4, 5; 4, 10 and 4, 17.

28 *Op. cit.* (note 21) *f*. 5, v.

29 *Magni Hippocratis Coaca Praesagia, opus plane divinum, et verae Medicinae tanquam Thesaurus, cum Interpretatione et Commentariis Jacobi Hollerii . . . nunc primum Desiderii Jacotii . . . opera in lucem editis. Eiusdem . . . Jacotii . . . Commentariorum ad idem opus libri tredecim* (Lyons, apud Gulielmum Rovillium, 1576).

30 The publisher Rouille in his address to the reader writes that he has not included Jacot's commentary upon the third part of the text, since that would have made the volume altogether too bulky. He also promises a smaller edition, 'so that it can be the more easily carried about as a manual by those who are being initiated into the rites of medicine, for without (this book) the whole subject of diagnosis cannot be complete.' This piece of publisher's propaganda reflects the Parisian belief in the practical importance of the work.

31 *Claudii Galeni Opera Omnia*, 22 vols. (Leipzig, 1821–33), XVII(A), pp. 507 and 574–5. Galen stated that *Coan Prognoses* was a spurious work and not to be trusted, except for the material in it which also occurs in *Prognostics, Aphorisms*, and *Epidemics*. Although Galen wrote no commentary upon it, he did on *Prorrhetics 1*, most of which text also occurs in *Coan Prognoses*. Hence the Parisians had Galen's guidance, at least for these passages, and they made use of it. But in most cases Duret is obliged to disagree with Galen, since Galen regarded *Coan Prognoses* as unreliable while Duret's brief was to demonstrate its truth. Although the Parisians regarded Galen with profound respect as a commentator upon Hippocrates, they made no scruple about disagreeing with him when they thought it necessary.

32 E. Littré, *Oeuvres complètes d'Hippocrate*, 10 vols. (Paris, 1839–61), V, pp. 588–733. The history of the textual tradition, and the part in it played by the Parisians, is thoroughly discussed by O. Poeppel, *Die hippokratische Schrift* Κωακαὶ προγνώσεις *und ihre Ueberlieferung* (Dissertation, Kiel, 1959).

33 See in general Wesley D. Smith, *The Hippocratic Tradition* (Ithaca and London, 1979), ch. 2, 'Galen's Hippocratism.' Galen's anti-empiricist bias in interpreting Hippocrates is expressed most clearly in his commentary upon the *Aphorisms*, and was therefore perfectly familiar to scholars of the sixteenth century.

34 The idea is expressed in the subtitle of Jacot's edition, which echoes the words of his dedication to Henri III: 'Ac mihi . . . hoc divinum opus Hippocraticae doctrinae totiusque Medicinae thesaurum esse quendam a maioribus relictum visum est.' Anuce Foes, in his introduction to *Coan Prognoses* in his edition of the *Opera* (Frankfurt, 1595), calls it a 'compendium of medicine' in which all the observations relevant to diagnosing the diseases of the parts of the body are gathered together from the whole of the Corpus and placed as it were into one 'repository'. Foes thus regarded it as a diagnostic text. He mentions in particular the wealth of detail in the descriptions of 'peripneumonia' and 'pleuritis', and says that nowhere else can such a detailed picture of these diseases be found (p. 117).

35 *Hippocratis Coacae Praenotiones . . . interprete et enarratore Ludovico Dureto* (Paris, apud Baptistam du Puys, 1588), book III, sect. iv, no. 7: p. 493 of the Paris, 1658 edn from which all subsequent quotations are taken.

36 *Op. cit.* (note 34), 117: 'multi sunt cooptati viri celebres et summa eruditione clari, qui dissipatas undique parentis reliquias, ex adversariis et schedis in unum veluti doctrinae corpus componerent. Ex quo existit haec quae hodic omnium manibus teritur absolutissima artis Medicae encyclopaedia . . .' Foes' justification of the practical advantages of his arrangement and his hope that his edition will be used at the bedside of the sick is given in his second dedication – which is addressed to the Paris faculty (*sig.* a, 4, v).

37 See note 10 above.

38 'Ἱπποκράτους Ἀφορισμῶν . . .' (Paris, apud Gul. Morelium, 1557). The edition includes Greek texts and Latin translations of *Aphorisms*, *Prognostics*, *Coan prognoses*, *Dreams*, and *Oath*. The translations are those of Cornarius, taken from his 1546 translation of the *Opera Omnia*; the Greek text is also that of Cornarius, taken from his 1538 Basel edition, but corrected from his 1546 translation. The corrector is unknown. See Poeppel, *op. cit.* (note 32), p. 189.

39 Houllier's comments are brief explanations of the content. He worked on the Greek text (see Poeppel, *op. cit.* (note 32), p. 189) and made a new translation.

40 The story is told by Jean Duret in a letter to Pierre Droet which, together with Droet's reply, is prefixed to the 1588 edition of Duret's commentary. Droet confirms that both he and Jacot had attended Duret's lectures in 1570. (According to Duret *fils*, Jacot was a well-organized lecture-room shark who employed the services of shorthand writers, not only at Paris but at Montpellier and other universities as well.) Someone else who heard Duret lecture on *Coan Prognoses* was Joannes Opsopoeus, who refers to this fact in his notes on the text in an edition which he published in 1587. (*Hippocratis Iusiurandum . . .*, (Frankfurt, 1587), p. 743.) Opsopoeus seems to have been in Paris between 1575 and 1582. If this is true, Duret must have lectured on *Coan Prognoses* more than once.

41 *Biographie Universelle*, vol. xii, 97–8. The source for biographies of Duret is J.-B.-L. Chomel, *Elogé de Louis Duret* (Paris, 1764).

42 *Liber prior de Morbis Mulierum Mauricio Cordaeo Rhemo interprete et explicatore* (Paris, apud Dionysium Duvallium, 1585):

> 'Unde hoc etiam documentum capere charitas quidem iubet et cogit (hinc enim consurget auditoribus saltem Hippocratismus) tanti facere me Lodoicum Duretum de re cuiusque Hippocratea meritissimum, quum siquidem ante triginta annos in Regia Cameracensi exedra Hippocratis περίπατον elegerit et tamdiu continuarit, praesente me interea ante annos septem et viginti, et adsiduo totum quinquennium auditore . . .' (sig. c, ij, r).

This is, incidentally, the first occurrence of the word 'Hippocratism' known to me.

43 For the date of the lectures on Houllier see above; the dates for the lectures on *Humours* and *Regimen in Acute Diseases* are given in Girardet's edition of these (below, note 46), 'Address to the reader'.

44 Opsopoeus, *op. cit.* (note 40), p. 743.

45 *Op. cit.* (note 16), dedication.

46 *In magni Hippocratis librum de Humoribus Purgandis, et in libros tres de diaeta Acutorum Ludovici Dureti Segusiani Commentarii . . . a Petro Girardeto . . . primum in lucem prolati* (Paris, apud Joannem Jost, 1631).

47 *Op. cit.* (note 46), p. 6. This is Duret's definition of the Hippocratic word *tekmarsis*, which appears at the beginning of *Regimen in Acute Diseases*. This definition was taken up and enthusiastically developed by Duret's pupil Guillaume de Baillou.

48 *Op. cit.* (note 14), dedication.

49 *Op. cit.* (note 35), p. 1.

50 *Ibid.*, p. 164.

51 *Ibid.*, pp. 365–6.

52 *Ibid.*, pp. 368–70.

53 *Ibid.*, p. 202.

54 See p. 156 and note 6 above.

55 Vesalius' opinion was expressed in his letter on venesection, published at Basel in 1539. On this letter and on Vesalius' part in the controversy see C. D. O'Malley, *Andreas Vesalius of Brussels 1514–1564* (Berkeley and Los Angeles, 1964), pp. 68 and 95–7.

56 *Op. cit.* (note 35), p. 388.

57 To those who have an ear for such things, the slightly affected complacency of the Paris group, the sense of belonging to a *cénacle*, will be conveyed by the house-that-Jack-built hendecasyllabics which Baillou wrote for Liébault's edition of Houllier's *Aphorisms* (note 21):

> Laus est Hippocrati, quod eruditos
> de rebus medicis libros reliquit
> in quibus brevitas nitet Laconum
> sed multos revocans ab his legendis

> Laus est Hollerio, quod explicavit
> de rebus medicis librum eruditum
> in quo totius artis involutae
> latent divitiae segesque rerum

> Laus Coi genio alteri Dureto
> magistri, quod et elegantiore
> et praestanti magis modo explicavit
> (Regis regie ita intonat Cathedra)
> de rebus medicis libros relictos
> in quibus brevitas nitet Laconum
> sed multos revocans ab his legendis

> Laus est et Liebauto . . .
> nam leges aphoristicas brevesque
> in quibus brevitas nitet Laconum
> edito scolio edit atque promit . . .

58 See the papers 'Medicine in the age of Montaigne' and 'Montaigne and Medicine' by Vivian Nutton and Margaret Brunyate respectively in K. Cameron (ed.) *Montaigne and his Age* (Exeter, 1981), pp. 15–25 and 27–38.

59 E. W. Goodall, 'A French Epidemiologist of the Sixteenth Century', *Annals of Medical History*, N.S., vii (1935), 409–27.

60 *Comparatio Medici cum Chirurgo, ad Castigandam quorundam Chirurgorum audaciam qui nec possunt tacere nec bene loqui, Gulielmo Ballonio auctore* (Paris, D. Vallensis, 1577).

61 The works edited and published by Thévart are as follows. *Consiliorum Medicinalium libri II* (Paris, J. Quesnel, 1635–6) (*Liber tertius et postremus*, 1649); *Definitionum Medicarum liber* (Paris, J. Quesnel, 1639); *Commentarius in libellum Theophrasti de Vertigine* (Paris, J. Quesnel, 1640); *Epidemiorum et Ephemeridum libri duo* (Paris, J. Quesnel, 1640); *De Convulsionibus libellus* (Paris, J. Quesnel, 1640); *De Virginum et Mulierum Morbis liber, in quo multa ad mentem Hippocratis explicantur* (Paris, J. Quesnel, 1643); *Opuscula Medica de Arthritide, de Calculo, et de Urinarum hypostasi. In quibus omnibus Galeni et Veterum Authoritas contra J. Fernelium defenditur. Item . . . de Rheumatismo et Pleuritide Dorsali* (Paris, J. Quesnel, 1643).

62 *Biographie Universelle* (Paris, 1854), II, pp. 642–3. *Dictionnaire des Sciences Médicales* (Paris, 1820). The article is by Reydellet. The ultimate source for Baillou is the life by Réné Moreau which Girardet prefixed to the *Epidemics*, taken from Moreau's *De Illustribus Medicis Parisiensibus*. On B. and Sydenham, see Goodall, *op. cit.* (note 56), pp. 421–2.

63 Ἐπιδημιαι   Morbi populares
   Ἐφημερίδες   Diaria
   Πάρεργα   Appendices
   Τετηρημένα   Observata
   Ἐρωτήματα αξιολόγα   Quastiones memorabiles
   Συμμιχτά   Miscellanea
                        -*Op. cit* (note 61), p. 1.

64 *Ibid.*, sig. e, iij, r.

65 *Ibid.*, pp. 2–3.

66 *Ibid.*, pp. 55–67.

67 *Ibid.*, pp. 75–87.

68 Galen had distinguished between those works of Hippocrates which were written in 'hypomnematic' (memoranda) form and those which were more discursive. This distinction was often quoted by renaissance scholars, who found the memoranda style of the *Epidemics* enormously difficult, and were correspondingly impressed by it. There is a modern study of its syntactical characteristics by Volker Langholf, *Syntaktische Untersuchungen zu Hippokrates-Texten* (Mainz, Akademie der Wissenschaften, 1977). Baillou's imitation of it is particularly clear in *Paradigmata et Historiae Morborum ob Raritatem observatione dignissimae*, which Thévart printed with the third book of the *Observationes*, e.g. no. 22: 'Magdalenae ad aedes habitanti' (A favourite type of address in the Hippocratic *Epidemics*) 'pes palpitare vehementer ex pollice dextro coepit. Haec palpitatio hinc recta ascendebat per crus, femur, et lumbos, donec

ad caput perveniret, quo contacto desipiebat, postea statim convellebatur spuma ad os facta.' I do not suggest that such pastiche is incompatible with a serious purpose, only that it is a significant factor in our estimation of what Baillou was about.

69 Lexical work was a characteristic of the school. Apart from Baillou's own brief *Definitiones Medicae* (not a lexicon but a series of lexical essays on 47 Greek words), there was Jean de Gorris' *Definitionum Medicarum libri XXIV* (Paris, 1564), and Anuce Foes' great *Oeconomia Hippocratis* (Frankfurt, 1588). The atmosphere for such lexicographical work in Paris was set by Henri Estienne's two enormous *Thesauri* of the Greek and Latin tongues.

70 The Parisian doctors' consciousness of style appears very plainly in Moreau's life of Baillou. Moreau describes Baillou's prowess in the disputations which were a regular part of faculty life ('he was second to none in composing and embellishing theses, whether you look at the richness of his *sententiae*, the polish of his language, the variety of his learning, or the orderly arrangement of his subject matter'), and explains how Paris theses differ from those of other medical schools in their literary elegance:

> 'Thesium apud Medicos Parisienses compositio ut varium et eruditum opus, sic difficile, arduum, et argutum: concisa dictio sed comta, artificium singulare, sed de industria involutum, multiplices rerum et verborum ad gratiam non ad lasciviam comparatae deliciae, eruditio mascula non elumbis, condita sententiis non lenociniis epicheiremata'

(quoted from the Venice, 1735, edn of the *Opera Omnia*, vol. 1, sig. b, 3, r). Such disputations with the applause they could evoke and the vices as well as the virtues which they must have encouraged no doubt go a long way to explain the characteristics of Baillou's work. His essays are, however, not theses, although they may be related to them. His thesis *De Arthritide* is quite different from the essay of the same title to which Thévart published it as an appendix (Venice, 1736), IV, p. 293–6), although it is full of literary graces (*flosculi*).

71 I have discussed this in 'Literacy and the development of Greek Medicine', *Formes de pensée dans la Collection hippocratique* (Geneva, 1983), pp. 145–61.

72 The *consilia* are arranged in chronological order, many though not all are dated, and Baillou wrote for each of the first two books an address to the reader, dated August 1572 and October 1574, respectively.

73 (Venice, 1735), II, pp. 236–45.

74 *Op. cit.* (note 61 above).

75 Arcolani died in 1484. His *Expositio in Nonum librum Almansoris* was first printed at Padua in 1480.

Notes to Chapter 9, L. Deer Richardson

1 This work is presented in Linda Allen Deer, 'Academic Theories of Generation in the Renaissance: the Contemporaries and Successors of

Jean Fernel (1497–1558)', unpublished Ph.D. thesis, University of London, 1980.

2 As Vivian Nutton and Faye Getz, among others, have reminded me, Fernel was by no means the first or the only medical writer to introduce the concept of diseases of the total substance. Andrew Wear touches on the same topic in his chapter in this book, and Dr Nutton has published his conclusions in the first of a series of articles: 'The Seeds of Disease: an Explanation of Contagion and Infection from the Greeks to the Renaissance', *Medical History*, XXVII (1983), 1–34.

3 Jean Fernel. *De Abditis Rerum Causis Libri Duo* (Venice, 1550); *Jo. Fernelii Ambiani, Medicina* (Paris, 1554). (Hereafter Fernel, *DARC* and Fernel, *Medicina*, respectively.) Sherrington lists nineteen sixteenth- and sixteen seventeenth-century editions of the *Medicina*, and twenty seven editions and reprintings of *DARC* (pp. 189–200); Jacques Roger claims ninety-seven complete editions or translations of his medical works between 1554, when the *Medicina* was first printed, and 1680, and sixty-three re-editions of *DARC* (pp. 6, 23). Charles Sherrington, *The Endeavour of Jean Fernel, with a list of the editions of his writings* (Cambridge, 1946). Jacques Roger, 'Jean Fernel et les Problèmes de la Médecine de la Renaissance', *Conferences du Palais de la Découverte*, séries D, no. 70 (1960).

4 *Ad Librum Fernelii de Spiritu et Calido Innato, Jo. Riolani Commentarius* (Paris, 1576), ch. three, fo. 7b. (Hereafter Riolan, *De Spiritu et Calido Innato*.) Joannes Argenterius, *De Somno et Vigilia* (Florence, 1556), book two, ch. six, p. 273.

5 Joannes Bronzerius, *De Innato Calido et Naturali Spiritu disputatio* (Padua, 1626), ch. three, p. 56: 'In qua sententia, uno excepto Fernelio, et paucis novitatum amatoribus, plerosque alios omnes veritatis studiosos concordes reperio.'

6 D. P. Walker. 'The Astral Body in Renaissance Medicine.' *Journal of the Warburg and Courtauld Institutes* XXI (1958), 119–33.

7 Guillaume Plancy, *Vie de Fernel*, transl. by Sherrington in *The Endeavour of Jean Fernel*.

8 *Cl. Galeni Pergameni Libri Tres. Primus, de Facultatum Naturalium Substantia . . . Guinterio Joanne Andernaco interprete* (Paris, 1528) (hereafter, Galen, *De Facultatum Naturalium Substantia*). *Claudii Galeni De Elementis . . . Victore Trincavelio Interprete. Adiecimus in calce Hippocratis librum de Elementis, una cum commentario in eudem Jacobi Sylvii medici* (hereafter Galen, *De Elementis*). *Claudii Galeni de Temperamentis Libri III . . . Cum Isagoge . . . & scholiis marginalibus . . . per Jacobum Sylvium* (hereafter Galen, *De Temperamentis*). Sylvius's commentaries were published with these editions of *De Elementis* and *De Temperamentis*. *Methodus Joannis Baptistae Montani De Elementis . . .* (Vienna, 1554), includes Montanus's other two commentaries as well. (Hereafter Montanus, *Methodus*.)

9 Montanus, *Methodus* (Methodus de facultatibus naturalibus), p. 10v.

10 Galen, *De Temperamentis*, pp. 64–5; pp. 68–9; p. 73 and pp. 97–100.

11 Galen, *De Naturalium Facultatum Substantia*, pp. 2r–3r.

12 Galen, *De Temperamentis*, p. 121.

13 Sylvius, in Galen, *De Temperamentis*, ch. three, p. 141. ('In temperamento est facultatum essentia, ut in natura diximus'.)

14 *Physiologia* book III, ch. five, p. 90, in Fernel, *Medicina*.

15 *Ibid.*, book V, ch. one; ch. two, pp. 122–5; Fernel, *DARC* book I, ch. four, p. 45.

16 Fernel, *DARC* book I, p. 5; bk II, p. 143.

17 *Ibid.*, p. 56. 'Plurima enim cernimus quae cum sint eiusdem temperamenti, dissimiles tamen figuras acceperunt rursumque; aliis consimiles esse figuras, quorum sit dissimilimum inter se temperamentum; quod ex medicorum sententiis plenius postea & uberius probabitur.'

18 *Physiologia*, book IV, pp. 102–3, in Fernel, *Medicina*.

19 Fernel, *DARC* book II, ch. eight, p. 195.

20 *Ibid.*, p. 198. Needless to say, the term 'occult' as in the phrase 'occult causes' had none of the associations with the cult of the irrational that it has today. It is used by Fernel simply to mean 'hidden' and as the opposite of 'manifest'.

21 *Ibid.*, p. 203.

22 Jacques Aubert, *Progymnasmata, in Joan. Fernelii Med. Librum de Abditis Rerum Naturalium et Medicamentorum causis: quibus adduntur quorundam gravisimorum morborum curationes* (hereafter Aubert, *Progymnasmata*) (Basel, 1579) ch. five, pp. 68–72.

23 *Claudii Galeni Pergameni De Simplicium Medicamentorum Facultatibus Libri Undecim. Theodorico Gerardo Gaudano interprete* (Paris, 1545); Fernel, *DARC* book II, ch. ten, p. 219.

24 Fernel, *DARC* book II, ch. eleven, p. 224.

25 *Ibid.*, p. 228.

26 *Ibid.*, p. 229: '. . . alii caeca symptomata, quae venenatus humor inferre consuevit.'

27 *Ibid.*

28 *Ibid.*, book II, ch. eleven, esp. pp. 230–6.

29 Fernel, *Medicina* (the seven books on pathology), bk. I, esp. ch. three 'Morbum omnem in corporis partisve substantia consistere'; ch. seven, 'Similaris morbis differentiae', esp. pp. 7 & 8 on diseases of the total substance; ch. nine, which includes a section on illnesses whose causes are 'trans naturam' which parallels bk. II, ch. sixteen of *DARC*; ch. eleven, on the types of causes of disease; bk. IV, esp. ch. seventeen 'De maligna pestilenteque febre, quae totius substantiae morbus est'; ch. nineteen, on elephantiasis; ch. twenty on lues venerea.

30 *C. Galeni Pergameni Methodus Medendi, vel de morbis curandis libri quatuordecim. Thoma Linacro Anglo interprete* (Paris, 1530), bk. XIII, ch. six. The passage is cited by Brutus, Fernel, *DARC* ch. nineteen, p. 305, and prefigured in the argument of earlier chapters. Caesalpino also quotes it in his discussion of the operation of the occult quality and the action of poisons: Andreas Caesalpino, *Quaestionum Medicarum libri II*, in *Quaestionum Peripateticarum, Libri V* (Venice, 1593), ch. thirteen, pp. 198v–199v. (Hereafter Caesalpino, *Quaestionum Medicarum.*)

31 Fernel, *DARC* book II, ch. sixteen, esp. p. 277.

32 *Ibid.*, ch. seventeen, p. 281.

33 Hippocrates, *The Nature of the Child*, ch. 17. I have used Iain Lonie's translation in the Penguin Classics edition: *Hippocratic Writings*, ed. G. E. R. Lloyd (1978).

34 Fernel, *DARC*, ch. seventeen. pp. 284–8.

35 *Ibid.*, ch. nineteen, pp. 304–10; also in ch. seventeen.

36 Aubert, *Progymnasmata*. Praefatio ad Lectorem, p. 5v: 'Denique nihil sit in huius scriptus, quod vere Fernelianum non sit.'

37 *Ibid.*, ch. fifteen , p. 68. His discussion on these points continues in chapters eighteen and nineteen, on diseases of the total substance; twenty one and twenty two in which he gives temperamental causes for scabies and phthisis; twenty four on plague, and twenty nine on epilepsy and hysteria.

38 Personal communication concerning 'Explorations in Renaissance Writings on the Practice of Medicine.'

39 Those relevant to this topic are Riolan, *De Spiritu et Calido Innato*, already mentioned; *Joannis Riolani in Libros Fernelii partim Physiologicos, partim Therapeuticos Commentarii* . . . (Mompelgarti, 1588); *Ad libros Fernelii de Abditis Rerum Causis, Joannes Riolani commentarius* (Paris, 1602?) (hereafter Riolan, *De Abditis Rerum Causis*). The information on editions comes from Sherrington, *The Endeavour of Jean Fernel*.

40 Riolan, *De Spiritu et Calido Innato*, *passim*.

41 Riolan, *De Abditis Rerum Causis*, ch. eleven, pp. 71–2: 'neque . . . morbus dicitur contagiosus nisi excretione morbida morbum congenerem in altero possit genere.'

42 *Ibid.*, the final chapter, p. 116.

43 *Ibid.*, ch. seventeen, p. 99.

44 Cesalpino, *Quaestionum Medicarum*, note 30; Andrea Bacci, *De Venenis, et Antidotis, seu communia praecepta ad humanum vitam tuendam saluberrima* . . . *De Canis Rabiosi Morsu, et eius curatione*. Rome, 1586; Giuseppi degli Aromatari, *Disputatio de Rabie Contagiosa, cui praeposita est Epistola de generatione plantarum ex seminibus* . . . (Venice, 1625).

45 *Ibid.* (Aromatari), book IV, p 30.

46 Laurent Joubert, *Medicinae Practicae in Operum Latinorum Tomus Primus* (Lyons, 1582).

47 Horatio Augenio . . . *Epistolarum et consultationum Medicinalium Libri XXIX* (Frankfurt, 1597); *Epistolarum Medicinalium Tomi Tertii Libri in Duodecim* (Frankfurt, 1600); *De Vera Ratione, qua quisque vitae suae amans periculosissimo pestis tempore sese praeservare possit* (Leipzig, 1593) (also in Italian, 1627 edn). (Hereafter Augenio, *De Vera Ratione*.)

48 Augenio, *De Vera Ratione*, ch. seven, 'Quomodo a coelo fiat pestis', p. 28.

49 Antonius Lodovicus, *De Occultis Proprietatibus, Libri quinque* (Lisbon, 1540); Joannes Franciscus Ulmus, *De Iis quae in Medicina agunt ex Totius Substantiae Proprietate* (Augsburg, 1576); *De Occultis in re medica Proprietatibus, libri quatuor*. Brescia, 1597. (Hereafter Ulmus, *De Occultis*.)

50 Ulmus, *De Occultis*, ch. four, pp. 8–12 for discrimination between things

of similar temperaments. In the earlier work, he appears to accept Fernel's deriving of these powers from the heavens (e.g. p. 17r on the action of the magnet) but in *De Occultis* (ch. seven, p. 21 'Qualitates rerum occultas non provenire ex astris . . .') he disagrees: magnets work anywhere, whatever the caelestial combinations.

51 Grevin, Jacques. *Deux Livres des Venins, Ausquels il est amplement discouru des bestes venimeuses, theriaques, poisons et contrepoisons* (Anvers, 1568).

52 *Ibid.*, pp. 9–10, 'Venins de trois natures'.

53 Julius Palmarius, *De Morbis Contagiosis libri septem* (Paris, 1578).

54 *Ibid.*, p. 13.

Notes to Chapter 10, A. Cunningham

General note: All translations are my own, except where otherwise mentioned. First editions of all the works have been used here, except where noted. A caution is in order about the use of one of the editions: the *Opera Omnia* edited by Bohnius, and published at Leipzig in 1687. Apart from the omission of the prefatory matter, and the re-arrangement of the treatises and their contents, this edition forces Fabricius to suffer the ultimate indignity of being portrayed as a Vesalian anatomist! Unfortunately, this is the edition chosen to be reproduced in microprint in the Landmarks of Science series.

1 J. H. Randall, Jr, 'The Development of Scientific Method in the School of Padua', *J. Hist. Ideas*, I (1940), 177–206.

2 See his essay in this volume.

3 D. M. Balme, 'Aristotle's use of Differentiae in Zoology', as reprinted in J. Barnes, M. Schofield and K. Sorabji (eds.) *Articles on Aristotle 1. Science* (London, 1975), pp. 183–93. The quotations are from pp. 190–2. The paper was originally published in 1962.

4 Aristotle, *History of Animals*, 487 a 10; Balme, p. 185.

5 Howard B. Adelmann, *The Embryological Treatises of Hieronymus Fabricius of Aquapendente*, 2 vols. (New York, 1942, repr. 1967). The quotations are from vol. 1, pp. 76, 87, and 86 respectively.

6 Jerome J. Bylebyl, 'The School of Padua: Humanistic Medicine in the sixteenth century', in C. Webster (ed.) *Health, Medicine and Mortality in the sixteenth century* (Cambridge, 1979), pp. 335–70; see esp. pp. 362–7.

7 Antonio Favaro, *Atti della Nazione Germanica Artista nello Studio di Padova*, 2 vols. (Venice, 1911), vol. 1, p. 286. Translation slightly modified from that offered by Adelmannn, vol. 1, p. 17.

8 For instance, even an order from the Praetor of the university could not get Fabricius to lecture on the dissection of the abdomen on the occasion cited; only student uproar compelled him to lecture on what the students wanted.

9 Not that Fabricius was the first to use 'Theatre' as a title: I am pointing to the significance of the fact that he built one theatre and wrote another one, both devoted to the displaying of anatomy.

10 On many of these aspects of Fabricius' intentions, see the Dedication to *De Venarum Ostiolis*.

11 The records of the German Nation reveal many of the topics on which Fabricius actually lectured over the years: their correspondence with the topics on which he later published is remarkable.

12 See Dedication to *De Venarum Ostiolis*.

13 The exception is *On the Formation of the Egg and the Chick*.

14 The 'Galenic' dimensions of this three-fold account will be dealt with at the end of the present chapter.

15 In addition he has mentioned a work of his, 'Anatomical Method' (dedication to *On the Larynx*); this was not printed. The existence of two manuscripts bearing this title, and attributed to Fabricius, has been brought to my attention by Dr Vivian Nutton, and I hope to deal with them at a later date.

16 F. J. Cole, *A History of Comparative Anatomy from Aristotle to the Eighteenth Century* (London, 1949), see pp. 99–112.

17 I have used the 1624 Frankfurt edition of these two treatises.

18 That is, *History of Animals*; *Parts of Animals*; *Generation of Animals*, etcetera.

19 I use the 1624 Frankfurt edition.

20 I use the 1604 edition as reprinted by Adelmann.

21 See Part II, c. 1 for this argument.

22 Obviously, therefore, it does not possess a particular 'similar part' within it which is the site of such a unique action.

23 See the dedication (above).

24 *Pars prima*, cap. 2.

25 Balme, *op. cit.*

26 I have omitted treatment of *De Musculi Artificio*; *De Ossium Dearticulationibus*, both published in 1614, but everything I say in this chapter applies to them too.

27 Reading *utilem* for *utilitatem*.

28 For this and the next translation from Aristotle's Greek, I am most grateful to my colleague Gary Rubinstein.

29 See dedication to *De Voce*.

30 *On the Usefulness of the Parts*; see esp. Book I, 15, 18–19; Book XVII.

31 See *On the Usefulness of the Parts*, Book I, 19, where the term is used.

32 The present chapter is preliminary to a book on Harvey's activity, on which I am presently engaged.

Notes to Chapter 11, J. J. Bylebyl

1 Walter Pagel, *William Harvey's Biological Ideas* (New York, 1967), pp. 90–3, 214–19; *idem, New Light on William Harvey* (Basel, 1976), pp. 67–72, 152–5; Gweneth Whitteridge, *William Harvey and the Circulation of the Blood* (London, 1971), pp. 68–76; Jerome J. Bylebyl, 'The Growth of Harvey's *De Motu Cordis*', *Bull. Hist. Med.*, XLVII (1973), 434–7.

2 On late medieval medical scholasticism, see Nancy Siraisi, *Taddeo Alderotti and his Pupils* (Princeton, N.J., 1981).

3   On medical humanism and its impact, see R. J. Durling, 'Linacre and Medical Humanism', in Francis Maddison, Margaret Pelling, and Charles Webster (eds.), *Linacre Studies. Essays on the Life and Work of Thomas Linacre c. 1460–1524* (Oxford, 1977), pp. 76–106; and J. J. Bylebyl, 'The School of Padua. Humanistic Medicine in the Sixteenth Century', in Charles Webster (ed.), *Health, Medicine, and Mortality in the Sixteenth Century* (Cambridge, 1979), pp. 335–70.

4   Bylebyl, 'School of Padua', pp. 363–5.

5   Lloyd G. Stevenson, 'Anatomical Reasoning in Physiological Thought', in C. Mc. Brooks and P. F. Cranefield (eds.), *The Historical Development of Physiological Thought* (New York, 1959), pp. 27–38, discusses the links between structural and functional knowledge up through the nineteenth century. W. R. Albury discusses a major turning point in the severing of those links in 'Experiment and Explanation in the Physiology of Bichat and Magendie', *Stud. Hist. Biol.*, I (1977), 47–131.

6   Siraisi refers to this topic *passim* in her contribution to this volume. See also K. E. Rothschuh, 'Das System der Physiologie von Jean Fernel (1542) und seine Wurzeln', *Verh. XIX int. Kong. Geschichte der Med.*, *Basel 1964* (Basel, 1966), pp. 529–36; Bylebyl, 'School of Padua', pp. 338–9, 368–70; and, e.g., Giovanni Costeo, *Disquisitionum physiologicarum . . . in primam primi Canonis Avic. sect. libri sex* (Bologna, 1589).

7   The three Galenic categories of structure, action, and use were pervasive to renaissance anatomical literature, although not all anatomists fully understood the distinction between action and use.

8   French, in this volume.

9   See Bylebyl 'School of Padua', pp. 357–9, and further refs. cited there.

10 These principles are enunciated in Vesalius, *De Humani Corporis Fabrica* (Basel, 1543), preface, and are also reflected in the verdicts on anatomical and physiological authors in Jean Riolan, *fils. Anthropographia* (Paris, 1626), esp. pp. 50–6.

11 Among Galenic works newly available in the sixteenth century, two were especially rich in exemplifying this point, namely *On Anatomical Procedures* and *On the Teachings of Hippocrates and Plato*. For early editions, see R. J. Durling, 'A Chronological Census of Renaissance Editions and Translations of Galen', *J. Warb. and Court. Insts*, XXIV (1961), pp. 283 (no. 17) and 285–6 (no. 51).

12 Vesalius, *Fabrica*, p. 658.

13 Charles Sherrington, *The Endeavour of Jean Fernel* (Cambridge, 1946); Rothschuh, 'Das System'. My references are to the edition of the *Physiologia* in Fernel, *Opera Medicinalia* (Venice, 1566).

14 Plancy, 'Life', transl. Sherrington, *The Endeavour*, p. 155.

15 Rothschuh, 'Das System', p. 533.

16 Fernel, *Opera*, pp. 62–3.

17 *Ibid.*, pp. 13–14, 68–9.

18 See esp. *ibid.*, p. 30: 'Quoniam igitur non functiones ususque partium hoc loco sed meram corporis historiam persequimur. . . .' However, Fernel's anatomical description is actually replete with references to the functions of the organs, showing how deeply engrained was the tradition

of keeping structure and function united. The result is considerable overlap between book I, *De partium corporis humani descriptione*, and book VI, *de functionibus et humoribus*.

19 *Ibid.*, p. 68.

20 *Ibid.*, p. 69.

21 Laurentius, *Historia anatomica Humani Corporis & singularum eius partium multis controversiis & observationibus novis illustrata* (Paris, 1600).

22 *Ibid.*, '*Studioso lectori*'.

23 Harvey, *Exercitatio Anatomica de Motu Cordis et Sanguinis in Animalibus* (Frankfurt a.M., 1628), p. 20, referring to Laurentius, p. 472. Earlier works bearing this title include two thirteenth-century tracts *De Motu Cordis* by Alfred of Saraschel and Thomas Aquinas, discussed by Pagel in *Harvey's Biological Ideas*, pp. 90–3; Gentile da Foligno, *Tractatus de Corde . . . Pars prima in qua disputatur de Motu Cordis a qua virtute fiat*, in his *Quaestiones et tractatus extravagantes* (Venice, 1520), fos. 89–101; Nicolò Falcucci, chapter '*De motu cordis*' in *Sermo quartus de Membris spiritualibus* (Venice, 1533), fos. 92v–93v; and Battista Fiera, *Quaestio . . . de Motu Cordis et Arteriarum*, published with his *Commentaria . . . in Artem Medicinalem diffinitivam Galeni* (Mantua, 1515?). In *Margarita Philosophica* Gregor Reisch included the heading '*de motu cordis*' as one of the subdivisions of natural philosophy; see Lisa Jardine, *Francis Bacon. Discovery and the Art of Discourse* (Cambridge, 1974), p. 103, where she reproduces the outline of philosophy from the Freiburg, 1504, edn of the *Margarita*.

24 Galen, *De Pulsuum Differentiis*, IV, ii; in Galen, *Opera quae exstant*, ed. C. G. Kühn, 20 vols. (Leipzig, 1821–33), VIII, p. 714. Subsequent references will be to 'K' and the volume of the Kühn edition.

25 *De Respiratione*, xx; ed. and transl. W. S. Hett in Aristotle, *On the Soul. Parva Naturalia. On Breath*, Loeb Classical Library (London, 1964), pp. 474–9.

26 Averroës, *Commentarium magnum in Aristotelis de Anima libros*, ed. F. Stuart Crawford (Cambridge, Mass., 1953), p. 265: 'Et locus . . . est suus tractatus quem facit de Anhelitu, et iste tractatus non pervenit ad nos.'

27 Averroës, *Colliget* (Lyons, 1531), fos. 18v–19r.

28 Aristotle, *De Anima*, III, x; ed. and transl. Hett, p. 191.

29 In the text of *De Anima* accompanying the Latin version of Averroës' commentary (ed. Crawford, p. 525), '*gigglymos*' is rendered as '*motus girativus*'. The meaning 'circular movement' seems to be systematically assumed in the accompanying commentary, so the error may already have occurred in Averroës' Arabic version of *De Anima*. In William of Moerbeke's version, '*gigglymos*' comes out as '*circulatio*' (text incl. in Thomas Aquinas, *In libros de Anima Aristotelis expositio* [Venice, 1507], fo. 61r). Cf. also Pagel, *New Light on Harvey*, pp. 152–3.

30 Averroës, *Commentarium*, p. 526, already relates the circular motion to the heart in a general way, but it seems to have been Aquinas who first hit on the idea that the movement of the heart might itself be circular or quasi-circular, analogous to that of the heavens. See Aquinas, *In libros de*

Anima expositio, fo. 61; *idem, De Motu Cordis*, 19–25, transl. V. R. Larkin, in J. *Hist. Med.*, XV (1960), pp. 28–30; and also Pagel, *Harvey's Biological Ideas*, pp. 90–3.

31 Falcucci, *Sermo quartus*, fo. 92v.

32 On these disputes, see Galen, *De Anatomicis Administrationibus*, VII, iv (K2, p. 597); *De Pulsuum Usu*, iv (K5, pp. 162–9; and *De Puls. Diff.*, IV, ii and vi (K8, pp. 702–3, 732–3).

33 Galen, *An in Arteriis Natura Sanguis Contineatur*, viii (K4, pp. 734–5); *De Locis Affectis*, V, iii (K8, p. 316); and *De Puls. Diff.*, I, xxv (K8, p. 552).

34 In addition to the preceding refs., see *An sang.*, vi and vii (K4, pp. 725–6, 729–30); and *De Puls. Diff.*, IV, vi (K8, pp. 732–3).

35 *An sang.*, vii (K4, pp. 730–1); *De Puls. Usu*, v (K5, p. 168).

36 *De Anat. Admin.*, VII, xvi (K2, pp. 645–8); *An sang.*, viii (K4, pp. 733–6).

37 *De Anat. Admin.*, VII, xii (K2, pp. 626–41).

38 *De Pulsibus ad Tyrones*, i (K8, p. 453; *De Puls. Diff.*, IV, vi (K8, pp. 732–3).

39 *De Anat. Admin.*, VII, xii (K2, p. 641).

40 The Greek text is included in the *Oeuvres* of Rufus of Ephesus, ed. and transl. Daremberg and Ruelle (Paris, 1879), pp. 219 ff. The Latin version is included in the volume of *Spuria* in the various edns of the Giunta Galen. I am grateful to Richard Durling for sharing with me his rich knowledge of the medieval tradition of this text.

41 Rufus, *Oeuvres*, p. 222.

42 *Ibid.*, p. 223.

43 Pietro d'Abano, *Conciliator Controversiarum, quae inter Philosophos et Medicos versantur* (Venice, 1565), fos. 120v–121v.

44 *Ibid.*, fo. 121r.

45 *Ibid.*

46 *Ibid.*

47 Torrigiano, *Plus quam commentum in parvam Galeni artem* (Venice, 1557), fo. 58r.

48 *Ibid.*, fos. 36–37, 58v–60r.

49 *Ibid.*, fo. 59v.

50 *Ibid.*, fo. 60.

51 Jacopo da Forlì, *Expositio in Artem medicinalem Galeni* (Venice, 1547), fos. 126–7.

52 *Ibid.*, fos. 132–3.

53 Falcucci, *Sermo quartus*, fo. 93v; Benzi, *Expositio super libros Tegni Galieni* (Venice, 1498), fos. 37v–38r; Savonarola, *De Pulsibus*, ch. 1, published with his *Practica Canonica de Febribus* (Venice, 1552), fo. 94. See also Lynn Thorndike, 'A Medical Manuscript of the Fourteenth Century', J. *Hist. Med.*, X (1955), p. 393, regarding discussions of these questions by Angelo da Siena and Gentile da Foligno.

54 Falloppia, *Tractatus de partibus similaribus* in *Operum tomus secundus* (Frankfurt, 1600), p. 144.

55 Teodosi, *Medicinales Epistolae LXVIII* (Basel, 1553), reprinted in *Epistolae Medicinales diversorum authorum* (Lyons, 1557); ep. XVI, *de*

ratione pulsuum, pp. 425–7. In ep. VIII (pp. 415–16) Teodosi takes up the related question of the cause of the arterial pulse.

56 *Ibid.*, p. 425.

57 *Ibid.*, p. 426.

58 *Ibid.*, p. 427.

59 Rogano, *In Galeni libellum De Pulsibus ad Tyrones Commentarius* (Naples, 1556), fos. 11r, 16–19.

60 *Ibid.*, fos. 14v–15r.

61 *Ibid.*, fo. 22r.

62 *Ibid.*

63 Fernel, *Opera*, p. 189.

64 *Ibid.*, pp. 189–90.

65 Riolan, *Praelectiones in libros Fernelii physiologicos* (Paris, 1602), p. 200.

66 Vesalius, *Fabrica*, p. 658.

67 Guinter, *Institutionum Anatomicarum . . . libri quatuor . . . Ab Andrea Wesalio . . . emendatiores redditi* (Wittenberg, 1585), p. 71.

68 Vesalius, *Epistola docens venam . . . secandam* in *Opuscula selecta Neerlandicorum de Arte Medica*, VIII (Amsterdam, 1930), p. 70.

69 Ruben Erikkson (ed. and transl.), *Andreas Vesalius' First Public Anatomy at Bologna* (Uppsala and Stockholm, 1959), p. 293.

70 *Fabrica*, p. 658 [for 662.]

71 *Ibid.* The full statement is: 'Inflato igitur semel atque iterum pulmone, cordis motum visu tactuque quantum lubet examinas, & arteriae magnae caudicem dorso explicatam, aut in thoracis cavitate, aut ad lumborum vertebras comprehendis, & spectas pariter, nihilque tibi manifestius occurrit, quam cordis & arteriarum pulsuum rhythmus.' Immediately adjacent is a marginal heading, 'Num cordis & arteriarum par pulsus sit, examen.' In the light of the latter, I was long inclined to take the 'spectas pariter' as reporting a conclusion, 'you will see [that the heart and arteries move] at the same time', but on further consideration it seems to me more likely that it should be linked with the preceding 'comprehendis' as part of the method of investigation: 'you will grasp the aorta, and you will see it at the same time', paralleling the earlier 'cordis motum visu tactuque quantum lubet examinas.' And even if the 'spectas pariter' is taken in the first sense, it still falls short of a flat assertion that the heart and arteries *dilate and contract* at the same time.

72 *Ibid.*, pp. 595, 7.

73 Colombo, *De Re Anatomica* (Venice, 1559), p. 257.

74 *Ibid.*, p. 176.

75 Pagel, in *Harvey's Biological Ideas*, pp. 155–6 and 215–18, proposed that Colombo had simply retained the traditional designation 'systole' for the phase of the heartbeat which he now understood to be dilatation. Whitteridge, in *Harvey and the Circulation*, pp. 70–2, implicitly rejected this in pointing out, correctly, that Colombo knew that systole means 'contraction'. Whitteridge proposed that a printer's error must have given us 'systole' where Colombo wrote 'diastole,' but this is the only usage of either term in the whole passage, and so I can see no reason why

a typesetter would make the substitution. The error, if there was one, must have been Colombo's, and I would suggest that an ambiguity of syntax would slip by him more easily than a semantic contradiction. And as Pagel points out in *New Light on Harvey*, p. 70, my interpretation also has 'the advantage of "saving" the original text.'

76 Of early efforts to interpret this passage, Pagel, in *Harvey's Biological Ideas*, pp. 216–18, discusses those of Coiter, Riolan, and Harvey, while in *New Light*, pp. 69–70, he adds Conring to the list. Yet another was Johann Guinter von Andernach, in *De medicina veteri et nova . . . commentarii* (Basel, 1571), vol. I, pp. 260–1. Elsewhere (p. 364) Guenter endorses the views of his former Paris colleague Fernel on the relationship between heartbeat and arterial pulse.

77 Coiter, *Observationum Anatomicarum Chirurgicarumque miscellanea varia*, reprinted from the 1572 Nuremberg edn in *Opuscula selecta Neerlandicorum de arte medica*, XVIII (Amsterdam, 1955), pp. 140–3.

78 *Ibid.*, p. 140.

79 *Ibid.*, p. 142.

80 Varoli, *Anatomiae, sive de Resolutione Corporis Humani . . . libri IIII* (Frankfurt, 1591), pp. 51–2. This statement, by way of of Bauhin and Riolan, turns up in chapter four of Harvey's *De Motu Cordis* (pp. 25–6), where he misinterprets it to mean that all four chambers of the heart move at different times.

81 Bauhin, *Anatomes, liber primus . . . liber secundus* (Basel, 1597), p. 441.

82 Flacius, *Commentariorum physicorum de Vita et Morte, libri III* (Frankfurt, 1584), pp. 153–6; Jessen, *Anatomiae Pragae anno MDC . . . administratae Historia* (Wittenberg, 1601), fo. 91.

83 Bauhin, *Theatrum Anatomicum* (Frankfurt, 1605), p. 437.

84 Capivacci, *Opera Omnia* (Frankfurt, 1603), pp. 173, 195. These statements occur in his *De Anatomica Methodo Commentarius* and his *Tractatus de Pulsibus*, respectively, and both are supported by citations from Galen.

85 *Fabrica*, p. 659.

86 *De Re Anatomica*, p. 180.

87 Scaliger, *Exotericarum Exercitationum liber* (Paris, 1557), p. 365.

88 Jacques Houllier, *De Morbis Internis . . . et L. Dureti scholis* (Paris, 1611), p. 287. This is a very late edition; Duret died in 1586.

89 Falloppia, *Tractatus de Partibus Similaribus* in *Operum tomus secundus* (Frankfurt, 1600), p. 138.

90 Falloppia, *Lectiones de Partibus Similaribus*, ed. Coiter (Nuremberg, 1575), cap. 13.

91 *Tractatus*, p. 139.

92 *Ibid.*, pp. 140–4.

93 *Ibid.*, p. 140.

94 *Ibid.*, p. 142.

95 Cesalpino, *Peripateticarum Quaestionum libri quinque* (Venice, 1571), fos. 107v–112v.

96 *Ibid.*, fo. 108v: 'Dicere autem diverso tempore pulsare cor & arterias est negare sensum & quaerere rationem.'

97 *Ibid.*, fo. 109r.

98 *Ibid.*, fo. 108v.

99 This is not to say that there was no immediate response. One contemporary who seems to have been stimulated by Cesalpino to outright acceptance of the ebullition theory was Christoph Rumbaum, in *De Partibus Corporis Humani Exercitationes quaedam* (Basel, 1586), pp. 139–51.

100 Sassonia, *De Pulsibus* (Padua, 1603), fos. 5v–11v.

101 *Historia Anatomica*, pp. 472–81.

102 *Ibid.*, p. 475.

103 *Anthropographia* (1626), p. 52.

104 *Ibid.*, pp. 657–9; see also pp. 371–2 for a closely related discussion. These passages are analysed by Pagel in *Harvey's Biological Ideas*, pp. 212–13 and 216–18, where he also notes (p. 212) that they first appeared in the 1618 edn of *Anthropographia*.

105 Some of these borrowings are fully acknowledged, but, e.g., Varoli's observation (note 80, above) is worked into Riolan's text as if it were his own (*ibid.*, p. 657).

106 *Ibid.*, p. 659.

107 William Harvey, *Prelectiones Anatomiae Universalis* [facsimile and transcript] (London, 1886), fos. 77r–80r; *The Anatomical Lectures of William Harvey*, ed. and transl G. Whitteridge (Edinburgh and London, 1964), pp. 264–73.

108 *Prelectiones*, fo. 77r and 77v. More precisely, Harvey found no difficulty in directly perceiving when the auricles contract and when the arteries dilate; but he could not be certain from simple ocular inspection what the ventricles were doing in relation to these other two movements, and therefore had to reach his conclusions in this regard from various lines of indirect inference.

109 See esp. *ibid.*, fo. 78v, where Harvey explicitly offers proofs from both '*autopsia*' and '*ratione*' in support of his conclusion on the cause of the arterial pulse; and fo. 79r where he has written the heading '*Rationabile etiam,*' under which he enumerates six indirect proofs of his overall thesis.

110 Most of these derivations are fairly clear from Harvey's own account, except for the last two. C. D. O'Malley, F. N. L. Poynter, and K. F. Russell, in their annotated transl., William Harvey, *Lectures on the Whole of Anatomy* (Berkeley and Los Angeles, 1961), have shown that elsewhere in the lectures Harvey drew on Falloppia's *De Partibus Similaribus* (e.g., pp. 46 and 47), and so it seems a reasonable inference that Harvey derived the example of the inflated glove (*Prelectiones*, fos. 78v, 79r, 79v) and other points concerning the cause of the arterial pulse from the same source. Direct evidence of Harvey's early familiarity with Coiter's description is more difficult to come by, but it seems to me highly unlikely that Harvey would have overlooked so important a source, especially since it was published together with another account that would have been of high interest to him, that of the developing chick embryo (*Opuscula Selecta* XVIII, pp. 26–55).

111 Harvey, *De Motu Cordis*, chs. 2–4, pp. 21–9. My point is not that *De Motu*

Cordis is entirely lacking in argumentative and polemical elements (e.g., the *Proem* is given over largely to such matters), but that when compared with the *Prelectiones*, chs. 2, 3, and 4 seem to reflect a very conscious effort by Harvey to present his conclusions about the movement of the heart as if they were facts which are inseparable from his observations. For example, his account in the *Prelectiones* begins with a conflict of opinion, namely a view that is 'vulgo creditur,' and the opposing (and somewhat confusing) view of Colombo. After emphasizing the great difficulty of resolving the issue through observation, Harvey states his own conclusion, 'Erectio systolen esse' (fo. 77v), and then lines up pieces of evidence, mostly observational, in support of it. But in chapter two of *De Motu Cordis* he *begins* with a series of observations in which his conclusions are already implicit, and on the basis of which the character of the heart's movement can then be declared to be '*manifestum*' '*rationi consentaneum*,' and, finally, '*contrarium vulgariter receptis opinionibus.*' Colombo, the chief literary inspiration of Harvey's position, drops out of the picture entirely, probably because he did not want to obfuscate his own account by tackling the verbal ambiguity that marred Colombo's.

112 Harvey, *De Motu Cordis*, p. 21; Cunningham, in this volume.
113 Bylebyl, '*De Motu Cordis*: Written in Two Stages? Response,' *Bull. Hist. Med.*, LI (1977), pp. 145–6.
114 Harvey, *De Motu Cordis*, pp. 21, 24, 25.
115 *Ibid.*, p. 21.
116 Galen, *De Anat. Admin.*, VII, xii (K2, p. 641).

Notes to Chapter 12, L. García-Ballester

1 cf. my works 'Una Posibilidad Frustrada en la España del Siglo XVI: el arabismo como vía de acceso a las fuentes médicas griegas', *Cuadernos de Historia de la Medicina Española* (Salamanca), XIII (1974), 219–32; 'The Minority of Morisco Physicians in the Spain of the 16th Century and their Conflicts in a Dominant Christian Society', *Sudhoffs Archiv*, LX (1976), 209–34; *Medicina, Ciencia y Minorías Marginadas: los Moriscos* (Granada, 1977); 'The Circulation and Use of Medical Manuscripts in Arabic in 16th Century Spain'. *J. Hist. Arabic Sci.*, III (1979), 190–213; *Los Moriscos y la Medicina* (Barcelona, 1984).
2 L. García-Ballester, *Historia Social de la Medicina en la España de los Siglos XIII al XVI* (Madrid, 1976).
3 L. García-Ballester, 'Los Orígenes de la Profesión Médica en Cataluña: el *Collegium* de dédicos de Barcelona (1342), in *Estudios dedicados a Juan Peset Aleixandre* (Valencia, 1982), II, pp. 129–49; *Arch. Mun. Valencia*, Tacha Real, K³, 3–6.
4 L. García-Ballester, 'The Minority of Morisco Physicians. . .', 216–20.
5 *Arch. Hist. Nac.* (A.H.N.), Madrid, Inquisición de Valencia, leg. 552, no. 33.
6 J. Ribera, *Disertaciones y Opúsculos*, 2 vols. (Madrid, 1928), I,, p. 427.
7 A. Castro, *Sobre el Nombre y el Quién de los Españoles* (Madrid, 1973), p. 276.

8 C. E. Dubler, *La 'Materia Médica' de Dioscórides: Transmisión medieval y renacentista*, 6 vols. (Barcelona, 1953–5).

9 L. García-Ballester, *Historia Social de la Medicina* . . ., p. 65–9.

10 J. M. López Piñero, 'Daza Chacón, Dionisio', in J. M. López Piñero *et al.* (eds.), *Diccionario Histórico de la Ciencia Moderna en España*, 2 vols. (Barcelona, 1983), I, pp. 272–4.

11 *Ibid.*, I, pp. 502–5.

12 T. Rothman, 'Laguna's Commentaries on Hallucinogenic Drugs and Witchcraft in Dioscorides' "Materia Medica"', *Bull. Hist. Med.*, XLVI (1972), 562–7.

13 A. Laguna, *Pedacio Dioscorides Anazarbeo Acerca de la Materia Medicinal y de los Venenos Mortíferos* (Amberes, 1555), book IV, ch. LXXV, fos. 42–2.

14 cf. J. M. López Piñero, *Ciencia y Técnica en la Sociedad Española de los Siglos XVI y XVII* (Barcelona, 1979).

15 P. Rossi, *Los Filósofos y las Máquinas, 1400–1700*, Spanish transl. (Barcelona, 1965).

16 J. M. López Piñero, *Ciencia y Técnica* . . ., pp. 154–63.

17 L. García-Ballester, 'La Cirugía en la Valencia del Siglo XV', *Cuadernos Historia Medicina Española* (Salamanca), VI (1977), 155–71.

18 D. Daza Chacón, *Práctica y Teórica de Cirugía en Romance y en Latín*, two parts (Madrid, 1678), 2nd part, p. 195.

19 *Ibid.*

20 L. García-Ballester, 'Las Obras Médicas de Luis Collado (*m.* 1589). Nota a propósito de un manuscrito del British Museum (Sloane MS. 2489), *Asclepio*, XXIII (1971), 263–70; J. M. López Piñeiro, 'Collado, Luis', in J. M. López Piñeiro *et al.* (eds.), *Diccionario Histórico* . . ., I, pp. 234–6.

21 A. H. N., Inquisición de Valencia, leg. 840. The emphasis is ours.

22 cf. L. Cardaillac, *Morisques et Chrétiens. Un affrontement polémique (1492–1640)* (Paris, 1977); A. Domínguez Ortíz and B. Vincent, *Historia de los Moriscos. Vida y tragedia de una minoría* (Madrid, 1978).

23 J. Ribera, 'Una Colección de Manuscritos Arabes y Aljamiados', in *Disertaciones y Opúsculos*, 2 vols. (Madrid, 1928), I, pp. 417–33; 'Supersticiones moriscas', in *ibid.*, I, 493–527.

24 F. Pons Boigues, 'La Inquisión y los Moriscos de Valencia', *El Archivo* (Denia), II (1887–88), pp. 230–2, 251–8, 309–14.

25 C. Lisón, 'Breve Historical Brujesco Gallego', in *Ensayos de Antropología Social* (Madrid, 1973), pp. 165–226.

26 J. Ribera, 'Supersticiones Moriscas', I, pp. 512–13.

27 Archivo Diocesano de Cuenca (A.D.C.), Inquisición, leg. 343, no. 48–76.

28 C. Lisón, 'Breve Historical Brujesco Gallego', pp. 216 ff.

29 A.D.C., Inquisición, leg. 343, no. 48.

30 *Ibid.*

31 A.H.N., Inquisición de Valencia, leg. 840.

32 'Ysti (medici) Morischi medentur infirmis, de quorum salute desperarunt medici Christiani', cf. J. Bleda, *Defensio Fidei in Causa Neophitorum sive Moriscorum Regni Valentiae* (Valencia, 1610), p. 368.

33 B. Malinowski, *Magic, Science and Religion and other Essays* (New York, 1955).
34 J. Ribera, 'Supersticiones Moriscas', I, pp. 512–13.
35 A.H.N., Inquisición de Valencia, leg. 549, no. 13.
36 *Ibid.*
37 *Ibid.*
38 J. Ribera, 'Supersticiones Moriscas', I, p. 512.
39 A.H.N., Inquisición de Toledo, leg. 192, no. 4.
40 A.H.N., Inquisición de Valencia, leg. 551.
41 *Ibid.*, leg. 551, no. 14.
42 *Ibid.*
43 *Constituciones Sinodales del Arzobispado de Granada hechas por el Ilustrísimo señor D. Pedro Guerrero . . . en el mes de octubre de 1572* (Granada, 1573), book V.
44 L. García-Ballester, *Medicina, Ciencia y Minorías Marginadas: los Moriscos* (Granada, 1977), pp. 22–3, 37–9.
45 A. Domínguez Ortíz and B. Vincent, *Historia de los Moriscos*, pp. 122–41.
46 *Actas Cortes de Castilla* (Madrid, 1607), November thirteenth, vol. XXIII, pp. 583–7.
47 *Ibid.*, p. 587. The French historian Le Flem in his researches on the Inquisition trial at Valladolid (1594) has found one morisco doctor and another morisco surgeon in Avila and only one morisco medical student registered in the faculty of medicine at the University of Valladolid. It is very difficult to find the name of a morisco student in the university registers because, as Le Flem says: 'the moriscos belonging to the upper classes resolved to conceal their "impure origin"'. J. P. Le Flem, 'Les Morisques du nord-ouest de l'Espagne en 1594 d'après un Recensement de l'Inquisition de Valladolid', *Melanges Casa de Velázquez*, I (1965), p. 233.
48 *Actas Cortes de Castilla*, p. 583.
49 *Ibid.*, pp. 583–4 and A.H.N. Inquisición de Valencia, leg. 840.
50 *Actas . . .*, p. 584.
51 *Ibid.*, p. 586.
52 *Ibid.*, p. 587.
53 *Ibid.*, p. 585.
54 L. S. Granjel, 'El Ejercicio de la Medicina en la Sociedad Española Renacentista', *Cuadernos Historia Medicina Española*, X (1971), 13–53.
55 *Actas . . .*, p. 585.
56 L. Alonso Muñoyerro, *La Facultad de Medicina en la Universidad de Alcalá de Henares* (Madrid, 1945), p. 152.
57 *Actas . . .*, p. 585.
58 B. Vincent, 'L'Expulsion des Morisques du Royaume de Grenade et leur Repartition en Castille (1570–1)'. *Melanges Casa de Velázquez*, VI (1970), 211–46.
59 B. Vincent, 'L'Albaicín de Grenade au XVI siècle (1527–87). *Melanges Casa de Velázquez*, VII (1971), 187–222.
60 B. Vincent, 'L'Expulsion . . .', p. 213.
61 A. Domínguez Ortíz, 'Los Moriscos Granadinos antes de su Definitiva

Expulsión, *Miscelánea Estudios Arabes y Hebreos* (Granada), XII–XIII (1963–4), p. 118.

62 *Ibid.*

63 *Tratado acerca de los Moriscos (1605–6)*, Bibl. Nac. Madrid, MS. 8888, fo. 54r.

64 'Quod autem hoc ita sit, constat de multis medicis, praesertim de illo Gandiensi Pachet (the Morisco physician), qui curavit dominum nostrum Regum adhuc infantulum'. J. Bleda, *Defensio Fidei* . . ., p. 368.

65 H. Lapeyre, *Géographie de l'Espagne Morisque* (Paris, 1559), p. 125.

66 B. Vincent, *L'Expulsion* . . ., p. 225.

67 L. de Toro, *De Febris Epidemicae et Novae, quae latinae puncticularis, vulgo Tavardillo, et Pintas dicitur, Natura, Cognitione, et Medela* (Burgos, 1574).

68 *Ibid.*, fos. 11v and 27r.

69 A.D.G., Inquisición, leg. 343, no. 48.

70 On the medical teaching in the Saragossa *madrasa* during the second half of the fifteenth century, cf. L. García-Ballester, *Historia social de la Medicina* . . ., p. 72–7.

71 On the relationship between morisco doctors and Christian apothecaries, cf. A.H.N., Inquisición de Valencia, leg. 551, no. 14 and leg 552, no. 9.

72 A.D.C., Inquisición, leg. 347, no. 48.

73 *Ibid.*

74 J. Huarte de San Juan, *Examen de Ingenios para las Sciencias. Donde se muestra la differencia de habilidades que ay en los hombres, y el género de letras que a cada uno responde en particular* (Baeza, 1575).

75 cf. L. García-Ballester, 'The Circulation and Use . . .'

76 J. Ribera, *Disertaciones y Opúsculos*, I, p. 228.

77 L. Cardaillac sustains the same opinion; cf. his book *Morisques et Chrétiens* . . ., p. 58.

78 A.H.N., Inquisición de Valencia, leg. 552, no. 9.

79 *Ibid.*

80 L. Cardaillac, *Morisques et Chrétiens* . . ., p. 58.

81 A.H.N., Inquisición de Valencia, leg. 549, no. 19.

82 L. García-Ballester, *Historia Social de la Medicina* . . ., p. 20 ff. and 'Los Orígenes de la Profesión Médica en Cataluña . . .', pp. 129–32.

83 L. Cardaillac, *Morisques et Chrétiens* . . ., p. 30.

84 Pascual's translation of Vigo's *Practica in Arte Chirurgica Compendiosa* appeared for the first time in Valencia (1537) entitled *Libro o Pratica in Cirurgia del muy famoso y experto doctor Juan de Vigo . . . Traducido de lengua latina en castellana por el doctor Miguel Juan Pascual, Valenciano*. The popularity of this translation is shown by the fact that it was reprinted three times in the sixteenth century (1548, 1564 and 1581). cf. J. M. López Piñero, 'Pascual, Miguel Juan', in J. M. López Piñero *et al.* (eds.), *Diccionario Histórico* . . ., II, pp. 144–5.

85 López Piñero emphasizes that Pascual, in opposition to those who denied the existence of the bile duct in the normal organism, states: 'This opinion is false because, whereas an abnormality is rarely found, we often see this duct. I, myself, have seen it'. M. J. Pascual, *Libro o Practica in Cirurgia . . .* (Valencia, 1548), book I: 'De la nothomia', ff. xiii–xiv.

86 *Di Pedacio Dioscoride Anazarbeo libri cinque. Dell'Historia, et Materia Medicinale tradotti in lingua volgare italiana da M. Pietro Andrea Mathiolo Sanese medico. Con amplissimi discorsi, et comenti, et doctrissime annotation, et censure del medesimo interprete* . . . (Venice, 1544). cf. B. Zanobio, 'Mattioli, P.A.G.', in Ch. C. Gillispie (ed.), *Dictionary of Scientific Biography*, 15 vols. (New York, 1970–80), ix, pp. 178–80.

87 cf. quotation above.

88 cf. B. Zanobio, 'Mattioli, P.A.G.', in DSB, vol. 9, p. 179.

89 *Discurso de las Cosas Aromáticas, Arboles y Frutales, y de otras muchas Medicinas Simples que se traen de la India Oriental, y que sirven al uso de la medicina* (Madrid, 1572). cf. J. M. López Piñero, 'Fragoso, Juan', in J. M. López Piñero *et al.* (eds.), *Diccionario histórico* . . ., I, pp. 355–6.

90 L. García-Ballester, 'La Cirugía en la Valencia del Siglo XV', *Cuadernos Historia Medicina Española*, VI (1967), 155–71.

Index